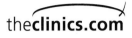

PSYCHIATRIC CLINICS OF NORTH AMERICA

Evidence-Based Geriatric Psychiatry

GUEST EDITOR
Stephen J. Bartels, MD, MS

December 2005 • Volume 28 • Number 4

SAUNDERS

An Imprint of Elsevier, Inc.
PHILADELPHIA   LONDON   TORONTO   MONTREAL   SYDNEY   TOKYO

W.B. SAUNDERS COMPANY
A Division of Elsevier Inc.

1600 John F. Kennedy Boulevard • Suite 1800 • Philadelphia, PA 19103-2899

http://www.theclinics.com

THE PSYCHIATRIC CLINICS OF NORTH AMERICA   Volume 28, Numbe
December 2005   ISSN 0193-95
Editor: Sarah E. Barth   ISBN 1-4160-268

The ideas and opinions expressed in *The Psychiatric Clinics of North America* do not necessarily refl
those of the Publisher. The Publisher does not assume any responsibility for any injury and/or dama
to persons or property arising out of or related to any use of the material contained in this periodical. T
reader is advised to check the appropriate medical literature and the product information currently p
vided by the manufacturer of each drug to be administered, to verify the dosage, the method and du
tion of administration, or contraindications. It is the responsibility of the treating physician or oth
health care professional, relying on independent experience and knowledge of the patient, to determi
drug dosages and the best treatment for the patient. Mention of any product in this issue should not
construed as endorsement by the contributors, editors, or the Publisher of the product or manufacture
claims.

The Psychiatric Clinics of North America (ISSN 0193-953X) is published quarterly by the W.B. Saund
Company. Corporate and editorial offices: Elsevier, Inc., 1600 John F. Kennedy Boulevard, Suite 18
Philadelphia, PA 19103-2899. Accounting and circulation offices: 6277 Sea Harbor Drive, Orlando,
32887-4800. Periodicals postage paid at Orlando, FL 32862, and additional mailing offices. Subscripti
prices are $180.00 per year (US individuals), $305.00 per year (US institutions), $90.00 per year (
students/residents), $215.00 per year (Canadian individuals), $370.00 per year (Canadian Institutior
$250.00 per year (foreign individuals), $370.00 per year (foreign institutions), and $125.00 per year (
ternational & Canadian students/residents). Foreign air speed delivery is included in all *Clinics'* su
scription prices. All prices are subject to change without notice. POSTMASTER: Send address chan
to *The Psychiatric Clinics of North America*, W.B. Saunders Company, Periodicals Fulfillment, Orlando,
32887—4800. **Customer Service: 1-800-654-2452 (US). From outside of the US, call 1-407-345-4000.**

The Psychiatric Clinics of North America is covered in *Index Medicus, Current Contents/Social and Behavic
Sciences, Social Science Citation Index, Embase/Excerpta Medica,* and PsycINFO.

Printed in the United States of America.

GUEST EDITOR

STEPHEN J. BARTELS, MD, MS, Director, Aging Services Research, New Hampshire-Dartmouth Psychiatric Research Center; Professor of Psychiatry and Community and Family Medicine, Dartmouth Medical School, Lebanon, New Hampshire

CONTRIBUTORS

GEORGE ALEXOPOULOS, MD, Professor of Psychiatry and Director, Weill-Cornell Institute of Geriatric Psychiatry, White Plains, New York

PATRICIA A. AREÁN, PhD, Department of Psychiatry and Langley Porter Psychiatric Institute, University of California, San Francisco, San Francisco, California

STEPHEN J. BARTELS, MD, MS, Director, Aging Services Research, New Hampshire-Dartmouth Psychiatric Research Center; Professor of Psychiatry and Community and Family Medicine, Dartmouth Medical School, Lebanon, New Hampshire

NIPALI BHARANI, MD, Acting Instructor, Department of Psychiatry and Behavioral Sciences, University of Washington, Seattle, Washington

MARTHA L. BRUCE, PhD, MPH, Professor of Sociology in Psychiatry, Department of Psychiatry, Weill Medical College of Cornell University, White Plains, New York

MARTIN G. COLE, MD, FRCP(C), Professor, Department of Psychiatry, St. Mary's Hospital and McGill University, Montreal, Quebec, Canada

ALLEN J. DIETRICH, MD, Departments of Psychiatry and Community and Family Medicine, Dartmouth Medical School, Lebanon, New Hampshire

ROBERT E. DRAKE, MD, PhD, Director, New Hampshire-Dartmouth Psychiatric Research Center; Andrew Thomson Professor of Psychiatry, Dartmouth Medical School, Lebanon, New Hampshire

REBECCA DRAYER, MD, Physician Investigator, Western Psychiatric Institute and Clinic, University of Pittsburgh, Pittsburgh, Pennsylvania

DILIP V. JESTE, MD, Department of Psychiatry, University of California, San Diego/VA San Diego Healthcare System, San Diego, California

JORDAN KARP, MD, Physician Investigator, Western Psychiatric Institute and Clinic, University of Pittsburgh, Pittsburgh, Pennsylvania

WAYNE KATON, MD, Professor and Vice Chair, Department of Psychiatry and Behavioral Sciences, University of Washington, Seattle, Washington

IRA R. KATZ, MD, PhD, Professor of Psychiatry; Director, Section of Geriatric Psychiatry, Department of Psychiatry, University of Pennsylvania; Mental Illness Research, Education and Clinical Center, Philadelphia Veterans Affairs Medical Center, Philadelphia, Pennsylvania

JULIE N. KLINGER, MA, University Center for Social and Urban Research, University of Pittsburgh, Pittsburgh, Pennsylvania

CHRISTOPHER LANGSTON, PhD, Senior Program Officer, John A. Hartford Foundation, New York, New York

ERIC J. LENZE, MD, Assistant Professor, Western Psychiatric Institute and Clinic, University of Pittsburgh Medical School, Pittsburgh, Pennsylvania

R. SCOTT MACKIN, PhD, Department of Psychiatry and Langley Porter Psychiatric Institute, University of California, San Francisco, San Francisco, California

LYNN M. MARTIRE, PhD, Department of Psychiatry and University Center for Social and Urban Research, University of Pittsburgh, Pittsburgh, Pennsylvania

DAVID W. OSLIN, MD, Associate Professor, School of Medicine, Geriatric and Addiction Psychiatry, University of Pennsylvania, Philadelphia; Philadelphia Veterans Affairs Medical Center (CESATE) and VISN 4 MIRECC, Philadelphia, Pennsylvania

THOMAS E. OXMAN, MD, Departments of Psychiatry and Community and Family Medicine, Dartmouth Medical School, Lebanon, New Hampshire

DIANE POWERS, MA, Research Scientist, Department of Psychiatry and Behavioral Sciences, University of Washington, Seattle, Washington

SARAH I. PRATT, PhD, New Hampshire-Dartmouth Psychiatric Research Center, Lebanon, New Hampshire

CHARLES F. REYNOLDS III, MD, Western Psychiatric Institute and Clinic, University of Pittsburgh, Pittsburgh, Pennsylvania

HERBERT C. SCHULBERG, PhD, Intervention Research Center for Late-Life Mood Disorders, Department of Psychiatry, Weill Medical College of Cornell University, White Plains, New York

RICHARD SCHULZ, PhD, Department of Psychiatry and University Center for Social and Urban Research, University of Pittsburgh, Pittsburgh, Pennsylvania

BINDU SHANMUGHAM, MD, MPH, Instructor of Psychiatry, Weill-Cornell Institute of Geriatric Psychiatry, White Plains, New York

MARK SNOWDEN, MD, MPH, Associate Professor, Department of Psychiatry and Behavioral Sciences, University of Washington, Seattle, Washington

MELINDA A. STANLEY, PhD, Professor and Head, Division of Psychology, Menninger Department of Psychiatry and Behavioral Sciences, Baylor College of Medicine; Houston Center for Quality of Care and Utilization Studies, Michael E. DeBakey Veterans Affairs Medical Center, Houston, Texas

JÜRGEN UNÜTZER, MD, MPH, MA, Professor and Vice Chair, Department of Psychiatry and Behavioral Sciences, University of Washington, Seattle, Washington

ARICCA D. VAN CITTERS, MS, Project Coordinator, Department of Community and Family Medicine, Dartmouth Medical School; New Hampshire-Dartmouth Psychiatric Research Center, Lebanon, New Hampshire

DANIEL WEINTRAUB, MD, Assistant Professor of Psychiatry and Neurology, Department of Psychiatry, University of Pennsylvania, Philadelphia; Parkinson's Disease Research, Education and Clinical Center and Mental Illness Research, Education and Clinical Center, Philadelphia Veterans Affairs Medical Center, Philadelphia, Pennsylvania

JULIE LOEBACH WETHERELL, PhD, Assistant Professor, Department of Psychiatry, University of California, San Diego, San Diego, California

ROBERT C. YOUNG, MD, Professor of Psychiatry, Payne Whitney Westchester and Institute of Geriatric Psychiatry, Weill Medical College of Cornell University; New York Presbyterian Hospital, Westchester, White Plains, New York

CONTENTS

as the third-line treatment option, numerous articles have reviewed the evidence base for psychotherapy research in older adults and have evaluated the efficacy of psychotherapy as a treatment for late-life depression. Most of these studies have focused on the evaluation of cognitive-behavioral therapy, brief dynamic therapy, interpersonal psychotherapy, reminiscence therapy, and the combination of these interventions with medication management. This updated review systematically evaluates the evidence base for psychotherapy as an empirically supported treatment of late life depression.

Evidence-Based Pharmacologic Interventions for Geriatric Depression

Bindu Shanmugham, Jordan Karp, Rebecca Drayer, Charles F. Reynolds III, and George Alexopoulos

Late-life depression is under-recognized and undertreated in older adults. Although the existing empirical treatment literature is limited, published studies and expert consensus recommendations find that antidepressants are effective. Treatment of psychotic depression has not been investigated adequately in older adults, although common practices include treatment with a selective serotonin reuptake inhibitor or serotonin-norepinephrine reuptake inhibitor in conjunction with an atypical antipsychotic. Treating with antidepressants augmented by psychotherapy can minimize relapse and disability in depressed patients. Continuation and maintenance treatment at an adequate dose and for an adequate length of time is critical in minimizing relapse. Empirical trials are needed that evaluate the selection and effectiveness of pharmacologic combination therapy and other treatment strategies for treatment resistant and partially responsive major depressive disorder in older adults.

Evidence-Based Pharmacological Treatment of Geriatric Bipolar Disorder

Robert C. Young

Despite the impact of bipolar disorder in late life, there is limited evidence to guide treatment in these patients. Pharmacotherapy is a cornerstone of management. Vulnerability to drug side effects and toxicity may be increased by pharmacokinetic factors and by other age-associated changes such as dementia. Lithium and valproate may be efficacious for manic elders, but drug selection, dosing, and duration are not based on randomized controlled trials. Similarly, newer anticonvulsants and atypical antipsychotics have received minimal investigation. Bipolar depression and long-term treatment also await systematic study in elders. Age-associated factors may also modify benefit. Treatment research is critically needed in this population.

treatment should include information that goes beyond the efficacy of individual agents in relatively short-term studies to include findings that validate algorithms for combining or sequencing treatments over time, depending on the individual patient's responses. However, until now, little research has been conducted to address questions about long-term management.

Evidence-Based Interventions for Nursing Home Residents with Dementia-Related Behavioral Symptoms

Nipali Bharani and Mark Snowden

Behavioral symptoms are common in dementia. Although there is no US Food and Drug Administration-approved indication, there are a growing number of randomized controlled trials of drug therapy to treat dementia-related agitation. In addition, numerous nonpharmacologic interventions for treating agitation in nursing home residents continue to be developed. The interventions most commonly studied in randomized controlled trials include activity and sensory therapies and staff training interventions. This article systematically reviews the literature on pharmacologic and nonpharmacologic treatments for dementia-related agitation in nursing home residents. The intent is to provide clinicians with an evidence-based guide for choosing among pharmacologic and nonpharmacologic interventions for behavioral symptoms in nursing home residents with dementia. The limitations of the available evidence and future research needs are also discussed.

Evidence-Based Caregiver Interventions in Geriatric Psychiatry

Richard Schulz, Lynn M. Martire, and Julie N. Klinger

The primary goal of this article was to identify recent randomized, controlled trials that evaluated the efficacy of psychosocial and behavioral interventions for family caregivers of patients often seen by geriatric psychiatrists and to describe and synthesize the findings of these studies. Caregiving studies for Alzheimer's disease, stroke, and mental illness are included that, together, account for a large proportion of the published caregiver intervention studies. Discussion focuses on intervention studies that involved psychosocial treatment for caregivers and also included environmental and behavioral interventions for the care recipient.

Evidence-Based Mental Health Services for Home and Community

Martha L. Bruce, Arrica D. Van Citters, and Stephen J. Bartels

Current evidence provides promising support for home-based mental health services for older adults whose access to traditional practice-based models of care is limited. Observational, uncontrolled studies report that mental health outreach services may be associated with greater access for mentally ill older people. More rigorous studies report that home and community-based treatment is associated with a reduction in psychiatric symptoms. However, additional studies are needed using rigorous, standardized approaches to measure mental health outcomes and to characterize the intervention. Well-designed, controlled studies may help identify effective and sustainable approaches to providing evidence-based mental health treatment to frail or homebound older adults.

FORTHCOMING ISSUES

RECENT ISSUES

ELSEVIER
SAUNDERS

Psychiatr Clin N Am
28 (2005) xiii–xv

PSYCHIATRIC
CLINICS
OF NORTH AMERICA

Preface

Evidence-Based Geriatric Psychiatry

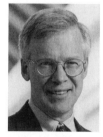

Stephen J. Bartels, MD, MS
Guest Editor

In 2003, the President's New Freedom Commission on Mental Health directed clinicians and systems to adopt evidence-based practices across the life span as one of the most important steps to fixing a mental health system judged to be "in shambles." Previous issues of the *Psychiatric Clinics of North America* have been dedicated to describing the practice of evidence-based psychiatry for children and adults. To date, however, the field of geriatric psychiatry has been neglected in initiatives aimed at identifying and implementing evidence-based practices (EBPs). Skeptics have suggested that evidence for effective geriatric mental health practices is sparse, and recommendations for an initiative to implement EBPs for older adults is premature. Like many opinions voiced by experts, this is a testable hypothesis that can be addressed by a critical appraisal of the empirical evidence. In this issue of the *Psychiatric Clinics of North America*, the contributing authors have asked and answered the question, "Is there a substantial evidence base supporting effective practices and programs for mental health disorders affecting older adults?"

This issue takes the first step toward improving mental health services for older adults by providing a critical overview of geriatric EBPs. We begin with a general overview that provides working definitions of evidence-based medicine and evidence-based practices and describes principles used in evaluating scientific evidence. We also justify the need for a treatment literature that is specific to older adults and provide an overview of the practice of evidence-based geriatric psychiatry. Next, systematic reviews evaluate the effectiveness of interventions for a variety of mental health disorders. First,

0193-953X/05/$ - see front matter © 2005 Elsevier Inc. All rights reserved.
doi:10.1016/j.psc.2005.10.001   *psych.theclinics.com*

several reviews consider geriatric depression and the evidence base for prevention, psychosocial interventions, and pharmacologic treatments. These articles are followed by a series of systematic reviews appraising the evidence for treatments of geriatric bipolar disorder, geriatric anxiety disorder, late-life substance use disorders, schizophrenia in older adults, and psychosis associated with dementia and Parkinson's disease. The next set of articles considers evidence-based practices related to specific settings or models of care. This group of articles begins with an evidence-based review of treatments for psychiatric disorders in nursing homes, followed by a review of caregiver support interventions, home and community-based care, and integrated mental health services for older adults in primary care. The final article in this issue ties together the process of bridging science and services by describing a case history of developing, testing, and disseminating an evidence-based geriatric mental health intervention based on the IMPACT model of depression care management in primary care.

This issue is well-timed to respond to several major recent events. First, many mental health providers and consumers have become aware of the importance of evidence-based medicine in improving the quality of mental health care. Second, states and mental health organizations are engaged in strategic planning, in response to the Commission's directive to transform services by implementing evidence-based practices. For example, the State of Oregon has passed a statute requiring that 75% of state-supported mental health services consist of EBPs by the year 2009. Third, federal funding has been allocated to technical assistance to support dissemination of evidence-based practices for older adults with mental health and substance use disorders. Fourth, the White House Conference on Aging will convene this year to develop national policy recommendations aimed at addressing the needs of older Americans over the coming decade. Mental health and aging has been identified as a priority topic in a series of preconference forums.

Finally, the timing of this issue marks the end of an extraordinary era of accomplishment and leadership for aging research at the National Institute of Mental Health (NIMH). After almost three decades as Chief for Geriatric Research, Dr. Barry Lebowitz departed this year from the NIMH to return to academic life as Professor of Psychiatry at the University of California at San Diego. Much of the field of geriatric psychiatry and psychology owes a debt of gratitude for his tireless advocacy, enthusiasm, critical advice, and skillful mentoring. Many of the studies and content areas represented in this issue were developed, implemented, and completed under his watchful eye and sponsorship. As demonstrated by the articles in this issue, the field of geriatric psychiatry and mental health services has matured and flourished during his tenure. The senior authors requested that this collection of research reviews be introduced with an appreciation of Dr. Lebowitz's invaluable contributions to the field. In a fitting recognition of the legacy of the Lebowitz era, this issue delivers a clear response to the skeptic's question, "Is there a substantial evidence-base supporting effective practices and programs for mental health disorders affecting older adults?"

Stephen J. Bartels, MD, MS
New Hampshire Dartmouth Psychiatric Research Center
2 Whipple Place, Suite 202
Lebanon, NH 03766, USA

E-mail address: sbartels@dartmouth.edu

ELSEVIER
SAUNDERS

Psychiatr Clin N Am
28 (2005) 763–784

PSYCHIATRIC
CLINICS
OF NORTH AMERICA

Evidence-Based Geriatric Psychiatry: An Overview

Stephen J. Bartels, MD, MS*,
Robert E. Drake, MD, PhD

*New Hampshire-Dartmouth Psychiatric Research Center, 2 Whipple Place,
Suite 202, Lebanon, NH 03755, USA*

Despite unparalleled developments in medical science and a health care budget that spends more on health care for each person than any other country in the world, the American health care system is failing. As determined by the 2001 landmark study by the Institute of Medicine "Crossing the Quality Chasm," the American health care system is plagued by high expenditures for unnecessary procedures, varies widely in quality, fails frequently to provide basic treatments supported by scientific evidence, and is "in need of fundamental redesign and reform" [1]. The more recent President's New Freedom Commission on Mental Health made a similar determination based on a study of the mental health system, concluding, "America's mental health service system is in shambles" [2] and that "State-of-the-art treatments, based on decades of research, are not being transferred from research to community settings. Meanwhile, many outdated and ineffective treatments are currently being actively supported" [3]. The Subcommittee on Older Adults similarly has identified serious concerns regarding quality, access, and workforce capacity, and recommended the dissemination and implementation of evidence-base practices (EBPs) as one of the most important initiatives for improving quality of care for older persons with mental disorders [4].

This article provides an overview of evidence-based medicine (EBM) and EBPs in the treatment of psychiatric disorders in older adults. The following topics are address:

- Why an evidence-based approach is important to improving outcomes for older persons with mental disorders

---

* Corresponding author.
E-mail address: sbartels@dartmouth.edu (S.J. Bartels).

- Defining evidence, evidence-based medicine, and evidence-based practices
- Evaluating the evidence
- Improving clinical practice as an evidence-based clinician
- Limitations and caveats in applying evidence-based medicine and evidence-based practices to geriatric psychiatry

Why is an evidence-based approach important to improving outcomes for older persons with mental disorders?

Older adults with mental disorders are more likely to receive inappropriate or inadequate treatment compared with younger adults who have mental disorders [5] and compared with other older adults who do not have mental disorders [6,7]. There are a variety of potential reasons for poorer quality of geriatric mental health services compared with the treatment of younger adults. Some of these reasons relate to endemic problems in the system of care, including economic barriers, physical barriers to care, fragmented services, and a workforce that is inadequately trained in geriatric mental health interventions [4,8]. Almost half of older adults with a recognized mental disorder do not seek or receive mental health services [9]. Barriers to care include a lack of economic resources, the stigma associated with mental health services, poor recognition of mental disorders in older persons, and a lack of accessible, affordable, and age-appropriate services [10–12]. Other problems in the quality of care may be related to the lack of providers with training or expertise in the assessment and treatment of geriatric mental disorders.

The challenge of providing quality mental health care for older persons is exemplified by geriatric depression in primary care. Over one third of older adults in primary care have clinically significant symptoms of depression or anxiety [13,14], and primary care physicians are the largest provider of geriatric mental health services [15]. However, the many demands in a busy primary care practice present substantial challenges to providing comprehensive and effective health care to the older patient who, typically, has multiple medical problems that demand attention and receives prescriptions of multiple medications that can interact [16]. It is in this context that the older primary care patient has an increased risk of receiving inappropriate psychiatric medications and is also less likely to be treated with psychotherapy compared with younger patients with psychiatric treatment needs [5].

One potential solution to improving the quality of psychiatric care to older adults is to escalate the training of geriatric specialists and to develop more specialty clinics. However, future projections of the geriatric specialty workforce predict a dramatic shortfall of clinicians with training in geriatrics, even under the best of circumstances [4,17]. Furthermore, even when specialized mental health clinics are available and referrals from primary care are supported by providing transportation and timely appointments, fewer than half of older adults referred to specialty mental health clinics follow through with a referral to engage in active mental health or substance abuse treatment under these optimal circumstances [18]. A proven solution to this dilemma can be found in a quick review of the evidence base for the effective treatment approaches of geriatric depression in primary care. Integrated models of collaborative care and depression care management that apply depression treatment algorithms are now considered an evidence-based practice with broad application. A systematic review of this approach is provided by Oxman and colleagues [19], complemented by a case history presented by Unützer [20] that describes the development and implementation of evidence-based integrated models of mental health services in primary care.

In addition to problems in quality associated with shortcomings in the system of mental health care for older persons, other potential reasons for suboptimal outcomes may relate to a lack of knowledge in geriatrics. Whereas few clinicians would debate that the field of pediatrics supports a knowledge base and clinical approach that differs from adult medicine, a similar appreciation for geriatrics is not assumed widely in the treatment of older adults. Nonetheless, it is well documented that the process of aging is associated with a variety of changes in physiologic, cognitive, and social functioning that influence tolerability, safety, and outcomes of treatment. For example, responses to psychotherapeutic and psychosocial interventions vary widely in the context of age-related cognitive impairment disorders [21]. Similarly, pharmacotherapy is complicated by age-associated differences in sensitivity to medication side effects and pharmacologic response rates [22]. Further complicating the psychiatric treatment of older adults is the common presence of medical comorbidity and the increased risk of drug-drug interactions in older persons [23]. Older adults consume an average of six prescribed medications and 3.4 nonprescribed medications on a regular basis [24], increasing the risk of adverse reactions with each additional drug [25]. All of these age-associated factors argue for providing clinical services and treatments that are based on empirical studies of treatment effectiveness specifically tested in geriatric populations.

How do research findings apply to the real-world practice of geriatric psychiatry?

Efficacy versus effectiveness

Until the recent growth in geriatric mental health interventions research, clinicians were forced to extrapolate from studies with uncertain relevance to the treatment of older persons. For many years, standard drug trials typically excluded people over the age of 65 in an effort to select individuals who had the fewest confounding or complicating conditions and the lowest risk of adverse events and withdrawals from pharmaceutical trials [22]. The past several decades have witnessed a significant growth in research on geriatric mental health interventions and services research, including treatment efficacy and effectiveness studies [19,20,26–36]. Efficacy research commonly refers to studies conducted under highly controlled conditions, using carefully selected populations, and often comparing a single active treatment to a placebo or a fixed alternative. A major aim of efficacy studies is to maximize internal validity by controlling for as many variables as possible to focus the study on a single research variable or question. For example, a study designed to test the efficacy of a new antidepressant drug in reducing symptoms of depression might first evaluate the drug in a homogeneous population of carefully selected patients with similar characteristics who have no co-occurring psychiatric or medical illnesses and who are not taking other medications. The administration of fixed doses of the experimental medication might be observed to ensure adherence and consistency, and the prescribing physician, study participants, and research raters would be blinded to any information that might include knowing if the administered drug is the experimental agent or placebo control. The prescribing physician might be a highly trained specialist with expertise in clinical trials research, providing free treatment in a university clinic, including access to experts in the field. Rigorously designed efficacy studies are considered a critical first step in establishing the likelihood that an intervention will result in the desired outcome, in comparison with placebo or a well-defined alternative under highly controlled conditions.

In contrast, a major aim of effectiveness research is to maximize external validity (or generalizability) by conducting studies under conditions that include usual patients, routine practice settings, and routine clinical providers. Effectiveness studies minimize the number of exclusionary criteria and strive to produce findings that will generalize to other people, settings, and circumstances. For example, a recent generation of effectiveness studies of geriatric mental health interventions have been undertaken to test the outcomes of treatments in routine practice settings provided by routine clinical providers. Examples of this type of study include the Clinical Antipsychotic Trials in Intervention Effectiveness (CATIE) [37], the Sequenced Treatment Alternatives to Relieve Depression (ie, STAR*D) [38], and the Improving Mood: Providing Access to Collaborative Treatment (ie, IMPACT) trials for late-life depression [20,39]. These studies have few exclusionary criteria and include older individuals with medical comorbidity and multiple medical medications and an evaluation of different treatment options provided in routine clinical practice settings. In practice, efficacy and effectiveness research lie on a continuum. For example, the CATIE study uses a randomized, controlled trial (RTC) design that emphasizes standardized implementation but also allows for a stepped approach that includes the choice of an open trial phase for individuals that have failed to respond to the randomly assigned, blinded condition. The study settings consist of university and community clinics with patients who have a variety of comorbid conditions but have exclusion criteria beyond routine practice conditions to increase the likelihood of participation for the duration of the experimental trial.

Despite these recent advances in research methods and a growing empirical literature documenting treatment efficacy and effectiveness, an urgent need remains to accelerate the growth and investment in geriatric mental health interventions and services research. Recent evaluations of funding trends in aging-related research at the National Institute of Mental Health have shown that the number of newly awarded aging-related grants have either declined or failed to grow at a time when demographic projections predict an impending public health crisis associated with geriatric mental disorders in America [4]. It is also noteworthy that federally funded research studies require inclusion of children (or a specific explanation justifying why children are excluded from a proposed study), yet they do not require inclusion of persons over 65 years old [40]. Despite these limitations, the systematic reviews in this volume attest to how far the field has come in producing a substantial geriatric treatment literature that is well supported by scientific evidence.

What constitutes evidence?

Scientific evidence is the cornerstone of EBM, and it provides the criteria for identifying EBPs. The term evidence refers to scientific information that is produced from well-designed empirical experiments in which outcomes are carefully measured for a well-defined treatment compared with a placebo treatment, no treatment, or an alternative treatment. Well-designed empirical experiments are those in which data are collected under specified conditions that allow for clear differentiation between treatments and their comparisons, that control for differences between the study participants or recipients of the treatments, and that control for bias that study participants, practitioners, and researchers may bring to the observations collected in the experiment. The double-blind RCT is often described as the gold standard for a well-designed treatment study. Randomization of study participants is used to balance observed (measured) and unknown (unmeasured) differences that might otherwise occur between participants assigned to the intervention and comparison conditions. "Blinding" means that the raters do not know if the study participant has been assigned to the intervention or control condition, ensuring that the raters are unbiased in rating outcomes. Well-conducted RCTs include close monitoring of the interventions for fidelity to ensure that different participants in the same condition receive the same intensity, dose, and quality of the intervention, regardless of whether they receive the intervention from different providers or at different times. Finally, RCTs use reliable and valid instruments and include ongoing supervision and checks for the accuracy of assessments by different raters.

Although the double-blind, placebo-controlled RCT is considered the optimal method for establishing treatment efficacy, some of the features of this design are not possible or appropriate for some studies of interventions, and they rarely apply to the evaluation of services. First, blinding of the participants is generally impossible in psychosocial interventions in which the study participant is aware of being assigned to either the intervention or control group. Second, it is neither practical nor feasible to evaluate the large number of available interventions and the numerous combinations of two or more interventions using RCTs. Third, many RCTs that are designed to establish the efficacy of a treatment (eg, a new medication) compare the active treatment to an inactive placebo. Although this is an important step in establishing efficacy, these studies do not address the more common clinical dilemma of choosing between two alternative active treatments. More commonly, the treating clinician needs data on a head-to-head comparison of two competing treatments, yet these studies are often unavailable. Fourth, there may be significant limitations to the generalizability of data obtained in RCTs when only specific types of individuals may consent to participate in a demanding experimental protocol that requires a willingness to be randomized to very different treatment alternatives. RCTs intentionally select patients, practitioners, conditions, and settings that are highly constrained to enhance internal validity, and thus, they are limited in how well they generalize to situations of routine care [41]. Finally, double-blind, RCTs are usually expensive, difficult to conduct, and not available for most clinical situations [42]. In instances in which standard double-blind RCTs are not appropriate or available, the quality of alternative experimental data needs to be considered in the evaluation of the evidence base. A basic premise of evidence-based medicine is the use of the best available evidence in making clinical decisions. In this respect, the concept of evidence includes a spectrum of evidence from randomized clinical trials to quasi-experimental designs, observational outcome studies, and single case reports.

What is evidence-based medicine?

Sackett and colleagues [43] have defined evidence-based medicine as "the conscientious and judicious use of current best evidence from clinical care research in the management of individual patients." In contrast to a tradition of clinical decisions based on professional experience, case anecdotes, and accumulated medical facts, EBM emphasizes the use of a systematic approach to formulating and answering clinical questions by quickly finding and evaluating the current best evidence. In medical education, this has translated into training practitioners in the real-time use of technology to find the answers to clinical questions and to critically appraise the scientific evidence supporting the effectiveness of tests, treatments, and services. Broadly defined, EBM is the use of the best available evidence by providers and consumers and involves a collaborative process of informed clinical decision making [43–45]. More recently, the concept of EBM has been elaborated to emphasize three critical components in making clinical decisions: (1) using the current best evidence; (2) applying and adapting evidence to meet the specific circumstances and clinical needs of the patient, based on an experienced clinical evaluation; and (3) incorporating the specific values and preferences of an informed patient in a process of shared decision making. These additional distinctions are critical to understanding EBM as a process that incorporates the clinical experience of the provider and the health care preferences and values of the consumer [46–49].

Using the best available scientific evidence

The history of medicine contains numerous examples of harmful or ineffective treatments that endured as standard practice in the absence of scientifically valid evidence. Wide practice variation still exists in the rates and types of treatment for common disorders that cannot be explained by differences in illness severity or patient-based factors [50,51]. EBM assumes that treatments can be characterized accurately along a hierarchy of evidence that informs clinical decision making and supports the development of evidence-based standards for treatment [46]. This hierarchical evaluation of evidence helps to guide decisions and is complimented by clinical experience and judgment of the clinician and informed by the preferences of the health care consumer [46]. For example, a commonly used approach to ranking treatment studies defines the following hierarchy: (1) meta-analyses, systematic evidence-based reviews, or direct evidence from several double-blind randomized trials or an N of 1 controlled trial; (2) single properly designed RCTs; (3) case-controlled studies, pre-post studies or quasi-experimental studies from more then one research group; and (4) expert recommendations based on descriptive studies or clinical case reports [52]. In addition to the evaluation of the quality of study designs, the hierarchy of evidence should incorporate an assessment of the number of replications, the magnitude of treatment effects, the relevance of outcomes, and the generalizability of the findings (Box 1) [52].

An alternative approach to evaluating evidence for psychotherapy interventions is offered by Chambless and Hollon [53,54]. In this classification hierarchy, effective interventions are defined by the evidence of superior outcomes from at least two well-designed prospective randomized, controlled studies by different investigators, with clearly described or manualized interventions, or by a large series (≥ 9) of single case design experiments. Interventions that are classified as having probable effectiveness are defined by two studies showing that treatment was superior to a waiting-list control group, a small series (≥ 3) of single case design experiments, or one or more studies that meet criteria for the highest level of evidence but have not yet been replicated by different investigators.

Box 1. Hierarchical classification of evidence for effectiveness for research studies

1. "N of 1" randomized study
2. A properly conducted meta-analysis or a rigorous, systematic review of well-designed RCTs
3. Two or more well-designed RCTs conducted by different investigators involving different study samples
4. A single properly designed RCT
5. Studies without randomization (ie, single group pre-post, cohort, time series or matched case-control studies)
6. Other quasi-experimental studies from more than one center or research group
7. Expert reports and authorities' recommendations based on descriptive studies or clinical evidence

---

Individualizing the evidence

Contrary to common misconceptions regarding the practice of evidence-based medicine, EBM does not encourage or support the unqualified application of treatment protocols or algorithms or an otherwise "cookbook" treatment approach. Once the best available evidence is identified for a specific clinical problem, the clinician must then evaluate how data from a given study population applies to the unique situation of a specific patient. In this respect, the clinician's skills are critical to the important task of interpreting the available evidence base in the light of the individual consumer's health status, disabilities, comorbidities, and circumstances. For example, data supporting the selection of atypical antipsychotic medications to treat symptoms of psychosis need to be interpreted in the context of the clinician's evaluation of clinical indications and associated risk factors. Whereas the use of the atypical antipsychotic olanzapine may be appropriate for the treatment of psychosis in a young adult who is otherwise healthy, the treatment of the older person with comorbid diabetes and Alzheimer's dementia could be associated with an increased risk of worsening diabetic control and a greater risk of cerebrovascular accidents [31]. Individualizing the evidence is especially important in the field of geriatrics, in which medical comorbidity is the rule rather than the exception. In these instances, patients need to be provided with information that is immediately relevant to their own risks and benefits and to make truly informed choices regarding health care [55].

Incorporating patients' preferences

The early beginnings of patient-centered health care were introduced by Balint [56], who studied the patient's perspective on illness and the doctor-patient relationship, and by Engel [57], who proposed the biopsychosocial model of illness. These perspectives underscore that effective clinical practice needs to include an understanding of the patient's experience of illness and how the patient values different treatment effects, side effects, and risks. These principles evolved into the patient-centered view of medicine in the 1980s [58–60].

Patient-centered health care incorporates the patient's personal experience of illness, values, and preferences for being involved in decision making [61]. EBM has adopted the philosophy and principles of patient-centered care in a process called shared decision making [62]. In this model, the clinician and patient act in a partnership to consider the evidence and discuss the risks and benefits of different treatment options. After he or she explores the different treatment options, the patient is then encouraged to take as much responsibility as possible in making an informed choice. In this respect, EBM assumes that informed choices by patients that consider individual preferences outweigh the scientific evidence [63]. For example, a patient with psychotic depression may be informed that the scientific evidence supports the superior efficacy of electroconvulsive therapy (ECT) or the combination of an antipsychotic and an antidepressant over treatment consisting of an antidepressant alone. However, when the information on the relative risks and side effects associated with ECT and antipsychotic medication are carefully considered, the patient may prefer to begin treatment with the less effective alternative consisting of antidepressant monotherapy. According to the model of shared decision making, the clinician is a consultant to the patient, helping to provide information and to clarify choices in the context of their personal values and preferences. In this respect, both the clinician and the patient become consumers of the evidence in the process of EBM.

In summary, EBM is the use of the current best evidence, adapted by the experienced clinician to address the specific circumstances of the individual patient, incorporating the preferences and values of the patient in a process of shared decision making. Another systematic application of the scientific evidence to inform clinical practice pertains to identifying those clinical interventions and services that are proven to be effective, defined as evidence-based practices or EBPs.

What are evidence-based practices?

Although it is generally accepted that the scientific evidence can be conceptualized along a hierarchy, the precise criteria or cut-off point used to define a given mental health intervention as "evidence-based" have been subjected to considerable discussion and debate. For example, the American Psychological Association defines a treatment as evidence-based when sufficiently rigorous evidence of efficacy exists, consisting of at least two RCTs or 10 single-case experimental studies with patients fitting diagnostic criteria of the Diagnostic and Statistical Manual of Mental Disorders, revised

Fourth Edition, using interventions that are administered according to treatment manuals [53,54].

An alternative approach to defining evidence-based practices is exemplified by the National Registry of Evidence-based Programs and Practices (NREPP) (www.modelprograms.samhsa.gov). In this schema, quantitative ratings are applied to different components of the evidence base to develop rating scores that define the level of evidence for specific treatments and services. The NREPP process consists of ratings of 16 domains to obtain an overall rating that establishes specific practices as promising, effective, or model programs. Whereas the criteria for an effective program consists of an intervention supported by well designed, replicated studies, a model program meets these criteria for effectiveness and is also accompanied by step-by-step manuals to guide practitioners in implementing the intervention. Although the NREPP process holds promise as a resource for clinicians, NREPP is focused largely on evaluating models of care and service interventions (rather than discrete treatments) and has had very limited application to geriatrics.

Other systematic efforts to identify mental health EBPs using standardized and transparent criteria are in early stages. Teams assembled to review and synthesize the evidence for mental health interventions include the American Psychological Association [54], the Cochrane Collaborative [64], the British Medical Journal Publishing Group [65], Evidence-based Mental Health [66], the Schizophrenia Patient Outcome Research Team [67], the Texas Medication Algorithm Project [68], and the National Evidence-based Practices Project [69]. To date, none of these efforts has focused specifically on mental health interventions for older adults, and they have a limited direct application to geriatrics. Nonetheless, the principles embedded in these approaches can inform future initiatives to identify mental health EBPs for older adults. Regardless of the specific criteria used, the principles underlying these approaches to classifying EBPs reflect Cochrane's assertion made several decades ago that limited health care resources should be prioritized for interventions with proven effectiveness, based on well-designed studies that emphasize randomized clinical trials [70].

Evidence-based practices in geriatric mental health

To date, the present authors are unaware of any ongoing, comprehensive, and systematic efforts dedicated specifically to reviewing and defining evidence-based geriatric mental health interventions. An early approximation is provided by a recent survey of the available literature of meta-analyses and systematic evidence-based reviews of geriatric mental health interventions and services [44]. In this review of geriatric mental health evidence-based practices, 11 evidence-based reviews and 37 meta-analyses evaluating the effectiveness of pharmacologic and nonpharmacologic interventions for mental disorders in older adults were identified. Not surprisingly, this summary found the greatest support based on multiple studies of pharmacologic and nonpharmacologic interventions for dementia and major depression. In contrast, few systematic reviews exist for treatments of geriatric alcohol use disorders and anxiety disorders, and no meta-analyses or evidence-base reviews were found for geriatric bipolar disorder or for geriatric schizophrenia. These published systematic reviews can be helpful in defining the published literature when there are adequate numbers of studies to support a meta-analysis or aggregate systematic review, but they are less helpful for treatments in which only a small number of studies have been conducted. The systematic reviews in this issue of *Psychiatric Clinics of North America* take the next step in describing the evidence base for geriatric mental health interventions across a spectrum of disorders and service models.

Practicing as an evidence-based clinician

Despite a rapidly growing body of research describing empirically supported treatments, the typical busy clinician rarely has the time to keep up with the constant stream of newly published research findings. However, a revolution in information technology in the field of medicine is changing the landscape of education and practice. Whereas conventional medical knowledge relied on outdated general knowledge gained from textbooks and augmented by selective skimming of the content of favorite journals, the contemporary clinician relies on immediate electronic access to the most current information on specific clinical questions. The skills for accessing these sources of data are now a common component of undergraduate medical education, but they are also available to the clinician in practical summaries. For example, practical guide books by Guyatt and Rennie [44] and Strauss and colleagues [71] provide excellent step-by-step manuals with detailed instruction on using and appraising the evidence base, conducting web-based searches, and locating and evaluating individual research studies.

The core elements of locating the best available information consist of first "asking an answerable question," and then using the most efficient approach to locate the answer [71]. Formulating a focused question that is most likely to yield an answer is an acquired skill, but it can be guided by structuring the inquiry around four components, patient or problem, intervention, comparison, and outcome, which are summarized by the acronym PICO [72]. The PICO question first identifies the specific *p*atient population or *p*roblem. The next step clearly designates the *i*ntervention (or exposure) of interest and the alternative choice or *c*omparison (if relevant). Finally the specific *o*utcome should be identified. Once this clinical question has been articulated, then a focused search for the answer can be conducted [71].

A practical approach to evaluating the evidence is to first consult electronic databases consisting of systematic reviews conducted previously. For example, reports from the Cochrane Collaboration, Evidence-Based

Mental Health, or Best Evidence provide summaries and evaluations of the published evidence for well-specified clinical questions [44]. An alternative approach is to specify searches in PubMed or MEDLINE to first identify any available meta-analyses that might have been conducted [73]. Finally, if a previously conducted systematic review is not available, a direct search of the primary research literature can be conducted. First searching through the use of the "Clinical Queries" search engine in PubMed allows for the focused identification of published RCTs, before expanding the search to include studies that are lower in the hierarchy of evidence, such as open-label, case-control, or naturalistic outcome studies [74]. Tips for improving the quality of PubMed or MEDLINE searches are available in a number of recent publications [43–45,75,76].

Limitations and caveats in applying EBM and EBPs to geriatric psychiatry and geriatric mental health services

The recent recommendations by the President's Commission on Mental Health highlight the implementation of evidence-based practices as the keystone for improving the quality of mental health services in America [3]. However, a number of limitations and caveats are important to acknowledge in the context of recommendations for broad-based adoption of EBM and EBPs (Box 2).

Adequacy of the scientific evidence

One source of tension in the field of evidence-based psychiatry is the extent to which there is empirically based data available to inform specific clinical situations and problems. Despite significant progress in the field of geriatric psychiatry, there are substantial areas that lack extensive data to guide clinical decision making. For example, gaps in the treatment literature include a lack of studies ranging from pharmacologic treatment of late-life bipolar disorder and geriatric anxiety disorders to the effectiveness of psychosocial rehabilitation in older adults with schizophrenia. Although the highest level of evidence for a particular intervention is considered to be findings from meta-analyses, systematic evidence-based reviews, or

---

Box 2. Limitations and caveats

1. Adequacy of the scientific evidence
2. Limits of data based on conventional RCTs
3. Individualizing the evidence
4. Selection and definition of EBPs
5. Limits of pooled data and meta-analyses
6. Potential bias in reporting the evidence by researchers

replicated randomized controlled trials [46], it is important to recognize that evidence-based medicine is based on using the best *available* evidence in directing the decision-making processes. In areas in which the amount and quality of research varies widely for different disorders, the range of sources of evidence should be considered.

Despite these limitations, it is also the case that the field of geriatric psychiatry and mental health research has developed rapidly over the last decade to support large numbers of studies, especially for common disorders such as depression and cognitive impairment disorders. An up-to-date indication of the remarkable growth of the clinical evidence base is reflected in the impressive array of studies and content areas systematically reviewed in articles included in this issue of *Psychiatric Clinics of North America* on evidence-based geriatric psychiatry.

Limits of data based on conventional randomized controlled trials

The double-blind RCT constitutes a gold standard as an optimal method for objectively establishing the scientific evidence of treatment efficacy. However, this approach also contains some inherent limitations when it is applied to the clinical practice of geriatric psychiatry. First, efficacy trials are designed generally to emphasize internal validity by limiting potential experimental confounding factors and imprecision that might be caused by variations in the treatment population, treatment setting, or providers of the intervention. Although this approach is often necessary to establish the efficacy of an intervention, it may present problems in interpreting the generalizability of the findings or effectiveness when applied to heterogeneous populations, usual care treatment settings, and routine providers. This is a concern especially in the field of geriatrics, in which comorbidity and variation in health status and functioning are the rule rather than the exception. Similarly, older adults with mental health needs are most likely to receive or accept mental health services in busy primary care settings [15]. It is not always clear how findings from studies conducted in controlled experimental settings such as academic research centers apply to these settings, where relatively few studies of treatment effectiveness have been conducted. These settings also vary with respect to provider expertise, training, and professional discipline, possibly limiting confidence that the same results may be found when an intervention is applied by nonexpert providers. For these reasons, there have been calls for a greater emphasis on effectiveness and health services research that use methods designed to maximize generalizability of findings to heterogeneous populations, settings, and providers. In many instances, these studies may preserve the advantages of randomization but emphasize usual care populations, settings, and providers using an approach that has been termed "practical clinical trials" (or PCTs) [77].

Conventional experimental designs may also be limited in informing complex clinical questions because of the nature of RCTs that compare single interventions. In this respect, they are limited in complex situations such as determining the next best agent in a series of failed trials or in deciding on different combinations of therapies. The sheer number of possible sequences and combinations of available treatments for different clinical conditions makes it impossible to provide clinical recommendations based entirely on data from RCTs [78,79]. An alternative approach to address this gap uses standardized surveys and quantitative methods to derive expert consensus [80]. Although this approach inevitably carries many of the limitations of expert opinions that are not directly based on experimental evidence, advantages over conventional group consensus procedures include the use of blinded ratings and presentations of aggregate confidence intervals for each treatment recommendation. An example of this approach is provided by guidelines on the pharmacotherapy of geriatric depression by Alexopoulos and colleagues [81]. Using a nine-point rating of the appropriateness of different treatment choices, 100 experts were asked to rate different assessment scales, acute and maintenance treatment strategies, dosing and duration of treatment, strategies for managing treatment-resistant conditions, the use of combination therapy, and drug selection in the context of medical comorbidity. Aggregate analyses were then conducted to determine the degree of consensus among the experts and to calculate confidence intervals for each treatment recommendation. As such, this approach represents an alternative for situations when empirically derived data are unavailable or not feasible.

Individualizing the evidence

Evidence alone is inadequate to guide treatment selections. As described previously in this overview, the proper application of EBM does not support or advocate the indiscriminate application of treatment protocols or the use of "cookbook" medicine. Data from empirical trials need first to be interpreted or adjusted in the context of a competent clinical assessment of the unique circumstances, clinical presentation, risk factors, and needs of the individual patient. Although data-based adjustments of anticipated risks and expected outcomes can often be individualized to specific patients for well-studied medical interventions [71], comparable approaches are relatively weak in the field of mental health. However, the clinician can still use clinical knowledge of the individual patient to interpret and apply findings from research populations. For example, after a brief search of the most recent research literature, a clinician may locate a comprehensive meta-analysis, finding similar efficacy of first-generation and atypical antipsychotic medications in the treatment of psychosis. However, data from longitudinal observational studies demonstrate that the risks of tardive dyskinesia are significantly greater for older persons, women, and for those who have many years of exposure to first-generation antipsychotic medications [82]. These factors would be important information in considering treatment recommendations for a 75-year-old woman who has a psychotic relapse and who has a history of extensive exposure to antipsychotic medications. In another example, a clinician may locate a study reporting similar efficacy of an antidepressant that can be administered once per week, compared with an alternative agent requiring daily dosing. This would be important information in treating a depressed, cognitively impaired older person who lives alone but receives weekly visits from a home care nurse.

An additional component of individualizing the evidence consists of incorporating patient values or preferences. This important element of EBM is elaborated in current models of shared decision making [83]. Although the research on shared decision making has developed substantially over the last decade, little is known about approaches that are optimized specifically to meet the needs of the older patient. It is likely that older adults vary considerably with respect to the extent that they prefer to rely on the physician's recommendation compared with weighing treatment options on their own. In addition, older persons with different degrees of cognitive impairment present challenges in evaluating decisional capacity and the ability to engage in an informed process of weighing the merits of different treatments. Further research is needed on approaches that support shared decision making specific to the older person with different degrees of functional ability, cognitive capacity, and personal preferences.

Selection and definition of mental health EBPs

The Institute on Medicine report "Crossing the Quality Chasm" [1] and the more recent recommendations of the Present's Commission on Mental Health [3,4] have stimulated broad-based calls for the dissemination and implementation of EBPs in health care. Policy makers and payers have joined in this call to action, reflecting Cochrane's early admonition that limited health care dollars should be prioritized for treatments with proven effectiveness [70]. Many states and mental health care provider organizations are engaged in processes to identify specific EBPs for targeted implementation and dedicated resource allocation. This movement is exemplified by a recent law passed by the state of Oregon that mandates 75% of state-supported mental health services be required to consist of EBPs by the year 2009 [84,85].

In the midst of these initiatives, consumers have voiced concerns regarding the application of an evidence-based approach to the field of mental health. Among the many issues voiced by consumers is the lack of research conducted on mental health service alternatives (eg, peer support and other recovery-based services), which is perceived as a reflection of a research agenda driven by the scientific research community rather than consumers' needs and preferences [86]. At the center of this critique is the concern that valued services will not be reimbursed because the research community has not selected these services for study in a randomized clinical trial or because certain interventions may not be amenable to a test of effectiveness by an RCT.

Expressing a related concern, some health policy researchers object that decisions identifying specific treatments for priority funding should not rely on findings derived primarily from RCTs. For example, Tanenbaum [87] notes that current workgroups formulated to identify specific lists of evidence-based mental health practices tend to use RCTs as the gold standard, yet they fail to differentiate between treatments that lack evidence because of a finding of ineffectiveness, versus those that lack evidence because they have not been studied. Additional concerns include the position that some forms of psychotherapy and socially complex services are ill suited to RCT research designs, that sound clinical practice is not necessarily consistent with the direct implementation of findings from science, and that different definitions of effectiveness are being used, sometimes in the service of minimizing expenditures or cost effectiveness [87]. These concerns and caveats regarding EBPs challenge researchers and policy makers to engage in an informed dialogue on the appropriate use, interpretation, application, and definition of scientific evidence in relation to health policy. The need for these discussions may be especially important for the field of geriatrics because of the common use of multicomponent interventions and the complex challenge of evaluating treatment outcomes for chronic and degenerative disorders.

Limits of pooled data and meta-analyses

Although there are significant advantages to seeking meta-analyses as a source for evaluating the level of evidence to support the efficacy or safety of a given intervention, there are inherent limitations that need to be considered in interpreting results based on pooled data. These approaches can be overly conservative in excluding informative studies, or, alternatively, they may cluster studies with inadequate attention to major differences. For example, common problems associated with conclusions about the aggregate efficacy or safety of a given intervention from different studies include small sample sizes and lack of power, heterogeneity of study subjects and methods, lack of interchangeable measures and outcomes, and differences in the quality and duration of studies [88,89]. Hence, there may be instances in which data from a single, large, well-designed RCT may be more valid than pooled analyses from a large number of different smaller studies with varying methods and outcomes.

An additional limitation to relying on aggregate analyses of published reports pertains to the problem of unpublished data. This issue is recently of particular relevance to the field of geriatric psychiatry in relation to recent reports on the safety of atypical antipsychotics in the treatment of dementia. An increased risk of cerebrovascular accidents and mortality associated with atypical antipsychotics in the treatment of patients with Alzheimer's dementia was only recognized after years of prescribing atypical antipsychotics in the context of initially favorable reports on the safety and effectiveness of these agents in geriatric patients. After aggregating unpublished data from a number of different industry-supported clinical trials, 15 of 17 placebo-controlled studies of olanzapine, risperidone, quetiapine, and risperidone showed increases in mortality, compared with placebo, for older adults with behavioral disorders of dementia. Together, these studies involved 5106 patients and identified mortality rates of 4.5% among those receiving atypical antipsychotics, compared with 2.6% among those receiving placebo. Overall, aggregate analyses demonstrated a 1.6- to 1.7-fold increase in mortality, most commonly because of cardiovascular events, sudden death, or infections [90,91]. In this respect, it is important to consider if the available data are comprehensive and fully representative or comprise a select subset of results. The implementation of a new policy requiring the registration of all clinical trials as a prerequisite to being eligible for publication may help to reduce the likelihood that only selected data are being released for publication [92].

Potential bias in the report of the evidence by researchers

Approximately 70% of the funding for clinical drug trials conducted in the United States is procured from industry [93]. In addition to the possibility of bias in study designs and selective reporting of findings, contractual agreements with academic investigators may include provisions to control publication of findings or ensure that scientific reports occur in publications sponsored by industry with minimal input by the academic investigator [93]. Lucrative honoraria and gifts from industry have also been implicated in influencing attitudes and behaviors of investigators [94,95]. In addition to potential bias in the reporting of individual research studies, caution is warranted in relying on reviews of the literature in expert consensus guidelines. Conventional expert consensus guidelines are often assembled under the sponsorship of professional organizations that are invested in promoting specific treatment modalities. Of particular concern, expert panels developing treatment guidelines are composed largely of participants who have a relationship with industry. For example, review of 44 clinical guidelines for medical disorders published between 1991 and 1999 found that 87% of the authors had a financial relationship to at least one pharmaceutical company, although 42 of the 44 guidelines did not specify the existence of potential conflicts of interest [95].

Summary

Despite various limitations and caveats in the application of an evidence-based approach to the practice and delivery of geriatric psychiatry, the future of EBM holds tremendous promise for improving the quality and effectiveness of services provided by practitioners. Effective training of clinicians in evidence-based practices will be an essential component of mainstreaming these practices into usual care and enhancing the quality of mental health services for older adults. In translating an evidence-based approach into daily practice, clinicians will need to develop the skills to quickly access and communicate findings on treatment outcomes, while also tailoring these findings to the unique clinical situation. Finally, clinicians will need to increase their familiarity and comfort with the process of shared decisions that actively incorporates the preferences and values of individual patients. In using an evidence-based approach to improve systems of care, scientific evidence will need to be synthesized in a transparent, standardized manner so that health care organizations and systems ensure that effective practices are provided and supported. In this respect, the principles of EBM should inform implementation of EBPs and the policies for creating evidence-based health care systems.

The field of geriatric psychiatry is in the early stages of embracing EBM, mostly through the promotion of selected EBPs. As evidenced by this issue, the field is beginning to synthesize evidence in the form of systematic reviews and evidence-based treatment recommendations. Procedures and workgroups are underway to identify core evidence-based practices for widespread implementation. However, the field of geriatric psychiatry is challenged by a variety of issues and inherent limitations that complicate the application of an evidence-based approach in daily clinical practice. Although great strides have been made in developing the evidence base for effective treatments of a wide spectrum of geriatric mental disorders, we are still hampered by a lack of knowledge on the best approach to implementing these practices and the supporting principles of EBM in routing practice settings. In particular, the field of geriatric psychiatry lacks adequate information needed to individually adapt findings on outcomes and risks from research studies to individual patients with different degrees of medical comorbidity, functional abilities, and cognitive capacities. Other significant challenges include how to best engage in the process of shared decision making in the context of varying levels of cognitive capacity and decision-making preference. Finally, there is an urgent need to develop effective approaches to train practitioners in the necessary skills to practice EBM and to change systems of care to effectively implement and deliver evidence-based practices.

References

[1] Institute of Medicine. Crossing the quality chasm: a new health system for the 21st century. Washington (DC): Institute of Medicine; 2001.
[2] Interim report of the president's new freedom commission on mental health: 2002. Available at: http://www.mentalhealthcommission.gov/reports/Interim_Report.htm. Accessed August 25, 2005.
[3] Hogan MF. The president's new freedom commission: recommendations to transform mental health care in America. Psychiatr Serv 2003;54(11):1467–74.

[4] Bartels SJ. Improving the United States' system of care for older adults with mental illness: findings and recommendations for the president's new freedom commission on mental health. Am J Geriatr Psychiatry 2003;11(5):486–97.

[5] Bartels SJ, Horn S, Sharkey P, Levine K. Treatment of depression in older primary care patients in health maintenance organizations. Int J Psychiatry Med 1997;27(3):215–31.

[6] Druss BG, Bradford WD, Rosenheck RA, et al. Quality of medical care and excess mortality in older patients with mental disorders. Arch Gen Psychiatry 2001;58(6):565–72.

[7] Giron MS, Wang HX, Bernsten C, et al. The appropriateness of drug use in an older non-demented and demented population. J Am Geriatr Soc 2001;49(3):277–83.

[8] Jeste DV, Alexopoulos GS, Bartels SJ, et al. Consensus statement on the upcoming crisis in geriatric mental health: research agenda for the next 2 decades. Arch Gen Psychiatry 1999; 56(9):848–53.

[9] George LK, Blazer DG, Winfield-Laird I, et al. Psychiatric disorders and mental health service use in later life. In: Brody JA, Maddox GL, editors. Epidemiology and aging. New York: Springer; 1988. p. 189–221.

[10] Pace WD. Geriatric assessment in the office setting. Geriatrics 1989;44(6):29–35.

[11] Fields SD. Clinical practice guidelines: finding and appraising useful, relevant recommendations for geriatric care. Geriatrics 2000;55(1):59–63.

[12] Administration on Aging. Older adults and mental health: issues and opportunities. Rockville (MD): Department of Health and Human Services; 2001.

[13] Hybels CF, Blazer DG. Epidemiology of late-life mental disorders. Clin Geriatr Med 2003; 19(4):663–96.

[14] Olfson M, Shea S, Feder A, et al. Prevalence of anxiety, depression, and substance use disorders in an urban general medicine practice. Arch Fam Med 2000;9(9):876–83.

[15] Klap R, Tschantz K, Unützer J. Caring for mental disorders in the United States: a focus on older adults. Am J Geriatr Psychiatry 2003;11(5):517–24.

[16] Klinkman M. Competing demands in psychosocial care: a model for the identification and treatment of depressive disorders in primary care. Gen Hosp Psychiatry 1997; 19(2):98–111.

[17] Van Citters AD, Bartels SJ. Caring for older Americans: geriatric care management and the workforce challenge. Geriatric Care Management Journal 2004;14(1):25–30.

[18] Bartels SJ, Coakley E, Zubritsky C, et al. Improving access to geriatric mental health services: a randomized trial comparing treatment engagement with integrated versus enhanced referral care for depression, anxiety, and at-risk alcohol use. Am J Psychiatry 2004;161(8): 1455–62.

[19] Oxman TE, Dietrich AJ, Schulberg HC. Evidence-based models of integrated management of depression in primary care. Psychiatr Clin North Am 2005;28(4):1061–77.

[20] Unützer J, Powers D, Katon W, et al. From establishing an evidence-based practice to implementation in real world settings: IMPACT as a case study in the use of evidence-based medicine. Psychiatr Clin North Am 2005;28(4):1079–92.

[21] Bates J, Boote J, Beverley C. Psychosocial interventions for people with a milder dementing illness: a systematic review. J Adv Nurs 2004;45(6):644–58.

[22] Banerjee S, Dickinson E. Evidence based health care in old age psychiatry. Int J Psychiatry Med 1997;27(3):283–92.

[23] Beyth RJ, Shorr RI. Epidemiology of adverse drug reactions in the elderly by drug class. Drugs Aging 1999;14(3):231–9.

[24] Larsen PD, Hoot Martin JL. Polypharmacy and the elderly. AORN J 1999;69(3):619–28.

[25] Beers MH, Ouslander JG. Risk factors in geriatric drug prescribing. Drugs 1989;37(1): 105–12.

[26] Mackin RS, Areán PA. Evidence-based psychosocial interventions for geriatric depression. Psychiatr Clin North Am 2005;28(4):805–20.

[27] Oslin DW. Evidence-based treatment of geriatric substance abuse. Psychiatr Clin North Am 2005;28(4):897–911.

[28] Schulz R, Martire LM, Klinger JN. Evidence-based caregiver interventions in geriatric psychiatry. Psychiatr Clin North Am 2005;28(4):1007–38.

[29] Shanmugham B, Karp J, Drayer R, et al. Evidence-based pharmacological interventions for geriatric depression. Psychiatr Clin North Am 2005;28(4):821–35.

[30] Cole M. Evidence-based review of risk factors for geriatric depression and brief preventive interventions. Psychiatr Clin North Am 2005;28(4):785–803.

[31] Weintraub D, Katz IR. Pharmacologic interventions for psychosis and agitation in neurodegenerative diseases: Evidence about efficacy and safety. Psychiatr Clin North Am 2005;28(4):941–83.

[32] Van Citters AD, Pratt SI, Bartels SJ, Jeste DV. Evidence-based review of pharmacological and non-pharmacological treatments for older adults with schizophrenia. Psychiatr Clin North Am 2005;28(4):913–39.

[33] Bruce ML, Van Citters AD, Bartels SJ. Evidence-based home and community-based mental health services. Psychiatr Clin North Am 2005;28(4):1039–60.

[34] Bharani N, Snowden M. Evidence based interventions for nursing home residents with dementia related behavioral symptoms. Psychiatr Clin North Am 2005;28(4):985–1006.

[35] Wetherell JL, Lenze EJ, Stanley MA. Evidence-based treatment of geriatric anxiety disorders. Psychiatr Clin North Am 2005;28(4):871–96.

[36] Young RC. Evidence-based treatments for geriatric bipolar disorder. Psychiatr Clin North Am 2005;28(4):837–69.

[37] Schneider LS, Ismail MS, Dagerman K, et al. Clinical Antipsychotic Trials of Intervention Effectiveness (CATIE): Alzheimer's disease trial. Schizophr Bull 2003;29(1):57–72.

[38] Lavori PW, Rush AJ, Wisniewski SR, et al. Strengthening clinical effectiveness trials: equipoise-stratified randomization. Biol Psychiatry 2001;50(10):792–801.

[39] Unützer J, Katon W, Callahan CM, et al. Collaborative care management of late-life depression in the primary care setting: a randomized controlled trial. JAMA 2002;288(22):2836–45.

[40] National Institutes of Health. NIH Policy and guidelines on the inclusion of children as participants in research involving human subjects. Available at: http://grants.nih.gov/grants/guide/notice-files/not98-024.html. Accessed August 25, 2005.

[41] Essock SM, Drake RE, Frank RG, et al. Randomized controlled trials in evidence-based mental health care: getting the right answer to the right question. Schizophr Bull 2003; 29(1):115–23.

[42] Woolf SH, DiGuiseppi CG, Atkins D, et al. Developing evidence-based clinical practice guidelines: lessons learned by the US Preventive Services Task Force. Annu Rev Public Health 1996;17:511–38.

[43] Sackett DL, Rosenberg WM, Gray JA, et al. Evidence based medicine: what it is and what it isn't. BMJ 1996;312(7023):71–2.

[44] Guyatt G, Rennie D. Users' guides to the medical literature: a manual for evidence-based clinical practice: the Evidence-Based Medicine Working Group. Chicago: AMA Press; 2002.

[45] Friedland DJ, Go AS, Davoren JB, et al. Evidence-based medicine: a framework for clinical practice. Stamford (CT): Appleton and Lange; 1998.

[46] Guyatt GH, Rennie D. Users' guides to the medical literature: a manual for evidence-based clinical practice. Chicago, IL: AMA Press; 2002.

[47] Sackett DL, Scott Richardson W, Rosenberg W, et al. Evidence-based medicine: how to practice and teach EBM. New York: Churchill Livingstone; 1997.

[48] Edwards E, Elwyn G. Evidence-based patient choice. New York: Oxford University Press; 2001.

[49] Haynes RB, Devereaux PJ, Guyatt GH. Clinical expertise in the era of evidence-based medicine and patient choice. ACP J Club 2002;136(2):A11–4.

[50] Wennberg JE. Practice variations and health care reform: connecting the dots. Health Aff (Millwood) 2004;(Suppl Web ExclusiveVAR):S140–4. Available at: http://content.healthaffairs.org/cgi/reprint/hlthaff.var.140v1. Accessed October 21, 2005.

[51] Wennberg JE. Unwarranted variations in healthcare delivery: implications for academic medical centres. BMJ 2002;325(7370):961–4.

[52] Gray JAM. Evidence-based healthcare: how to make health policy and management decisions. New York: Churchill Livingston; 1997.

[53] Chambless DL, Hollon SD. Defining empirically supported therapies. J Consult Clin Psychol 1998;66(1):7–18.

[54] Chambless DL, Ollendick TH. Empirically supported psychological interventions: controversies and evidence. Annu Rev Psychol 2001;52:685–716.

[55] Edwards A, Hood K, Matthews E, et al. The effectiveness of one-to-one risk communication interventions in health care: a systematic review. Med Decis Making 2000;20(3):290–7.

[56] Balint M. The Doctor, the patient, and his illness. London: Tavistock; 1957.

[57] Engel GL. A unified concept of health and disease. Perspect Biol Med 1960;3:459–85.

[58] Ellwood PM. Shattuck lecture: outcomes management: a technology of patient experience. N Engl J Med 1988;318(23):1549–56.

[59] Laine C, Davidoff F. Patient-centered medicine: a professional evolution. JAMA 1996; 275(2):152–6.

[60] Levenstein JH, McCracken EC, McWhinney IR, et al. The patient-centred clinical method: 1. a model for the doctor-patient interaction in family medicine. Fam Pract 1986;3(1):24–30.

[61] Stewart M, Brown JB. Patient-centredness in medicine. In: Edwards A, Elwyn G, editors. Evidence-base patient choice. New York: Oxford University Press; 2001. pp. 97–117.

[62] Charles C, Gafni A, Whelan T. Decision-making in the physician-patient encounter: revisiting the shared treatment decision-making model. Soc Sci Med 1999;49(5):651–61.

[63] Ashcroft R, Hope T, Parker M. Ethical issues and evidence based patient care. In: Edwards E, Elwyn G, editors. Evidence-based patient choice. New York: Oxford University Press; 2001.

[64] Centre for Reviews and Dissemination. Available at: http://www.york.ac.uk/inst/crd/crddatabases.htm. Accessed October 21, 2005.

[65] BMJ Publishing Group. Clinical Evidence: Mental Health. issue 7. Kingsport (TN): Quebecor; 2002.

[66] Evidence Based Mental Health. EBMH Website. Available at: http://ebmh.bmjjournals.com/. Accessed October 21, 2005.

[67] Lehman AF, Steinwachs DM. At issue: translating research into practice: the Schizophrenia Patient Outcomes Research Team (PORT) treatment recommendations. Schizophr Bull 1998;224(1):1–10.

[68] Miller AL, Chiles JA, Chiles JK, et al. The Texas Medication Algorithm Project (TMAP) schizophrenia algorithms. J Clin Psychiatry 1999;60(10):649–57.

[69] Drake RE, Goldman HH, Leff HS, et al. Implementing evidence-based practices in routine mental health service settings. Psychiatr Serv 2001;52(2):179–82.

[70] The Cochrane Collaboration. Why the "Cochrane" collaboration? [internet]. June 21, 2002. Available at: http://www.cochrane.org/cochrane/archieco.htm. Accessed August 1, 2002.

[71] Straus SE, Richardson WS, Glasziou P, et al. Evidence-based medicine: how to practice and teach EBM. 3rd edition. Edinburgh: Churchill Livingstone; 2005.

[72] Bartkowiak BA. Searching for evidence-based medicine in the literature part 1: the start. Clinical Medicine and Research 2004;2(4):254–5.

[73] PubMed. National Library of Medicine. http://www.ncbi.nlm.nih.gov/entrez/query.fcgi?db=PubMed. Accessed October 21, 2005.

[74] PubMed Clinical Queries. National Library of Medicine. http://www.ncbi.nlm.nih.gov/entrez/query/static/clinical.shtml. Accessed October 21, 2005.

[75] Greenhalgh T. How to read a paper: the Medline database. BMJ 1997;315(7101):180–3.

[76] Gray JAM. Evidence-based healthcare: how to make health policy and management decisions. New York: Churchill Livingston; 1997.

[77] Tunis SR, Stryer DB, Clancy CM. Practical clinical trials: increasing the value of clinical research for decision making in clinical and health policy. JAMA 2003;290(12):1624–32.

[78] Djulbegovic B, Hadley TR. Evaluating the quality of clinical guidelines: linking decisions to medical evidence. Oncology 1998;12(11A):310–4.

[79] Shekelle PG, Kahan JP, Bernstain SJ, et al. The reproducibility of a method to identify the overuse and underuse of medical procedures. N Engl J Med 1998;338(26):1888–95.

[80] Brook RH, Chassin MR, Fink A, et al. A method for the detailed assessment of the appropriateness of medical technologies. Int J Technol Assess Health Care 1986;2(1):53–63.

[81] Alexopoulos GS, Katz IR, Reynolds CF III, et al. The expert consensus guideline series: pharmacotherapy of depressive disorders in older patients. Postgrad Med 2001; October:1–86.

[82] Schatzberg AF, Cole JO, DeBattista C. Manual of clinical psychopharmacology. 3rd edition. Washington (DC): American Psychiatric Publishing Group; 1997.

[83] Tunis SR. A clinical research strategy to support shared decision making. Health Aff (Millwood) 2005;24(1):180–4.

[84] State of Oregon. Act: SB 267, Chapter 669 Oregon Laws: 2003. Available at: www.leg.state.or.us/orlaws/sess0600.dir/0669ses.htm. Accessed October 21, 2005.

[85] Oregon Office of Mental Health and Addiction Services. Proposed operational definition for evidence-based practices, final draft. Available at: www.dhs.state.or.us/mentalhealth/ebp/definition0722.pdf. 2004. Accessed October 21, 2005.

[86] Frese FJ III, Stanley J, Kress K, et al. Integrating evidence-based practices and the recovery model. Psychiatr Serv 2001;52(11):1462–8.

[87] Tanenbaum SJ. Evidence-based practice as mental health policy: three controversies and a caveat. Health Aff (Millwood) 2005;24(1):163–73.

[88] Schneider LS, Pollock VE, Lyness SA. A meta-analysis of controlled trials of neuroleptic treatment in dementia. J Am Geriatr Soc 1990;38(5):553–63.

[89] Flather MD, Farkouh ME, Pogue JM, et al. Strengths and limitations of meta-analysis: larger studies may be more reliable. Control Clin Trials 1997;18(6):568–79.

[90] Food and Drug Administration. FDA public health advisory: deaths with antipsychotics in elderly patients with behavioral disturbances. April 11, 2005. Available at: http://www.fda.gov/cder/drug/advisory/antipsychotics.htm. Accessed May 28, 2005.

[91] Kuehn BM. FDA warns antipsychotic drugs may be risky for elderly. JAMA 2005;293(20):2462.

[92] De Angelis C, Drazen JM, Frizelle FA, et al. Clinical trial registration: a statement from the International Committee of Medical Journal Editors. N Engl J Med 2004;351(12):1250–1.

[93] Bodenheimer T. Uneasy alliance: clinical investigators and the pharmaceutical industry. N Engl J Med 2000;342(20):1539–44.

[94] Wazana A. Physicians and the pharmaceutical industry: is a gift ever just a gift? JAMA 2000;283(3):373–80.

[95] Choudhry NK, Stelfox HT, Detsky AS. Relationships between authors of clinical practice guidelines and the pharmaceutical industry. JAMA 2002;287(5):612–7.

ELSEVIER
SAUNDERS

Psychiatr Clin N Am
28 (2005) 785–803

PSYCHIATRIC
CLINICS
OF NORTH AMERICA

Evidence-Based Review of Risk Factors for Geriatric Depression and Brief Preventive Interventions

Martin G. Cole, MD, FRCP(C)

*Department of Psychiatry, St. Mary's Hospital, 3830 Lacombe Avenue, Montreal,
Québec H3T 1M5, Canada*

Major depression occurs in at least 1% to 3% of the general elderly population [1,2], and an additional 8% to 16% of the elderly have clinically significant depressive symptoms [1,3]. The prognosis of these depressive states is poor [4]. A meta-analysis of outcomes at 24 months has estimated that only 33% of subjects were well, 33% were depressed, and 21% had died [5]. Moreover, studies of depressed adults report that those with depressive symptoms, with or without depressive disorder, have poorer functioning [6,7] comparable to or worse than chronic medical conditions such as heart and lung disease, arthritis, hypertension, and diabetes [8]. In addition to poor functioning, depression increases the perception of poor health [8], the use of medical services [9], and health care costs [10,11].

These findings suggest that depression in elderly community subjects is a serious problem [5]. Yet, among those who are detected and treated, the effectiveness of the available interventions is modest [12]. Even when acute-phase treatment and patient compliance are optimized, the rates of improvement and recovery at 12 months are low [13]. Even if acute-phase treatment is effective, the chances of relapse or recurrence are high [14]. Therefore, preventing depression is a priority.

In 1994, the Institute of Medicine (IOM) Report on Preventing Mental Disorders made a spirited call for increased research on preventive interventions [15]. This call was reiterated in the reports of the National Institute of Mental Health (NIMH) Psychosocial Intervention Development Workgroup on the Prevention and Treatment of Depression [16] and the NIMH Alliance Consensus Statement on Late-Life Mood Disorders [17]. The IOM report defined three levels of preventive interventions: (1)

E-mail address: martin.cole@ssss.gouv.qc.ca

universal preventive interventions targeted at communities, regardless of risk; (2) selective preventive interventions targeted at high-risk groups; and (3) indicated preventive interventions targeted at individuals with early signs or symptoms of mental disorder. Presently, the development of selective preventive interventions would seem to be appropriate. Thus, the present review identifies the risk factors for depression among elderly community subjects and explores the feasibility and effectiveness of brief preventive interventions. The review, presented in two parts (risk factors for depression and brief preventive interventions), is followed by an overall discussion of the findings and proposals for a research agenda. The review process, modified from the one described by Oxman and colleagues [18] involved a systematic selection of articles on each topic, an assessment of validity, the abstraction of data, and an examination of results.

Risk factors for depression

The first part of this article identifies the risk factors for depression among elderly community subjects by systematically reviewing original research on this topic.

Methods

Two computer databases, MEDLINE and PsychINFO, were searched for potentially relevant articles published from January 1966 to February, 2005 and from January 1967 to February 2005, respectively. For MEDLINE, the keywords depression, risk factor, aged, and community were used; for PsychINFO, the same words were used as text words. Relevant articles (based on the title and abstract) were retrieved for more detailed evaluation. The bibliographies of relevant articles, including a previous review by the present author's group [19], were searched for additional references. All articles retrieved were screened to meet the following six inclusion criteria: (1) original research published in English or French; (2) a study population of community residents; (3) subjects aged 50 years or more; (4) a prospective study that excluded subjects who were depressed at baseline (or controlled for baseline depression in the analysis); (5) studied at least one risk factor for depression; and (6) provided an acceptable definition of depression (either recognized diagnostic criteria or cut-off on a depression rating scale).

Next, the methods of each study were assessed according to the four primary criteria for risk factor studies described by the Evidence-Based Medicine Working Group [20]: the study clearly identified comparison groups that were similar with respect to important determinants of outcome, other than the one of interest (or differences in important determinants were controlled for in the analysis); exposures and outcomes were measured in the same way; there was a sufficiently long follow-up period (ie, 1 year); and a sufficient number of subjects completed the study (ie, 80% of inception cohort). Each study was scored with respect to meeting (+) or not meeting (−) each of the above criteria.

Finally, information about the sample size at baseline and follow-up, age, proportion of males, criteria for depression, exclusion criteria at baseline, length of follow-up, number of incident cases of depression, and risk factors was abstracted from each report. A qualitative meta-analysis was conducted by summarizing, comparing, and contrasting abstracted data. A quantitative meta-analysis was conducted for risk factors with usable data from two or more studies. To obtain an overall estimate of the odds ratio (OR) of depression associated with each risk factor, a meta-analysis was conducted using a Bayesian hierarchical (random effects) model [21]. In the Bayesian framework, information available before the analysis is combined with the observed data to obtain a posterior distribution for the parameters of interest [21]. It was assumed that no previous information was available. The variance between odds ratios from different studies is a measure of the heterogeneity between studies. A Bayesian 95% posterior credible interval may be interpreted in a straightforward manner as an interval that contains the parameter of interest with 95% probability, given the observed data. We also estimated the probability that the pooled odds ratio was greater than 1.

Results

The search strategy yielded 130 potentially relevant studies; 45 were retrieved for more detailed evaluation. Twenty studies met the inclusion criteria [22–41]. The other 25 studies were excluded for the following reasons: four did not meet the age criterion, 16 were not prospective, two did not study at least one risk factor, and three did not meet two or more of the inclusion criteria. The results of the validity assessment are presented in Table 1 [22–41]. Six studies met all of the criteria. Most studies had incomplete follow-up of the inception cohort.

The results of the 20 studies are summarized in Table 2 [22–38,41]. The 20 studies involved more than 23,058 subjects at baseline, more than 14,326 subjects at follow-up, and more than 1694 subjects with incident depression. The number of subjects at baseline and follow-up ranged from 141 to 3747 and 79 to 5449, respectively. Subjects' mean ages were reported in 11 studies (58–84.5 years). Seventeen studies reported a gender distribution in which 0% to 65% of subjects were men (median 41%). The length of reported follow-up ranged from 3 to 96 months (median 24 months). Nine studies used Diagnostic and Statistical Manual of Mental Disorders criteria or structured interview criteria to diagnose depression, nine studies used a cut-off on a depression rating scale, and two studies used both. Among the 17 studies that reported the frequency of incident depression, the frequencies ranged from 1.8% to 24.0%

Table 1
Validity of studies of risk factors for depression according to the primary criteria of the evidence-based working group

| | | | Follow-up | |
Study	Similar comparison groups	Same measures of depression	Length (12 mo)	Complete (80%)
Phifer and Murrell [22] 1986	+	+	−	−
McHorney and Mor [23] 1988	+	+	−	+
Kennedy et al [24] 1990	+	+	+	+
Harlow et al [25] 1991	+	+	+	−
Russell and Cutrona [26] 1991	+	+	+	+
Green et al [27] 1992	+	+	+	?
Livingston et al [28] 1993	+	+	+	−
Mendes et al [29] 1994	+	+	+	+
Beekman et al [30] 1995	+	+	+	−
Zeiss et al [31] 1996	+	+	+	?
Kivela et al [32] 1996	+	+	+	−
Prince et al [33] 1998	+	+	+	−
Turvey et al [34] 1999	+	+	+	?
Livingston et al [35] 2000	+	+	+	−
Schoevers et al [36] 2000	+	+	+	−
Geerlings et al [37] 2000	+	+	+	+
Forsell [38] 2000	+	+	+	−
Paterniti et al [39] 2000	+	+	+	+
Roberts et al [40] 2000	+	+	+	+
Kritz-Silvertein et al [41] 2001	+	+	+	−

+, meets criterion; −, does not meet criterion; ?, could not be determined.
From Cole MG, Dendukuri N. Risk factors for depression among elderly community subjects: a systematic review and meta-analysis. Am J Psychiatry 2003;160:1147–56; with permission.

(median 12.0%) and were generally higher in studies using cut-offs on rating scales as opposed to diagnostic criteria.

Forty-two different risk factors were studied by univariate analysis, 25 in two or more studies and 17 in one study each (Table 3). Disability, older age, new medical illness, poor health status, sleep disturbance, previous incidence of depression, low education, new disability, poor self-perceived health, poor social support, bereavement, and vision or hearing impairment were identified as risk factors for depression in at least two studies.

Forty-three risk factors were studied by multivariate analysis, 15 in two or more studies and 28 in one study each (Table 4) [42–50]. Disability, bereavement, new medical illness, poor health status, female gender, previous incidence of depression, and poor self-perceived health were identified as risk factors for depression in at least two studies each. Risk factors identified by both univariate and multivariate techniques in at least two studies each were disability, new medical illness, poor health status, previous incidence of depression, poor self-perceived health, and bereavement.

Only 13 risk factors had data that could be used in the quantitative meta-analysis (see Table 3). The combined odds ratios ranged from 1.0 to 3.3.

Table 2
Summary of prospective studies of risk factors for depression among community elderly

Study	Number of subjects		Age (y)		Male (%)	Criteria for depression	Exclusion criteria at baseline	Length of follow-up (mo)	Cases of incident depression	
	Baseline	Follow-up	Range	Mean					N	%
Phifer and Murrell [22] 1986	2937	1233	≥55	68	41	CES-D > 20	CES-D ≥ 16 psychiatric treatment in past 6 mo	6	66	5.4
McHorney and Mor [23] 1988	1754	1447		58	28	RDC	—	3–4	285	19.7
Kennedy et al [24] 1990	1243	1243	≥65	74	46	CES-D ≥ 16 + 5 pts above baseline	CES-D > 16	24	163	11.2
Harlow et al [25] 1991	600	445	65–75	—	0	CES-D	—	12	—	—
Russell and Cutrona [26] 1991	301	284	≥65	—	40	Zung depression scale	Poor health, psychiatric treatment in past 6 mo, dementia institutionalized	12	—	—
Green et al [27] 1992	1070	?	≥65	—	—	GMS-AGECAT (level 3.5)	GMS-AGECAT depression (level 3+)	36	44 (4.1)	4.1
Livingston et al [28] 1993	705	524	≥65	75	37	Short CARE (clinical depression)	—	24	22 (4.2)	4.2
Mendes et al [29] 1994	1046	731	≥65	73	65	CES-D ≥ 20	—	36	77	10.5
Beekman et al [30] 1995	340	238	55–89	—	50	CES-D ≥ 16	Depression MMSE < 16	12	38	16
Zeiss et al [31] 1996	?	680	≥50	—	41	CES-D ≥ 12 + SADS positive	Depression	24	95	14

(continued on next page)

Table 2 (continued)

Study	Number of subjects		Age (y)		Male (%)	Criteria for depression	Exclusion criteria at baseline	Length of follow-up (mo)	Cases of incident depression	
	Baseline	Follow-up	Range	Mean					N	%
Kivela et al [32] 1996	944	679	≥60	69	41	DSM-3	Depression	60	60	8.8
Prince et al [33] 1998	538	383	≥65	76	39	Short CARE (pervasive depression)	Depression	12	46	12
Turvey et al [34] 1999	?	5449	70–103	77	38	Modified CES-D ≥ 6 / CIDI case	— / —	24 / 24	327 / 193	6 / 3.5
Livingston et al [35] 2000	141	79	65–95	—	23	Short CARE (DPHS scale+)	ADL limitations, depression or dementia	36	19	24
Schoevers et al [36] 2000	3747	1940	65–84	—	38	GMS-AGECAT (level 3.5)	Depression, dementia	36	309	15.9
Geerlings et al [37] 2000	325	234	55–85	69	48	CES-D ≥ 16 + 5 pts above baseline	Depression	36	32	14.1
Forsell [38] 2000	1777	903	≥75	85	23	DSM-IV	Depression, anxiety, psychosis	36	29	3.2
Paterniti et al [39] 2000	1191	1014	59–71	65	41	CES-D (M > 16, F > 22)	Depression	224	64	6.3
Roberts et al [40] 2000	2370	2228	50–95	65	44	DSM-IV	Depression	12	—	—
Kritz-Silverstein et al [41] 2001	2029	944	50–89	71	46	BDI ≥ 13	Depression, severe disability	96	17	1.8

Abbreviations: ADL, Activities of Daily Living; BDI, Beck Depression Inventory; CES-D Scale, Center for Epidemiologic Studies Depression Scale; CIDI, Composite International Diagnostic Review; DPHS, Depression Homogeneous Scale; DSM, Diagnostic and Statistical Manual; GMS-AGECAT, Geriatric Mental State Schedule Automated Geratric Examination for Computer Assisted Taxonomy; MMSE, Mini-Mental State Examination; RDC, Research Diagnostic Criteria; SADS, Schedule for Affective Disorders and Schizophrenia; Short CARE, Shortened Comprehensive Assessment and Referral Evaluation.

From Cole MG, Dendukuri N. Risk factors for depression among elderly community subjects: a systematic review and meta-analysis. Am J Psychiatry 2003;160:1147–56; with permission.

Table 3
Results of meta-analysis

Risk factor	Combined odds ratio		Variance between studies		Probability odds ratio ≥ 1 (%)
	Posterior median	95% Credible interval (%)	Posterior median	95% Credible interval (%)	
Older age	1.2	0.9, 1.7	0.06	0.001, 0.64	91
Female	1.4	1.2, 1.8	0.01	≤0.001, 0.16	100
Lower education	1.5	0.8, 2.8	0.14	0.002, 2.20	95
Unmarried	1.0	0.8, 1.3	0.01	≤0.001, 0.30	50
Disability	2.5	1.6, 4.8	0.11	0.002, 1.49	100
Bereavement	3.3	1.7, 4.9	0.03	≤0.001, 1.57	99
Low socioeconomic status	1.2	0.5, 3.7	0.03	≤0.001, 5.87	80
Poor health status	1.8	0.5, 12.8	0.14	0.001, 10.71	91
Cognitive impairment	2.1	0.6, 8.6	0.39	0.008, 8.20	93
Sleep disturbance	2.6	1.9, 3.7	0.02	≤0.001, 0.52	100
Living alone	1.7	0.6, 4.7	0.03	≤0.001, 6.16	92
Prior depression	2.3	1.1, 7.1	0.11	0.001, 5.13	97
New medical illness	2.1	0.4, 10.1	0.71	0.08, 11.57	86

From Cole MG, Dendukuri N. The feasibility and effectiveness of brief interventions to prevent depression in older subjects: a systematic review. Int J Geriatr Psychiatry 2004;19:1019–25; with permission.

Greater heterogeneity was observed among studies evaluating lower education, disability, poor health status, cognitive impairment, previous depression, and new medical illness as risk factors for depression. Based on the combined odds ratios (and their 95% credible intervals) and the posterior distributions of the odds ratios ≥ 1, bereavement (OR 3.3; 95% CI, 1.7%, 4.9%), sleep disturbance (OR 2.6; 95% CI, 1.9%, 3.7%), disability (OR 2.5; 95% CI, 1.6%, 4.8%), previous depression (OR 2.3; 95% CI, 1.1%, 7.1%), and female gender (OR 1.4; 95% CI, 1.2%, 1.8%) were significant risk factors for depression. Older age, lower education, unmarried, and lower social class did not appear to be risk factors. Poor health status, cognitive impairment, living alone, and new medical illness were uncertain risk factors.

Discussion

This review proposed to determine risk factors for depression among elderly community subjects by systematically reviewing original research on this topic. There are, however, 10 potential limitations. First, the search of the literature was conducted by one author only. Second, the search was limited to articles published in English and French. Third, data were abstracted by one author only. Fourth, follow-up of the enrolled cohort was incomplete in most studies; however, the results of studies with or without complete follow-up were similar. Fifth, the examination of depression status was complicated by differences in the length of follow-up. Sixth, the examination of the results of the univariate and multivariate analyses were

Table 4
Validity of studies with respect to meeting (+) or not meeting (−) criteria

Study	Randomized	Similar groups at baseline	Equally treated groups	Blind-rated outcomes	Complete follow-up	Excluded or adjusted for depression at baseline
Parkes [44] 1981	+	−	+	−	−	−
Gilden et al [43] 1992	−	−	+	S/R	+	−
Haight [47] 1992	+	+	+	−	+	−
Lieberman et al [45] 1992	+	+	+	S/R	+	+
Levy et al [42] 1993	−	−	+	−	+	+
Muñoz et al [48] 1995	+	+	+	−	+	+
Haight et al [49] 2000	+	+	+	S/R	+	+
Phillips [50] 2000	+	+	+	+	+	−
Rybarczyk et al [46] 2001	+	+	+	S/R	+	−

Abbreviation: S/R, subject-rated depression scale.

From Cole MG, Dendukuri N. The feasibility and effectiveness of brief interventions to prevent depression in older subjects: a systematic review. Int J Geriatr Psychiatry 2004;19:1019–25; with permission.

complicated by differences in the definitions of some risk factors from one study to the next, and the examination of the results of the multivariate analyses were complicated by adjustments for different variables in different studies. Seventh, five factors were identified with some confidence that increased the risk of depression and four factors (older age, lower education, unmarried, and lower social class) that did not increase the risk of depression; many potential risk factors have not been studied adequately. Eighth, in these meta-analyses, it could not be determined whether the simultaneous presence of more than one risk factor resulted in a cumulative increase in the risk of depression; however, the results of four studies included in this meta-analysis [22,25,26,36] suggest that different risk factors play both additive and interactive roles. Finally, there was heterogeneity in the results for some risk factors (ie, lower education, disability, poor health status, cognitive impairment, previous depression, and new medical illness), perhaps related to definitions of these variables between studies and small sample size in some studies; consequently, the results of the meta-analysis for these risk factors must be interpreted cautiously. Nonetheless, despite the methodological limitations, bereavement, sleep disturbance, disability, previous depression, and female gender appear to be important risk factors for depression among elderly community subjects.

Brief preventive interventions

The following discussion determines the feasibility and effectiveness of brief interventions to prevent depression in older subjects by systematically reviewing all controlled trials on this topic.

Methods

Three computer databases, MEDLINE, PsychINFO, and HEALTH-STAR, were searched for potentially relevant articles published from January 1966 to February 2005, January 1974 to February 2005, and January 1975 to February 2005, respectively. For MEDLINE and HEALTHSTAR, the keywords depression (exploded) and prevention were used; for PsychINFO, depression (exploded) and primary mental health prevention were used.

Relevant articles (based on the title and abstract) were retrieved for more detailed evaluation. The bibliographies of relevant articles, including a previous review by the present author's group [51], were searched for additional references. All articles retrieved were screened to meet the following five inclusion criteria: (1) original research published in English or French; (2) subjects' mean age of 50 or more years; (3) a controlled trial study design (with a no-intervention or delayed intervention control group) of a brief (≤ 12 weeks) intervention to prevent depression; (4) the determination of depression status 12 months or more after enrollment ; and (5) the use of an acceptable definition of depression (either recognized diagnostic criteria or a depression rating scale). Studies of preventive interventions for post-stroke depression and interventions to prevent or relieve caregiver stress (and depression) were not included.

Next, the methods of each study were assessed according to six criteria, five described by the Evidence-Based Medicine Working Group [52] (ie, randomized study, no clinically significant difference between groups reported at baseline, equal treatment of groups except for the intervention, blind rating of outcomes, and all subjects enrolled in the trial are accounted for at follow-up) and one additional criterion (explicitly excluded subjects with depression at baseline or adjusted for depression at baseline in the analysis). Each study was scored with respect to meeting ($+$) or not meeting ($-$) each of the above criteria. Finally, information about the study design, patient population, risk of depression, numbers of subjects approached and enrolled in and completing the study, nature of the intervention, participation in the intervention, dropouts, outcome measures, and results was abstracted systematically from each report. To examine the feasibility of the interventions, the proportion of subjects who were approached and enrolled in the study (enrollment rate), completed the study (completion rate), and complied with the intervention (compliance rate) was tabulated. To examine the effectiveness of the interventions, differences were tabulated in depression symptom outcome scores between intervention and control groups or, when possible, the absolute risk reduction (ARR, difference in rates of depression between intervention and control groups) and the relative risk reduction (RRR, ratio of ARR to rate of depression in the control group) [53]. An ARR or RRR of 0% means that there is no difference between the intervention and control groups. A positive ARR or RRR with a magnitude of much more than 0% is indicative of a strong beneficial effect of the intervention. A qualitative meta-analysis was conducted by summarizing, comparing, and contrasting abstracted data.

Results

The search strategy yielded 474 potentially relevant studies, of which 89 were retrieved for more detailed evaluation. Nine trials met the inclusion criteria, two nonrandomized [42,43] and seven randomized [44–50] studies. The other 80 studies were excluded for the following reasons: four did not meet criterion 2; 46 did not meet criterion 3; seven did not meet criterion 4; two did not meet criterion 5; two did not meet criterion 6; and 19 did not meet two or more of the inclusion criteria. The results of the validity assessment are presented in Table 4. Five studies did not explicitly exclude subjects with depression at baseline or adjust for depression at baseline in the analysis; four studies did not have blind-rated outcomes.

A summary of information pertinent to the feasibility of the interventions is presented in Table 5 [42–50]. The populations, many of whom were older, were drawn from a wide range of settings. Subjects in eight studies were living in the community [42–50]. Among the five studies that reported enrollment, rates ranged from 21% to 100% (median 45%). Study completion rates ranged from 53% to 100% (median 76.5%). Compliance rates ranged from 29% to 100% (median 93.5%). The heterogeneity in study enrollment, completion, and compliance rates could not be explained by characteristics of the study population or type of intervention.

A summary of information pertinent to the effectiveness of the interventions is presented in Table 6 [42–50]. Six studies did not report the incidence rates of depression [44–47,49,50]. The authors of these studies were contacted, but they were unable to provide the rates; for these studies, evidence of significant differences in outcome depression symptom scores between groups are reported. Overall, there was a positive effect of the intervention shown in four studies [43,48–50]. There was a statistically significant difference in depression symptom outcome scores in two [52,53] of six studies favoring the intervention group. In the three studies for which data on incidence were available, ARRs ranged from −17% to 45%, and the RRRs ranged from −125% to 71%. The heterogeneity in effectiveness could not be explained by differences in trial design, study validity, patient population, type of intervention, or enrollment of only subjects at high risk of depression. In one study [43], the intervention was more effective in preventing mild to moderate than severe depression.

Discussion

This review proposed to determine the feasibility and effectiveness of brief interventions to prevent depression in older subjects. Despite an extensive literature search, only nine trials were identified that met the study inclusion criteria. Even then, five of these trials did not explicitly exclude depression at baseline or adjust for depression at baseline in the analysis; four did not have blind-rated outcomes; six did not report incidence rates of depression at follow-up; four did not report enrollment rates; and the sample size was small in many of the studies. Because of the heterogeneity of the study populations and interventions, no attempt was made to pool the results in a quantitative meta-analysis.

Nonetheless, it appears that many brief preventive interventions were feasible across a broad range of populations and settings. Median study enrollment and completion and compliance rates were 45%, 76.5%, and 93.5%, respectively. These rates would be considered acceptable for most interventions [53].

Given the methodological limitations of the trials and the inconsistent outcomes, the overall evidence of effectiveness was weak. Even so, three interventions appeared to have the potential to prevent depression in older subjects, including educational interventions for subjects with chronic illness [43,50], cognitive-behavioral interventions to reduce negative thinking [48], and life review [49].

Overall discussion

To reduce the incidence of depression in elderly populations, two different types of intervention models may be explored alone or in combination; namely, risk factor abatement models and brief preventive intervention models. As for risk factor abatement models alone, three of the five identified risk factors are potentially modifiable (ie, bereavement, sleep disturbance, and chronic illness and disability). Based on the pooled odds ratio data in this meta-analysis, the attributable risks for these 3 risk factors were 69.4% (95% CI, 42.2%, 79.5%), 57.0% (95% CI, 35.7%, 73.3%), and 56.5% (95% CI, 20.4%, 83.5%), respectively. Thus, a large proportion of depression in community elderly may be attributed to one of these risk factors. Because these risk factors are frequent in elderly community subjects, interventions to abate them could be expected to have an important public health impact.

The success of a recently described risk factor abatement program for preventing delirium among elderly medical inpatients [54] offers hope that such an intervention model may be useful in preventing depression among elderly community subjects. This program involved the identification of elderly medical inpatients with at least one of six targeted risk factors for delirium and the implementation of standardized intervention protocols for each of the risk factors present. The program attenuated the risk factors and reduced the incidence of delirium by 40%.

Individuals or populations that have one or more of the five risk factors for depression (eg, bereaved women with previous depression, disability, and sleep disturbance) could be identified. Subsequently, these individuals

Table 5
Summary of the feasibility of brief interventions to prevent depression

Study	Populations	Age range (mean)	Intervention	Duration of intervention (wk)	Follow-up (mo)	No. of subjects enrolled/approached (%)	No. of subjects enrolled in each group (%)		No. of subjects completing in each group (%)		Overall completion rate (%)	No. of intervention subjects who complied with the intervention (%)
							Intervention	Control	Intervention	Control		
Parkes [44] 1981	Bereaved referred by a hospice nurse	—(66)	At least one visit from a bereavement counsellor	?	20	67/67 (100)	32	35	27	29	85	32/32 (100)
Gilden et al [43] 1992	Attendees of a veterans' diabetes clinic	57–82 (68)	Weekly diabetes education classes	6	24	?	13	8	13	8	100	13/13 (100)
Haight [47] 1992	Homebound elderly receiving meals on wheels or home care	61–99 (76)	Life Review 1 hr/week	6	12	?	16	19	10	12	63	16/16 (100)
Lieberman et al [45] 1992	Consecutive widow(er)s 4–10 months after death of spouse from cancer	—(57)	Group therapy 80 min/week	8	12	78/78 (100)	58	20	34	19	53	34/58 (59)
Levy et al [42] 1993[a]	Bereaved from 6 oncology programs	—(61)	Weekly bereavement support group, 2–25 sessions	5 (median)	18	127/283 (45)	37	90	37	90	—	37/127 (29)
Muñoz et al [48] 1995	Disadvantaged primary care patients	18–69 (53)	2 hr/week course on CB depression prevention	8	12	150/707 (21)	72	78	66	72	92	7–8 sessions 36/72 (50) 1–6 sessions 22/72 (30)

Haight et al [49] 2000	Random sample from 13 nursing homes	60–104 (80)	Life Review 1 hr/week	6	12	?	60	60	37	27	53	60/60 (100) (est)
Phillips [50] 2000	Elderly with arthritis	65–74 (69)	1.5 hr/week arthritis education classes	10	12	?	101	101	99	98	98	—
Rybarczyk et al [46] 2001	Patients referred by HMO physicians	50–93 (66)	2 hr classes/week on mind/body wellness and CB techniques	8	24 / 12	302/905 (33)	140	162	96	108	68	7–8 sessions 64/140 (50) / 4–6 sessions 52/140 (37)

Abbreviations: CB, cognitive-behavioral; est, estimated; HMO, health maintenance organization.

[a] A nonrandomized trial in which the 37 subjects who participated in the intervention were compared with the 90 who refused the intervention.

From Cole MG, Dendukuri N. The feasibility and effectiveness of brief interventions to prevent depression in older subjects: a systematic review. Int J Geriatr Psychiatry 2004;19: 1019–25; with permission.

Table 6
Summary of the effectiveness of brief interventions to prevent depression

Study	Design	Enrolled subjects at high risk of depression	No. of subjects in each group		Measure of depression	Incidence of depression (%)		Absolute risk reduction (%)	Relative risk reduction (%)	Depression symptom scores at follow-up (favoring intervention group)
			Intervention	Control		Intervention	Control			
Parkes [44] 1981	RCT	Yes	32	35	Health questionnaire (depression)	—	—	—	—	No significant difference
Gilden et al [43] 1992	NRCT	No	13	8	SDS > 50	18	63	45	71	
Haight [47] 1992	RCT	No	16	19	SDS > 60	27	12	-15	-125	No significant difference
Lieberman et al [45] 1992	RCT	Yes/No	58	20	HSC	—	—	—	—	No significant difference
Levy et al [42] 1993	NRCT	No	37	90	CESD $\geq$ 16	45	28	-17	-61	
Muñoz et al [48] 1995	RCT	Yes	72	78	DIS	2.8	5.1	2.3	45	
Haight et al [49] 2000	RCT	No	60	44	BDI	—	—	—	—	Significant difference
Phillips [50] 2000	RCT	No	101	101	CESD	—	—	—	—	Significant difference at 12 and 24 mo
Rybarczyk et al [46] 2001	RCT	No	140	162	Modified CESD	—	—	—	—	No significant difference

Abbreviations: BDI, Beck Depression Inventory; CESD, Centre for Epidemiologic Studies Depression; DIS, Diagnostic Interview Schedule; HSC, Hopkins Symptom Checklist; NRCT, nonrandomized controlled trial; RCT, randomized controlled trial; SDS-Zung Depression Scale.

From Cole MG, Dendukuri N. The feasibility and effectiveness brief interventions to prevent depression in older subjects: a systematic review. Int J Geriatr Psychiatry 2004;19:1019–25; with permission.

could be targeted for interventions to abate the potentially modifiable risk factors and reduce the risk of depression. Such interventions may include education about the significance of the risk factors, bereavement counseling and support [55], new skills training, "maintenance of routines" protocols [56], enhancement of social supports [57], individual or group therapy to facilitate adjustment to loss of function [58], and sleep enhancement protocols [59].

As for the brief preventive intervention models alone, the present review suggests that these types of interventions are feasible. Although the overall evidence of effectiveness is weak, some types of brief interventions appear to have the potential to prevent depression in older subjects, such as educational interventions for subjects with chronic illness [43,50], cognitive-behavioral interventions to reduce negative thinking [51], and life review [52].

A common element of the latter three types of interventions was the use of cognitive-behavioral techniques to empower and reduce negative thinking, issues that are very relevant to depressive disorders in many older people [60]. Multiple losses, chronic disease and disability, and disenfranchisement often lead to a vicious cycle of disempowerment, negative thinking, feelings of helplessness, lowered self-esteem, and depression. Cognitive-behavioral interventions that empower and reduce negative thinking may well reduce the incidence of depression in this population. The use of similar types of interventions has already been reported to be effective in preventing depression in school-aged children [61] and younger adults [62–64].

Combinations of the two models could be categorized as selective brief preventative interventions (ie, preventive interventions targeted at high-risk groups). Presently, it would be useful to develop brief cognitive-behavioral, educational, or life review interventions for older, bereaved, and disabled women who have sleep disturbance and previous depression and to conduct randomized controlled trials of these interventions with sufficient power to detect an ARR of 2% to 4% in the incidence of depression at 1 year. Such trials should exclude subjects with clinical depression at baseline and record the use of any antidepressant therapy during the follow-up period. An alternative model might involve the development of similar types of brief preventive interventions for individuals with early symptoms of depression (ie, indicated preventive interventions).

To summarize, five risk factors for depression among elderly community subjects have been identified; some types of brief interventions appear to have the potential to prevent depression in older subjects. Despite the methodological limitations of the studies and these systematic reviews, these findings may guide efforts to develop and evaluate interventions to prevent depression in this population.

Proposal for a research agenda

The following are proposals for a research agenda on risk factors and brief preventive interventions.

Risk factors for geriatric depression

- A search of different databases in languages other than English or French to identify additional studies of risk factors
- Original studies that focus on identifying potential social risk factors
- Original studies that focus on identifying and clarifying physical health and disability as risk factors
- Original studies that examine combinations of risk factors and interactions between risk factors to identify groups at especially high risk of depression
- Original studies that focus on identifying potential protective factors
- All original studies should examine the interactions of age and gender with the risk factors

Brief preventive interventions

- A search of different databases in languages other than English or French to identify additional trials of brief preventive interventions
- A systematic review of studies involving abatement of risk factors for depression
- Controlled trials of interventions to abate risk factors for depression
- Controlled trials of brief preventive interventions for high risk groups
- Controlled trials of different intervention packages (eg, cognitive-behavioral and risk factor abatement) for different groups of seniors

References

[1] NIH Consensus Development Conference. Diagnosis and treatment of depression in late life. JAMA 1992;268:1018–24.
[2] Cole MG, Yaffe MJ. Pathway to psychiatric care of the elderly with depression. Int J Geriatr Psychiatry 1996;11:157–61.
[3] Blazer D. Depression in the elderly. N Engl J Med 1989;320:164–6.
[4] Beekman ATF, Geerlings SW, Deeg DJH, et al. The natural history of late-life depression. Arch Gen Psychiatry 2002;59:605–11.
[5] Cole MG, Bellavance F, Mansour A. Prognosis of depression in elderly community and primary care populations: a systematic review and meta-analysis. Am J Psychiatry 1999;156:1182–9.
[6] Steuten LMG, Vrijhoef HJM, van Merode GG, et al. The health technology assessment -disease management instrument reliably measured methodologic quality of health technology assessments of disease management. J Clin Epidemiol 2004;57:881–8.
[7] Von Korff M, Ormel J, Katon W, et al. Disability and depression among high utilizers of health care: a longitudinal analysis. Arch Gen Psychiatry 1992;49:91–100.
[8] Wells KB, Burman AM. Caring for depression in America: lessons learned from early findings of the Medical Outcomes Study. Psychiatr Med 1991;9:503–19.
[9] Katon W, Von Korff M, Lin E, et al. Adequacy and duration of antidepressant treatment in primary care. Med Care 1992;30:67–76.
[10] Unützer J, Patrick DL, Simon G, et al. Depressive symptoms and the cost of health services in HMO patients aged 65 years and older: a 4-year prospective study. JAMA 1997;277:1618–23.

[11] Katon WJ, Lin E, Russo J, et al. Increased medical costs of a population-based sample of depressed elderly patients. Arch Gen Psychiatry 2003;60:897–903.

[12] McCusker J, Cole M, Keller E, et al. Effectiveness of treatments of depression in older ambulatory patients. Arch Intern Med 1998;158:705–12.

[13] Unützer J, Katon W, Callahan CM, et al. Collaborative care management of late-life depression in the primary care setting. A randomized controlled trial. JAMA 2002;288:2836–45.

[14] Cole MG, Bellavance F. The prognosis of depression in old age. Am J Geriatr Psychiatry 1997;5:4–14.

[15] Mrazek P, Haggerty R. Reducing risks for mental disorders: frontiers for preventive intervention research. Washington (DC): National Academy Press; 1994.

[16] Hollon S, Muñoz RF, Barlow DH, et al. Psychosocial intervention development for the prevention and treatment of depression: Promoting innovation and increasing access. Biol Psychiatry 2002;52:610–30.

[17] Charney DS, Reynolds CF, Lewis L, et al. Depression and bipolar support alliance consensus statement on the unmet needs in diagnosis and treatment of mood disorders in late life. Arch Gen Psychiatry 2003;60:664–72.

[18] Oxman AD, Cook DJ, Guyatt GH. Users' guides to the medical literature: VI. how to use an overview. JAMA 1994;272:1367–71.

[19] Cole MG, Dendukuri N. Risk factors for depression among elderly community subjects: a systematic review and meta-analysis. Am J Psychiatry 2003;160:1147–56.

[20] Levine M, Walter S, Lee H, et al. Users' guides to the medical literature. IV. how to use an article about harm. JAMA 1994;271:1615–9.

[21] Gelman A, Carlin JB, Stern HS, et al. New York: Chapman & Hall; 1995.

[22] Phifer JF, Murrell SA. Etiologic factors in the onset of depressive symptoms in older adults. J Abnorm Psychol 1986;95:282–91.

[23] McHorney CA, Mor V. Predictors of bereavement depression and its health services consequences. Med Care 1988;26:882–93.

[24] Kennedy GJ, Kelman HR, Thomas C. The emergence of depressive symptoms in late life: the importance of declining health and increasing disability. J Community Health 1990;15: 93–104.

[25] Harlow SD, Goldberg EL, Comstock GW. A longitudinal study of the prevalence of depressive symptomatology in elderly widowed and married women. Arch Gen Psychiatry 1991;48: 1065–8.

[26] Russell DW, Cutrona CE. Social support, stress, and depressive symptoms among the elderly: test of a process model. Psychol Aging 1991;6:190–201.

[27] Green BH, Copeland JRM, Dewey ME, et al. Risk factors for depression in elderly people: a prospective study. Acta Psychiatr Scand 1992;86:213–7.

[28] Livingston G, Blizard B, Mann A. Does sleep disturbance predict depression in elderly people? a study in inner London. Br J Gen Pract 1993;43:445–8.

[29] Mendes de Leon CF, Kasl SV, Jacobs S. A prospective study of widowhood and the changes in symptoms of depression in a community sample of the elderly. Psychol Med 1994;24: 613–24.

[30] Beekman ATF, Deeg DJH, Smit JH, et al. Predicting the course of depression in the older population: results from a community-based study in the Netherlands. J Affect Disord 1995;34:41–9.

[31] Zeiss AM, Lewinsohn PM, Rohde P, et al. Relationship of physical disease and functional impairment to depression in older people. Psychol Aging 1996;11:572–81.

[32] Kivela SL, Kongas-Saviard P, Kimmo P, et al. Health, health behaviour and functional ability predicting depression in old age: a longitudinal study. Int J Geriatr Psychiatry 1996;11: 871–7.

[33] Prince MJ, Harwood RH, Thomas A, et al. A prospective population-based cohort study of the effects of disablement and social milieu on the onset and maintenance of late-life depression: The Gospel Oak Project VII. Psychol Med 1998;28:337–50.

[34] Turvey CL, Carney C, Arndt S, et al. Conjugal loss and syndromal depression in a sample of elders aged 70 years or older. Am J Psychiatry 1999;156:1596–601.

[35] Livingston G, Watkin V, Milne B, et al. Who becomes depressed? the Islington community study of older people. J Affect Disord 2000;58:125–33.

[36] Schoevers RA, Beekman ATF, Deeg DJH, et al. Risk factors for depression in later life; results of a prospective community based study (AMSTEL). J Affect Disord 2000;59:127–37.

[37] Geerlings SW, Beekman AT, Deeg DJ, et al. Physical health and the onset and persistence of depression in older adults: an eight-wave prospective community-based study. Psychol Med 2000;30:369–80.

[38] Forsell Y. Predictors for depression, anxiety and psychotic symptoms in a very elderly population: data from a 3-year follow-up study. Soc Psychiatry Psychiatr Epidemiol 2000;35: 259–63.

[39] Paterniti S, Verdier-Taillefer M-H, Geneste C, et al. Low blood pressure and risk of depression in the elderly: a prospective community-based study. Br J Psychiatry 2000;176:464–7.

[40] Roberts RE, Shema SJ, Kaplan GA, et al. Sleep complaints and depression in an aging cohort: a prospective perspective. Am J Psychiatry 2000;157:81–8.

[41] Kritz-Silvertein D, Barrett-Connor E, Corbeau C. Cross-sectional and prospective study of exercise and depressed mood in the elderly: The Rancho Bernado Study. Am J Epidemiol 2001;153:596–603.

[42] Levy LH, Derby JF, Martinkowski KS. Effects of membership in bereavement support groups on adaptation to conjugal bereavement. Am J Community Psychol 1993;21:361–81.

[43] Gilden JL, Hendryx MS, Clar S, et al. Diabetes support groups improve health care of older diabetic patients. J Am Geriatr Soc 1992;40:147–50.

[44] Parkes CM. Evaluation of a bereavement service. J Prev Psychiatry 1981;1:179–88.

[45] Lieberman MA, Yalom I. Brief group psychotherapy for the spousally bereaved: a controlled study. Int J Group Psychother 1992;42:117–32.

[46] Rybarczyk B, Demarco G, DeLaCruz M, et al. A classroom mind/body wellness intervention for older adults with chronic illness: comparing immediate and 1-year benefits. Behav Med 2001;27:15–27.

[47] Haight BK. Long-term effects of a structured life review process. J Gerontol B Psychol Sci 1992;47:312–5.

[48] Muñoz RF, Ying Y-W, Bernal G, et al. Prevention of depression with primary care patients: a randomized controlled trial. Am J Community Psychol 1995;23:199–222.

[49] Haight BK, Michel Y, Hendrix S. The extended effects of the life review in nursing home residents. Int J Aging Hum Dev 2000;50:151–68.

[50] Phillips RSC. Preventing depression: a program for African American elders with chronic pain. Fam Community Health 2000;22:57–65.

[51] Cole MG, Dendukuri N. The feasibility and effectiveness of brief interventions to prevent depression in older subjects: a systematic review. Int J Geriatr Psychiatry 2004;19: 1019–25.

[52] Guyatt GH, Sackett DL, Cook DJ. Users' guides to the medical literature II. how to use an article about therapy or prevention B: what were the results and will they help me in caring for my patients? JAMA 1994;271:59–63.

[53] Sackett DL, Haynes RB, Guyatt GH, Tugwell P. Clinical epidemiology. Boston: Little, Brown and Company; 1991.

[54] Inouye SK, Bogardus ST, Charpentier PA, et al. A multicomponent intervention to prevent delirium in hospitalized older patients. N Engl J Med 1999;340:669–720.

[55] Marmar CR, Horowitz MJ, Weiss DS, et al. A controlled trial of brief psychotherapy and mutual help group treatment of conjugal bereavement. Am J Psychiatry 1988;145:203–9.

[56] Brown LF, Reynolds CF, Monk TH, et al. Social rhythm stability following late-life spousal bereavement: associations with depression and sleep impairment. Psychiatry Res 1996;62: 161–9.

[57] Morgan DL. Adjusting to widowhood: do social networks really make it easier. Gerontologist 1989;29:101–7.
[58] Anderson BL. Psychological interventions for cancer patients to enhance quality of life. J Consult Clin Psychol 1992;60:552–68.
[59] Morin CM. Behavioural and pharmacological therapies for late-life insomnia: a randomized controlled trial. JAMA 1999;281:991–9.
[60] Blazer DG. Self-efficacy and depression in late life: a primary prevention proposal. Aging Ment Health 2002;6:315–24.
[61] Greenberg MT, Domitrovich C, Bumbarger B. The prevention of mental disorders in school-aged children: current state of the field. Prev Treat 2001;4:1–51.
[62] Seligman MEP, Schulman P, DeRubeis RJ, et al. The prevention of depression and anxiety. Prev Treat 1999;2:1–22.
[63] Vinokur A, Schul Y, Vuori J, et al. Two years after a job loss: long-term impact of the JOBS program on reemployment and mental health. J Occup Health Psychol 2000;5:32–47.
[64] Peden AR, Rayens MK, Hall LA, et al. Preventing depression in high-risk college women: a report of an 18-month follow-up. J Am Coll Health 2001;49:299–306.

PSYCHIATRIC
CLINICS
OF NORTH AMERICA

ELSEVIER
SAUNDERS

Psychiatr Clin N Am
28 (2005) 805–820

Evidence-Based Psychotherapeutic Interventions for Geriatric Depression

R. Scott Mackin, PhD*, Patricia A. Areán, PhD

Department of Psychiatry and Langley Porter Psychiatric Institute, University of California, San Francisco, 401 Parnassus Avenue, Box F-0984, San Francisco, CA 94143-0984, USA

In 1991, the National Institutes of Health consensus statement on the treatment of late-life depression ranked psychotherapy as third in a line of treatment options, with antidepressant medication first and electroconvulsive therapy second, indicating that there was insufficient evidence to recommend psychotherapy as a first-line treatment for depression in older adults [1]. Since that time, numerous articles have been written reviewing the evidence base for psychotherapy research in older adults and four meta-analyses of existing trials have been conducted (Table 1) [2–26]. In addition, several randomized clinical trials meeting guideline recommendations for evidence-based interventions [27] have evaluated the efficacy of psychotherapy as a treatment for late-life depression (Table 2) [28–43]. Most of these studies have focused on the evaluation of cognitive-behavioral therapy (CBT), brief dynamic therapy (BDT), interpersonal psychotherapy (IPT), reminiscence therapy (RT), and the combination of these interventions with medication management. This review systematically evaluates the evidence base for psychotherapy as an empirically supported treatment of late-life depression and is an update of the present authors' recent review of the literature [23].

Methods

Studies were selected through literature searches of MEDLINE (1966–2005) and PsychINFO (1840–2005) using the keywords psychotherapy, cognitive-behavioral therapy, interpersonal psychotherapy, reminiscence therapy, life review therapy, brief dynamic therapy, psychoeducation, depression, late-life depression, older adults, elderly, and geriatric depression. In addition, the studies used in earlier meta-analyses [7,12,21,26] were

---

* Corresponding author.
  E-mail address: scottm@lppi.ucsf.edu (R.S. Mackin).

Table 1
Literature reviews of psychotherapies for late-life depression

Study	Type of review	Therapies reviewed	Conclusions
Charatan [2] 1985	Summary	Antidepressants, ECT, psychotherapies	All modalities useful
Morris and Morris [3] 1991	Literature	CBT, RT, PST, skills training	Therapies efficacious; cognitive impairment special consideration
Reynolds [4] 1992	Literature	Antidepressants, IPT, CBT, combined treatment	Individual and combined treatments
Areán et al [5] 1993	Literature	CBT	Efficacious treatment
Clark and Vorst [6] 1994	Summary	Group	Need more research on group therapy with depressed elderly
Scogin and McElreath [7] 1994	Meta-analysis	BT, CT, psychodynamic RT, eclectic	Moderately or highly efficacious
Reynolds et al [8] 1995	Literature	Antidepressants, IPT	Both efficacious for long-term maintenance; review challenges in maintenance research
Koder et al [9] 1996	Literature	CT	Efficacious, insufficient evidence as to efficacy of adaptations
Thompson [10] 1996	Literature	CBT	CBT efficacious, minor adaptations for older adults
Lebowitz et al [11] 1997	Literature	CBT, IPT, PST	Efficacious
Engels et al [12] 1997	Meta-analysis	CBT, BT, RT	Efficacious
Zeiss and Breckenridge [13] 1997	Literature	CT, BT, IPT, BDT	CT and BT most cost effective
Gatz et al [14] 1998	Literature	CBT, IPT, BDT	CT, CBT, BDT probably efficacious; IPT promising
Niederehe and Schneider [15] 1998	Literature	Antidepressants, ECT, psychosocial	Efficacious
Klausner and Alexopoulos [16] 1999	Literature	CBT, PST, IPT, psychodynamic, RT	Acute treatment efficacious; probably efficacious for continuation, maintenance
Knight and Satre [17] 1999	Literature	CBT	Efficacious with suggested adaptations
Pachana [18] 1999	Literature	CBT, antidepressants, family, relaxation, combined	Efficacious; need more research on combined treatments, family, and substance abuse treatment

Table 1 (*continued*)

Study	Type of review	Therapies reviewed	Conclusions
Draper [19] 2000	Literature	Antidepressants, CT, CBT psychodynamic, exercise, music, ECT	Few studies; insufficient empirical evidence for efficacy of psychotherapies with medically ill elderly
Karel and Hinrichsen [20] 2000	Literature	CBT, IPT, psychodynamic, life review, group, family	CBT, IPT most empirical support; combined therapy and medications best for more severely depressed elderly
Pinquart and Sorensen [21] 2001	Meta-analysis	CBT, RT, BDT, ST, IPT	CBT produces above average effects on depression; individual more effective than group; weaker effects for older participants
Areán et al [22] 2001	Literature	CBT-PC, PST-PC, IPT-PC	All feasible and effectively adapted to primary care settings
Areán and Cook [23] 2002	Literature	CBT, PST, BDT, IPT, RT, CAMP	CBT, PST, CAMP-IPT effective; more research needed for BDT, IPT
Bartels et al [24] 2002	Literature	CBT, PST, BDT, IPT, CAMP	Empirical evidence supports psychosocial interventions for geriatric depression
Bartels et al [25] 2003	Literature	CBT, PST, BDT, IPT, CAMP	CT, BT, and CBT effective for tx of geriatric MDD
Bohlmeijer et al [26] 2003	Meta-analysis	RT, LR, CT, PST	RT and LR highly efficacious

Abbreviations: BDT, brief dynamic therapy; BT, behavioral therapy; CAMP, Combined antidepressant medication + psychotherapy; CBT, cognitive-behavioral therapy; CT, combined therapy; IPT, interpersonal psychotherapy; PST, problem-solving therapy; RT, reminiscence therapy; tx, treatment.

obtained. Studies were also included that pertain to the efficacy of psychotherapy and its combination with medication in the treatment of late-life depression (in individuals over the age of 60). Only those studies that used samples of sufficient size (25 or more participants per experimental condition) and compared the therapy against a wait-list or placebo control or the gold standard treatment at the time of the study were included in this review, to be consistent with previously published guidelines on defining empirically supported therapies [27].

More than 100 studies pertaining to the psychotherapeutic treatment of late-life depression were identified. Most studies were excluded based on the application of the Chambless and Hollon [27] criteria. Only 17 studies met the minimum sample size criteria. Four studies compared active

Table 2
Treatment outcome research: psychotherapies for late-life depression

Study	Number of subjects	Age (y)	Populations	Experimental conditions	Control condition	Outcome
Fry [28] 1983	162	65–82; mean = 68.5	MDD; community-dwelling,	Structured RT; unstructured RT	No treatment	Both treatments efficacious; structured RT more effective than unstructured RT
Fry [29] 1984	75	67–80	MDD; community-dwelling	Immediate vs delayed CBT Treatment package	NA	CBT efficacious in immediate and delayed treatment subjects
Thompson et al [30] 1987	91	60+; mean 67.1	MDD; outpatient	CT, BT, BDT	Wait list	All three therapies efficacious
Gallagher-Thompson et al [31] 1990	91	60+	MDD; outpatient, diagnosed patients 2-y follow-up	CT, BT, CT, or psychodynamic, BDT	NA	No difference in maintenance of gains by psychotherapy modality; All efficacious
Campbell [32] 1992	103	64–82	MDD; community dwelling	CBT	No treatment	CBT efficacious in reducing depression
Areán et al [5] 1993	75	55+	MDD; community dwelling	PST, RT	Wait list	PST and RT effective; PST showed greater benefit
Gallagher-Thompson and Steffen [33] 1994	66	Mean 62	MDD; depressed family caregivers	CBT, BDT	NA	BDT better for "new" caregivers; CBT better for "seasoned" caregivers
Blanchard et al [34] 1995	96	Mean 78.2	MDD; community screening	CT nurse intervention	Primary care control	Nurse CT intervention effective

Study	N	Age	Population	Intervention	Comparison	Results
Areán and Miranda [35] 1996	182	60+	Medically ill outpatients	Individual and group CBT	NA	Psychotherapies effective in medically ill elderly
Mossey et al [36] 1996	76	60+	Minor depression; recently released hospitalized elderly	IPC	Usual care	IPC more efficacious at 6-mo follow-up
Reynolds et al [37] 1999	187	Mean 67	Community elders with recurrent MDD	NT, NT + IPT, IPT + pill-placebo	Pill-placebo	NT + IPT most efficacious
Blanchard et al [38] 1999	64	Mean 78.2	MDD	Comprehensive intervention or medications + therapy	No treatment	Psychotherapeutic interventions effective for maintanence
Williams et al [39] 2000	415	Mean 71	Primary care patients with minor depression or dysthymia	Paroxetine, PST	Pill-placebo	Paroxetine moderately efficacious, PST more variable in efficacy
Thompson et al [40] 2001	102	60+	Veterans with MDD; VA outpatients	Desipramine alone, CBT alone, CBT plus desipramine	NA	All effective; combined therapy resulted in greater improvement; most effective for most severe depression
Unützer et al [41] 2002	1801	60+	Primary care patients with MDD	IMPACT intervention (PST, meds, or both)	Usual care	IMPACT collaborative care significantly more effective than usual care
Ciechanowski et al [42] 2004	138	60+	Minor depression dysthymia	PEARLS intervention (PST, meds, or both)	Usual care	PEARLS program significantly more effective than usual care
Wang [43] 2005	94	65	Tawainese elderly with depressive symptoms	RT	No treatment	RT more effective than control

Abbreviations: BDT, brief dynamic therapy; CBT, cognitive-behavioral therapy; CT, cognitive therapy; IMPACT, Improving Mood Promoting Access to Collaborative Treatment; IPT, interpersonal psychotherapy; MDD, major depressive disorder; NT, nortriptylene; PEARLS, Program to Encourage Active, Rewarding, Lives for Seniors; PST, problem-solving therapy; RT, reminiscence therapy; VA, Veterans Affairs.

treatments without a control group, two studies compared psychotherapy to a waiting list control, two studies compared psychotherapy to pill placebo, eight studies compared psychotherapy to usual care or no treatment, and one study was a 2-year follow-up. Two studies compared the effectiveness of psychotherapy to medication. Twelve studies focused on major depression, and five studies evaluated minor depression or dysthymia. Twelve studies evaluated CBT therapies, two evaluated IPT, three evaluated BDT, and three evaluated RT; several studies evaluated more than one treatment modality.

Results

Behavioral and cognitive-behavioral therapies

Behavioral therapy (BT) and CBT have received the most research attention of any psychotherapeutic interventions for late-life depression. These therapies conceptualize depression as the result of an inability to cope with life stressors, poor affect regulation skills, social isolation, and difficulty solving problems. Thus, cognitive-behavioral therapies treat depression by teaching patients methods for regulating their affect, remaining engaged in pleasant activities as a means of warding off depression, and changing depressogenic choices and behaviors through a problem-solving process [44]. Eleven randomized clinical trials or follow-up studies of cognitive or cognitive-behavioral interventions for the treatment of late-life depression meeting the criteria described previously have been published from seven different research centers. These studies have been conducted with individuals who have major depression, identified in clinical settings or through community screening, as well as with individuals who have minor depression or dysthymia. Three of these studies used comparisons with usual care, two used a wait-list control, two used a no-treatment control condition, and one study used a placebo-treatment condition. Some studies have included 1- to 2-year follow-up periods to determine the permanence of treatment outcome.

Major depression

Comparison with placebo or wait-list controls

Six randomized trials have compared CBT with usual care or wait-list control for individuals with major depression. All of the studies found that CBT was superior to usual care for depression [41], wait-list control [5,30], pill-placebo [39], and no treatment [32,34]. There is also evidence to suggest that these treatment gains persist over long periods of time. For instance, Gallagher-Thompson and colleagues [31] found that cognitive and behavioral interventions along with brief dynamic therapy maintained significant improvement of depressive symptoms over a 2-year period in comparison with a wait-list control condition. Overall, this research base suggests that CBT interventions are better than no treatment or usual care of late-life depression.

Comparisons with other psychotherapies

Research comparing CBT with other psychologic interventions has yielded mixed results. Studies comparing cognitive therapy, behavioral therapy, and brief dynamic therapy have found that all three treatments were efficacious, with no significant differences in treatment outcome [30,31, 33,45]. Only one other study has compared treatment modalities studies, and that study found that problem-solving therapy (PST) is more effective in reducing depressive symptoms than reminiscence therapy [5].

Comparison with antidepressant medication

Only one study has compared CBT with antidepressant medication in the treatment of major depression in older adults [40]. In this study, CBT was compared with the use of desipramine and a combination of CBT and desipramine in 100 older adults who had major depression. Results indicated that CBT and the combination of CBT and desipramine were more efficacious in treating depression symptoms than was desipramine alone [40]. However, to date, no geriatric research has compared CBT with the newer antidepressant medications (eg, selective serotonin reuptake inhibitors) for major depression.

Long-term effects and relapse prevention

Several studies by the same research group demonstrate that CBT along with cognitive therapy and brief dynamic therapy has positive effects 1 [30,45] and 2 years after treatment [31]. No other research groups have published long-term outcome results.

Dysthymia and minor depression

The literature on the efficacy of CBT for treating dysthymia or minor depression is emerging. These studies are important because these disorders are far more prominent in older adults than major depression. To date, two studies have investigated the effect of CBT on dysthymia or minor depression [39,42] . Williams and colleagues [39] used an abbreviated version of PST designed for primary care (PST-PC) medicine [46] that was compared with the administration of paroxetine and pill-placebo for the treatment of minor depression and dysthymia in older and younger adults in a primary care setting. The study found that both active treatments were effective in decreasing depressive symptoms and improving functioning; however, PST-PC was not as effective as paroxetine, had a slower onset of treatment effect, and was affected by the degree of therapist training in learning-based strategies [47]. A limitation of this study was that PST-PC is an abbreviated PST (four to six 30-minute sessions delivered over 8 weeks) and is much shorter in length than the traditional PST, which may not have been ideal for older adults [48]. Geropsychologists generally recognize that interventions should be modified for older adults by slowing the pace at which material is presented, emphasizing a repeated review of material and relying on multiple modes of information transmission to ensure that adequate exposure is achieved. These adaptations would, therefore, result in more treatment time with the patient than is needed with younger patients. Therefore, it is likely that participants in this study did not have adequate exposure to PST [39]. In a more recent study [42], a modified PST emphasizing social and physical activation over a longer time period (eight sessions over the course of 19 weeks) was shown to be more effective in reducing depressive symptoms, promoting remission of depression, and improving quality of life compared with usual care practices.

Summary and limitations

Research on the efficacy of CBT is compelling and suggests that these treatments are viable therapeutic treatment options for older adults suffering from major depression and, to a lesser degree, dysthymia and minor depression. The methodological strengths of this literature include the variety of investigators who have evaluated CBT, the sound implementation of the studies (use of Research Diagnostic Criteria or Diagnostic Statistical Manual Criteria, the use of manuals and therapist supervision, and control comparisons), and the use of long-term follow-up. Nevertheless, there are insufficient data on the efficacy of CBT for minority elderly, frail elderly, and older adults with mild cognitive impairment.

Interpersonal psychotherapy

Although IPT is considered generally to be commensurate with CBT as a psychotherapeutic intervention for depression in younger adults, there are fewer studies investigating the efficacy of IPT as a stand-alone therapy for older adults with depression. Interpersonal psychotherapy [49] consists of elements of psychodynamic-oriented therapies (exploration and clarification of affect) and CBT (behavior change techniques and reality testing of perceptions) that are used to address four areas of conflict: (1) unresolved grief; (2) role transitions; (3) interpersonal role disputes; and (4) interpersonal deficits. A major limitation of the IPT literature is that most research has studied IPT in conjunction with medication or pill-placebo, making it difficult to evaluate the stand-alone efficacy of the intervention. The generalizability of IPT research is further limited in that it has been evaluated primarily in healthy, ambulatory, white patients with major depression.

Major depression

Interpersonal psychotherapy plus pill-placebo versus wait list or placebo
Few studies have compared IPT with placebo or a wait-list control. However, in one study evaluating the treatment effects for chronic or recurrent major depression in late life, IPT plus pill-placebo was found to be better

than pill-placebo in preventing the recurrence of major depression [37]. Findings from this study suggest that the combined treatment with IPT and antidepressant medication may produce the best relapse prevention during the maintenance phase after acute treatment, whereas IPT plus pill-placebo produces the worst rates [37]. Therefore, IPT may be most effective as a maintenance treatment for severely depressed older adults when it is administered in combination with an antidepressant medication.

Dysthymia and minor depression

Only one study has evaluated the efficacy of IPT for minor depression in older adults. Mossey and colleagues [36] randomized 76 medically ill older adults with subdysthymia (Geriatric Depression Scale ≥ 10 and no current diagnosis of dysthymia or major depression) who had recently been discharged from acute hospital care to interpersonal counseling (IPC), a modified, shortened version of IPT, or usual care. Six months after treatment initiation, IPC was found to be superior to usual care in reducing depressive symptoms. Thus far, no studies have examined IPT for the treatment of individuals meeting the criteria for dysthymic disorder.

Summary and limitations

Interpersonal psychotherapy has not yet garnered support as a stand-alone intervention in the treatment of late-life depression. Although one study suggests that IPT could potentially be a useful stand-alone intervention for milder depression, the data from a larger clinical trial support a combined approach to treating late-life depression, particularly in chronic and recurrent types. As is also true for CBT, the generalizability of the IPT literature is somewhat limited by the fact that existing studies have tended to include small numbers of minority elderly, and most participants are healthy and ambulatory.

Brief psychodynamic therapy

The research support for BDT exists largely because of the research on CBT; this intervention has often been used as the comparison arm in these randomized trials. It has only been studied as an intervention for major depression, and as such, the present review is limited to that disorder. From a brief dynamic perspective, depression is often conceptualized from a psychodynamic perspective as being the result of unresolved, unconscious conflicts, usually stemming from childhood. The goal of this type of therapy is for the patient to understand and cope better with these feelings. As such, brief psychodynamic therapies focus on the reflection of past experiences, clarification of affect, the therapeutic relationship, and the confrontation of maladaptive interpersonal patterns, wishes, or conflicts [50,51].

As discussed previously in the review of CBT, BDT has been found to be an effective intervention for treating major depression in older adults [30,33]. In these studies, the BDT intervention was not manualized, but it did follow an outline to account for patient progress. There were no significant differences shown in the outcomes of brief dynamic therapy compared with other treatment modalities [30], and outcomes for major depression were maintained over 1- [30,45] and 2-year [31] periods.

Summary and limitations

BDT has a small evidence base as an efficacious intervention for late-life major depression. However, more research is needed to clarify its true efficacy because only one research group has conducted these trials. Brief dynamic therapy has not yet been compared with antidepressant medication in the elderly and also has not been investigated in individuals with minor depression or dysthymia. Future research is needed in these areas.

Reminiscence therapy

Like BDT, life review and reminiscence therapies are beginning to develop an evidence base. These interventions were studied decades ago as treatments for depression in nursing home patients but have not been studied rigorously for a number of years. More recently, there have been a number of reports evaluating their efficacy as a depression intervention; however, few meet the Chambless and Hollon standards for adding to the evidence base. Life review and reminiscence therapies are derived from Eriksonian developmental theory and have been developed specifically for older adults. Reminiscence therapies typically promote patients' recall of past events during the intervention, which can also include the use of photographs, music, and objects from the patient's past.

Reminiscence therapy has been proposed to counteract learned helplessness by promoting an individual's feeling of control over past and present life events [52]. Although several small open trials of RT in the treatment of late-life depression have been conducted, few larger randomized trials exist [5,28,43].

Both structured and unstructured life review therapies have been found to be effective interventions compared with a no-treatment control condition among older ambulatory community-based adults who have depression [28]. Similarly, findings reported by Wang and colleagues [43] have shown that an intervention consisting of a life review intervention resulted in a significant decrease in a report of selected depressive symptoms among elderly nursing home residents in Taiwan, compared with no-treatment control participants. In a third study that measured post-treatment and 3-month follow-up changes in depressive symptoms among community-dwelling older adults who had major depressive disorder, RT was found to be effective, although less effective than PST, in reducing depressive symptoms compared with a wait-list control group [5].

Summary and limitations

The research on RT suggests that it is a potentially useful intervention for the treatment of late-life depression; however, more research is needed to replicate these findings to evaluate the relative efficacy of this intervention compared with other therapies and to determine the efficacy of the intervention for minor depression and dysthymia. In addition, the prospects for using this type of intervention among minority elderly, frail elderly, and older adults who have mild cognitive impairment should be explored.

Combined antidepressant medication and psychotherapy

There has been a limited amount of research on the combined effects of antidepressant medication and psychotherapy compared with monotherapies for the treatment of late-life depression. Some preliminary data suggest that, for certain populations of older adults, combined treatments are better than monotherapies in the treatment of late-life major depression; however, these results are not equivocal. There is no research on combined treatments for dysthymia or minor depression.

Acute treatment of major depression

The research on combined medication and IPT has been described previously in detail. Antidepressant medication combined with IPT has been found to be most efficacious in treating major depression in ambulatory older adults who have chronic or recurrent depression [37], and the results seem to be as good in older adults as in younger adults [53]. In another study, Thompson and colleagues [40] investigated the efficacy of desipramine alone, CBT, and a combination of the two and found that all three conditions showed substantial improvement. The combined group showed greater improvement than desipramine alone, but there was little difference between CBT alone and the combined condition.

Summary and limitations

The evidence for combined treatments for late-life depression is still preliminary. Good support exists for the combination of medication and IPT as a means for preventing relapse and recurrence of major depression in older adults, particularly older adults who have recurrent major depression. Although promising, the research on medication with IPT suffers from the same set of limitations seen in the IPT literature; only one research group has studied this approach with adequately powered study designs, and as such, the generalizability of these findings is unclear. Similarly, with regard to CBT trials, in the one studied reviewed here, the finding that few differences between the CBT alone and a combined CBT and medication condition indicates that further research is necessary to evaluate the efficacy of combined interventions compared with specific monotherapies to determine the overall efficacy of these approaches.

Directions for future research

Although there have been studies of psychotherapy in specialized settings and with special populations, these studies did not meet the Chambless and Hollon evidence-based criteria. In particular, studies on the use of psychotherapy for people who have mild cognitive impairments, people living in rural areas, disabled elderly, and low-income minorities are either too small to provide any definitive information or are nonexistent.

Of particular importance for future study is the focus on older, depressed adults who have mild cognitive impairments (MCI). The majority of research on late-life depression has found a strong association with executive dysfunction [54–56] as well as memory deficits, slowed information processing speed, and visuospatial disturbances [56,57]. Although some of the variability in cognitive deficits associated with late-life depression may be attributed to the severity of depressive symptoms [58], much of the remaining variability is likely caused by comorbid neuropathologic conditions and their neuropsychologic sequelae. Furthermore, studies have shown that deficits in executive functions are associated with a poor and unstable response to antidepressant medications [59]. Given this, one alternative is to develop a more complex medication regime to address nonresponse in MCI individuals, and another alternative is to develop psychosocial interventions that address depression in individuals who have identified mild cognitive impairments. A small pilot study of PST [60] has shown that this latter alternative may be a viable one.

Another important area of study is increasing the access to psychotherapy for older people who cannot access this treatment, either because of disability or unavailability (eg, those living in rural areas). There is promising research on the efficacy of telephone-based psychotherapy for disabled adults [61] and bibliotherapy for distressed older patients living in rural areas [62]. More research of this nature should be conducted. Finally, research on the effects of psychotherapy for low-income minorities is also important to explore. Recent research on younger, poverty-level minorities has been mixed; some findings show psychotherapy to be very effective [63] and other findings show medications to be better than psychotherapy [64].

Based on the present review, the following conclusions and recommendations are made. First, CBT, RT, BDT, and the combination of medication and IPT are acutely efficacious in treating major depression in ambulatory older adults. More research is needed to determine long-term outcomes, the impact on functional outcomes (not just depressive symptoms), and the impact of these interventions on patients who have medical or psychiatric comorbid conditions. The present authors recommend that these interventions be evaluated using larger samples from multiple geographic sites so that their effectiveness in the typical older person with major depression can be evaluated appropriately. Single-site randomized trials on selected participants are no longer required.

Second, more controlled trials are needed to test the efficacy of BDT, IPT (without placebo), and the combined effects of CBT, PST, and BDT with antidepressant medication. It is anticipated that only a few more controlled trials are needed to clarify conflicting information from disparate studies. For instance, one additional trial of BDT for treating late-life major depression by another research group would meet the efficacy requirements set out by Chambless and Hollon [27]. Third, more research is needed on the efficacy of any psychotherapeutic intervention in the treatment of dysthymia and minor depression and in special populations such as frail elderly, cognitively impaired elderly, and older adults from minority groups. Additionally, because older adults are typically coping with more than depressive symptoms, that is, illness and quality of life issues, outcomes should focus more broadly on other functional domains such as quality of life, activity of daily living, and better management of illness, and not just on decrements in depressive symptoms.

Continued work in the area of psychotherapy for older adults is needed. There is a clear disparity in the number of geriatric psychotherapy and medication trials to date. Numerous studies documenting mental health treatment preferences show consistently that psychotherapy is considered by older adults to be a viable option and, in some studies, is preferred to antidepressant medication [65–67]. Given the results from preference studies, older adults may be accessing mental health treatments that have not been studied adequately. The elderly have the right to receive optimal, evidence-based mental health care, and psychotherapy is clearly an important aspect of that care in terms of scientific evidence and preference.

References

[1] NIH Consensus Development Conference. Diagnosis and treatment of depression in late life: November 4–6, 1991. NIH Consens State Sci Statements 1991;9(3):1–27.

[2] Charatan FB. Depression and the elderly: diagnosis and treatment. Psychiatr Ann 1985; 15(5):313–6.

[3] Morris RG, Morris LW. Cognitive and behavioural approaches with the depressed elderly. Int J Geriatr Psychiatry 1991;6(6):407–13.

[4] Reynolds CF III. Treatment of depression in special populations. J Clin Psychiatry 1992; 53(Suppl):S45–53.

[5] Areán PA, Perri MG, Nezu AM, et al. Comparative effectiveness of social problem-solving therapy and reminiscence therapy as treatments for depression in older adults. J Consult Clin Psychol 1993;61(6):1003–10.

[6] Clark WG, Vorst VR. Group therapy with chronically depressed geriatric patients. J Psychosoc Nurs Ment Health Serv 1994;32(5):9–13.

[7] Scogin F, McElreath L. Efficacy of psychosocial treatments for geriatric depression: a quantitative review. J Consult Clin Psychol 1994;62(1):69–74.

[8] Reynolds CF III, Frank E, Perel JM, et al. Maintenance therapies for late-life recurrent major depression: research and review circa 1995. Int Psychogeriatr 1995;7(Suppl):27–39.

[9] Koder DA, Brodaty H, Anstey KJ. Cognitive therapy for depression in the elderly. Int J Geriatr Psychiatry 1996;11(2):97–107.

[10] Thompson LW. Cognitive-behavioral therapy and treatment for late-life depression. J Clin Psychiatry 1996;57(Suppl 5):29–37.

[11] Lebowitz BD, Pearson JL, Schneider LS, et al. Diagnosis and treatment of depression in late life: consensus statement update. JAMA 1997;278(14):1186–90.

[12] Engels GI, Vermey M. Efficacy of nonmedical treatments of depression in elders: a quantitative analysis. Journal of Clinical Geropsychology 1997;3:17–35.

[13] Zeiss AM, Breckenridge JS. Treatment of late life depression: a response to the NIH consensus conference. Behav Ther 1997;28(1):3–21.

[14] Gatz M, Fiske A, Fox LS, et al. Empirically validated psychological treatments for older adults. J Ment Health Aging 1998;4:9–46.

[15] Niederehe G, Schneider LS. Treatments for depression and anxiety in the aged. In: Nathan PE, Gorman JM, editors. A guide to treatments that work. New York: Oxford University Press; 1998. p. 270–87.

[16] Klausner EJ, Alexopoulos GS. The future of psychosocial treatments for elderly patients. Psychiatr Serv 1999;50(9):1198–204.

[17] Knight BG, Satre DD. Cognitive behavioral psychotherapy with older adults. Clin Psychol Sci Pract 1999;6(2):188–203.

[18] Pachana NA. Developments in clinical interventions for older adults: a review. N Z J Psychol 1999;28(2):107–17.

[19] Draper BM. The mental health of older people in the community. Med J Aust 2000;173(2): 80–2.

[20] Karel MJ, Hinrichsen G. Treatment of depression in late life: psychotherapeutic interventions. Clin Psychol Rev 2000;20(6):707–29.

[21] Pinquart M, Sorensen S. How effective are psychotherapeutic and other psychosocial interventions with older adults? a meta-analysis. J Ment Health Aging 2001;7(2):207–43.

[22] Areán PA, Alvidrez J. Treating depressive disorders: who responds, who does not respond, and who do we need to study? J Fam Pract 2001;50(6):E2.

[23] Areán PA, Cook BL. Psychotherapy and combined psychotherapy/pharmacotherapy for late life depression. Biol Psychiatry 2002;52(3):293–303.

[24] Bartels SJ, Dums AR, Oxman TE, et al. Evidence-based practices in geriatric mental health care. Psychiatr Serv 2002;53(11):1419–31.

[25] Bartels SJ, Dums AR, Oxman TE, et al. Evidence-based practices in geriatric mental health care: an overview of systematic reviews and meta-analyses. Psychiatr Clin North Am 2003; 26(4):971–90.

[26] Bohlmeijer E, Smit F, Cuijpers P. Effects of reminiscence and life review on late-life depression: a meta-analysis. Int J Geriatr Psychiatry 2003;18(12):1088–94.

[27] Chambless DL, Hollon SD. Defining empirically supported therapies. J Consult Clin Psychol 1998;66(1):7–18.

[28] Fry PS. Structured and unstructured reminiscence training and depression among the elderly. Clin Gerontol 1983;1:15–36.

[29] Fry PS. Cognitive training and cognitive-behavioral variables in the treatment of depression in the elderly. Clin Gerontol 1984;1:15–36.

[30] Thompson LW, Gallagher D, Breckenridge JS. Comparative effectiveness of psychotherapies for depressed elders. J Consult Clin Psychol 1987;55(3):385–90.

[31] Gallagher-Thompson D, Hanley-Peterson P, Thompson LW. Maintenance of gains versus relapse following brief psychotherapy for depression. J Consult Clin Psychol 1990;58(3): 371–4.

[32] Campbell JM. Treating depression in well older adults: use of diaries in cognitive therapy. J Consult Clin Psychol 1992;66:7–18.

[33] Gallagher-Thompson D, Steffen AM. Comparative effects of cognitive-behavioral and brief psychodynamic psychotherapies for depressed family caregivers. J Consult Clin Psychol 1994;62(3):543–9.

[34] Blanchard MR, Waterreus A, Mann AH. The effect of primary care nurse intervention upon older people screened as depressed. Int J Geriatr Psychiatry 1995;10:289–98.

[35] Areán PA, Miranda J. The treatment of depression in elderly primary care patients: a naturalistic study. Journal of Clinical Geropsychology 1996;2:153–60.

[36] Mossey JM, Knott KA, Higgins M, et al. Effectiveness of a psychosocial intervention, interpersonal counseling, for subdysthymic depression in medically ill elderly. J Gerontol A Biol Sci Med Sci 1996;51(4):M172–8.

[37] Reynolds CF III, Frank E, Perel JM, et al. Nortriptyline and interpersonal psychotherapy as maintenance therapies for recurrent major depression: a randomized controlled trial in patients older than 59 years. JAMA 1999;281(1):39–45.

[38] Blanchard MR, Waterreus A, Mann AH. Can a brief intervention have a longer-term benefit? the case of the research nurse and depressed older people in the community. Int J Geriatr Psychiatry 1999;14(9):733–8.

[39] Williams JW Jr, Barrett J, Oxman T, et al. Treatment of dysthymia and minor depression in primary care: a randomized controlled trial in older adults. JAMA 2000;284(12):1519–26.

[40] Thompson LW, Coon DW, Gallagher-Thompson D, et al. Comparison of desipramine and cognitive/behavioral therapy in the treatment of elderly outpatients with mild-to-moderate depression. Am J Geriatr Psychiatry 2001;9(3):225–40.

[41] Unützer J, Katon W, Callahan CM, et al. Collaborative care management of late-life depression in the primary care setting: a randomized controlled trial. JAMA 2002;288(22):2836–45.

[42] Ciechanowski P, Wagner E, Schmaling K, et al. Community-integrated home-based depression treatment in older adults: a randomized controlled trial. JAMA 2004;291(13):1569–77.

[43] Wang JJ, Hsu YC, Cheng SF. The effects of reminiscence in promoting mental health of Taiwanese elderly. Int J Nurs Stud 2005;42(1):31–6.

[44] Wyman M, Gum A, Areán P. Psychotherapy with older adults. In: Maletta A, editor. Principles and practice of geriatric psychiatry. Philadelphia, PA: Lippincott Williams and Wilkins, in press.

[45] Thompson LW, Gallagher D, Czirr R. Personality disorder and outcome in the treatment of late-life depression. J Geriatr Psychiatry 1988;21(2):133–53.

[46] Mynors-Wallis L. Problem-solving treatment: evidence for effectiveness and feasibility in primary care. Int J Psychiatry Med 1996;26(3):249–62.

[47] Hegel MT, Barrett JE, Oxman TE. Training therapists in problem solving treatment of depressive disorders in primary care: lessons learned from the "Treatment Effectiveness Project". Fam Syst Health 2000;18:423–35.

[48] Gallagher-Thompson D, McKibbin C, Koonce-Volwiler D, et al. Psychotherapy with older adults. In: Snyder CR, Ingram RE, editors. Handbook of psychological change: psychotherapy processes and practices for the 21st century. New York: John Wiley and Sons; 2000. p. 614–37.

[49] Kerman G, Weissman MM, Rounsaville B, et al. Interpersonal psychotherapy for depression. In: Groves EJE, editor. Essential Papers on Short-Term Dynamic Therapy. New York: New York University Press; 1996. p. 134–48.

[50] Messer SB. What makes brief psychodynamic therapy time efficient? Clin Psychol 2001;8(1):5–22.

[51] Leichsenring F, Rabung S, Leibing E. The efficacy of short-term psychodynamic psychotherapy in specific psychiatric disorders: a meta-analysis. Arch Gen Psychiatry 2004;61(12):1208–16.

[52] Fry PS, Grover S. Cognitive appraisals of life stress and depression in the elderly: a cross-cultural comparison of Asians and Caucasians. Int J Psychol 1981;17(4):437–54.

[53] Reynolds CF III, Frank E, Kupfer DJ, et al. Treatment outcome in recurrent major depression: a post hoc comparison of elderly ("young old") and midlife patients. Am J Psychiatry 1996;153(10):1288–92.

[54] Kiosses DN, Klimstra S, Murphy C, et al. Executive dysfunction and disability in elderly patients with major depression. Am J Geriatr Psychiatry 2001;9(3):269–74.

[55] Lockwood KA, Alexopoulos GS, van Gorp WG. Executive dysfunction in geriatric depression. Am J Psychiatry 2002;159(7):1119–26.

[56] Butters MA, Whyte EM, Nebes RD, et al. The nature and determinants of neuropsychological functioning in late-life depression. Arch Gen Psychiatry 2004;61(6):587–95.

[57] King DA, Cox C, Lyness JM, et al. Quantitative and qualitative differences in the verbal learning performance of elderly depressives and healthy controls. J Int Neuropsychol Soc 1998;4(2):115–26.

[58] Elderkin-Thompson V, Kumar A, Bilker WB, et al. Neuropsychological deficits among patients with late-onset minor and major depression. Arch Clin Neuropsychol 2003;18(5): 529–49.

[59] Alexopoulos GS, Kiosses DN, Choi SJ, et al. Frontal white matter microstructure and treatment response of late-life depression: a preliminary study. Am J Psychiatry 2002;159(11): 1929–32.

[60] Alexopoulos GS, Raue P, Areán P. Problem-solving therapy versus supportive therapy in geriatric major depression with executive dysfunction. Am J Geriatr Psychiatry 2003; 11(1):46–52.

[61] Mohr D, Burke H, Merluzzi N. A preliminary report on skills-based telephone-administered peer support program for patients with multiple sclerosis. Mult Scler 2004;11(2):222–6.

[62] Floyd M, Scogin F, McKendree-Smith NL, et al. Cognitive therapy for depression: a comparison of individual psychotherapy and bibliotherapy for depressed older adults. Behav Modif 2004;28(2):297–318.

[63] Miranda J, Chung JY, Green BL, et al. Treating depression in predominantly low-income young minority women: a randomized controlled trial. JAMA 2003;290(1):57–65.

[64] Miranda J, Azocar F, Organista KC, et al. Treatment of depression among impoverished primary care patients from ethnic minority groups. Psychiatr Serv 2003;54(2):219–25.

[65] Landreville P, Landry J, Baillargeon L, et al. Older adults' acceptance of psychological and pharmacological treatments for depression. J Gerontol B Psychol Sci Soc Sci 2001;56(5): 285–91.

[66] Rokke PD, Scogin F. Depression treatment preferences in younger and older adults. Journal of Clinical Geropsychology 1995;1:243–57.

[67] Speer DC, Williams J, West H, et al. Older adult users of outpatient mental health services. Community Ment Health J 1991;27:69–76.

ELSEVIER
SAUNDERS

Psychiatr Clin N Am
28 (2005) 821–835

PSYCHIATRIC
CLINICS
OF NORTH AMERICA

Evidence-Based Pharmacologic Interventions for Geriatric Depression

Bindu Shanmugham, MD, MPH[a],*,
Jordan Karp, MD[b], Rebecca Drayer, MD[b],
Charles F. Reynolds III, MD[b],
George Alexopoulos, MD[a]

[a]Weill-Cornell Institute of Geriatric Psychiatry, 21 Bloomingdale Road,
White Plains, NY 10605, USA
[b]Western Psychiatric Institute and Clinic (WPIC), University of Pittsburgh,
3811 O'Hara Street, Pittsburgh, PA 15213-2593, USA

Geriatric depression is a growing public health problem [1,2]. The estimated prevalence of geriatric major depression in the general population is 1% to 2% [3,4]. Depressive symptoms not meeting the criteria for major depression occur in approximately 15% of older adults [5]. The prevalence of major depression in community-dwelling older adults is 1% to 3%, but the prevalence is at least 10% to 12% in primary care and hospital inpatient settings [6]. Despite the common prevalence of depression in older adults, late-life depression is often under-recognized and under-treated, particularly in nonpsychiatric settings [4].

Major depression is a leading cause of disability in adults [7]. In elderly patients, both depression and medical illness have an additive effect on disability and lead to an increase in mortality and nursing home placement [8,9]. Depression severity is a predictor of variance in instrumental activities of daily living [10]. The mechanisms linking depression and disability are still unclear, but it appears that the depressed state itself can be disabling, and depression increases the disability caused by chronic medical conditions [11]. Bruce and colleagues [12] have described a mutually reinforcing, downward-spiraling relationship between depression and disability. In contrast, treatment that results in a reduction in the severity of depression leads,

This work was supported by National Institutes of Mental Health Grants P13MH68638 (to Dr. Alexopoulos) and P30 MH52247 and P30 MH71944 (to Dr. Reynolds).

* Corresponding author.

E-mail address: bis2004@med.cornell.edu (B. Shanmugham).

1 year later, to a reduction of approximately 50% in the number of days burdened by disability.

A review of the evidence for the treatment of geriatric depression must be considered in the context of the considerable heterogeneity of late-life depression that inevitably complicates treatment outcomes. Recent attention has focused on the impact of underlying structural brain abnormalities and the presence of comorbid disorders as major factors affecting treatment response.

Cognitive impairment and structural abnormalities

Late-life depression is associated frequently with cognitive impairment [13] and may present with structural brain abnormalities such as ventriculomegaly and white-matter hyperintensities [14]. Structural brain abnormalities may define a subgroup of depressive disorders that are less likely to respond to treatment interventions. Preliminary findings suggest that white-matter microstructural abnormalities lateral to the anterior cingulate may be associated with a low rate of remission [15]. These underlying processes are an example of one of the many factors that may be associated with finding that major depression developing later in life tends to be more chronic and less amenable to treatment [14].

Psychiatric comorbidity

Co-occurring psychiatric disorders are also associated with poorer treatment responses to standard treatment for geriatric depression. The prevalence of anxiety disorders in elderly depressed patients is 10% to 20% [16,17]. Comorbid anxiety disorders are associated with decreased social functioning and increased somatic symptom severity [16]. Personality disorders co-occur with late-life depression or dysthymia 10% to 30% of the time. Patients with comorbid personality disorders are likely to have an onset of depression at an earlier age and multiple recurrent depressive episodes [18]. Elderly patients with major depression also have a three- to fourfold higher risk of having a comorbid alcohol use disorder compared with nondepressed elders [18]. These disorders are relatively common in older persons with depression and are associated with poorer treatment outcomes.

Medical comorbidity

Comorbid medical disorders are common among older adults with depression and complicate treatment response and outcomes. Medical illness is a risk factor for the development or worsening of depression, and depression itself is a risk factor for medical illness [19]. Depression in patients with chronic physical problems leads to a worsening of disability, higher rates of hospitalization and nursing home admission, and premature mortality [8,20–23]. Examples of comorbid medical disorders complicating the course and treatment outcome of geriatric depression include cardiovascular disease, cerebrovascular, endocrine, neurologic, and joint and connective tissue disorders, malignancy, and immunodeficiency disorders.

A substantial literature documents the complex relationship between depression and cardiovascular disease and between depression and cerebrovascular disease or stroke. Co-occurring depression has been associated with worse medical outcomes. For example, depression in cardiac patients is associated with a greater number of re-hospitalization days after angioplasty or coronary artery bypass grafting [24] and greater long-term mortality after myocardial infarction [25]. Co-occurring depression and treatment outcomes have also been associated with the type and location of vascular disease. For example, approximately 20% to 30% of post-stroke patients develop either minor or major depression. Left-sided stroke is more likely to lead to early onset (≤3 months) post-stroke depression, whereas right-sided stroke is more likely to lead to later-onset depression [26]. Depression after stroke is associated with cognitive impairment, especially when the lesions are left-sided [27]. Although there is only a limited literature on the treatment of post-stroke depression in geriatric patients, preliminary results are promising with respect to the prevention of relapse by early treatment with selective serotonin reuptake inhibitor (SSRI) antidepressants. For example, in a study of elderly post-stroke patients receiving fluoxetine or placebo for 3 months, the fluoxetine group had fewer depressive relapses compared with the placebo group within 3 to 18 months after stroke [28].

The association between endocrine disorders and depression in older adults is also well documented. For example, diabetes doubles the risk of comorbid depression [29]. Depression is also associated with poor treatment outcomes for diabetes. Depressed diabetics are less likely to adhere to dietary and medication recommendations than nondepressed diabetics are, and they use more medical and mental health services [30]. Hypothyroidism in the elderly has a prevalence rate of 5% to 20% in women and a prevalence rate of 3% to 8% in men [31]. Both overt and subclinical hypothyroidism is associated with depression [32]. However, diagnosis and treatment are complicated by the overlapping symptoms associated with both depression and hypothyroidism. For example, the symptoms of hypothyroidism include fatigue, psychomotor retardation, constipation, and mild weight gain. Similarly, common treatments for hypothyroidism can directly and indirectly affect the symptoms of depression, confounding assessments of treatment response.

Neurologic disorders that affect motor function are also associated with high rates of affective disorders in older adults. For example, Parkinson's disease has a rate of comorbid depression ranging from 40% to 50% [33]. Symptoms common to the two disorders are apathy, concentration and memory difficulties, and attention deficit. Patients with Parkinson's disease experience higher levels of dysphoria, irritability, and pessimism than individuals who are not suffering with the disorder [26]. The frontal lobe and basal ganglia dysfunction characteristic of Parkinson's disease may contribute to the development of depression in these patients, as do psychosocial factors such as social isolation and disability [33]. Multiple sclerosis is increasingly common in the elderly as treatment advances prolong survival. The prevalence of depression can be as high as 20% among patients with multiple sclerosis. The rate of completed suicide is over seven times that of the general population [26]. Lesions in the left anterior temporal and parietal regions have been associated with depression [34].

In addition to cardiovascular, cerebrovascular, endocrine, and neurologic disorders, other conditions that increasingly affect older adults have demonstrated associations with depression and treatment outcomes. Associations have been clearly documented between depression and a variety of disorders, including joint disease, connective tissue disorders, malignancy, and more recently, immunodeficiency disorders.

For example, fibromyalgia is a condition characterized by persistent diffuse pain, stiffness, fatigue, tender points, mood disturbances, and nonrestorative sleep. This illness occurs mainly in women, and the frequency increases with age. The prevalence of fibromyalgia in women between the ages of 60 and 79 years old is 7% to 10% [35,36]. Over half of the patients with fibromyalgia have major depressive disorder [37]. Pancreatic cancer is also a disease associated with aging, with a mean age of onset of 65 years [38]. Symptoms of depression and anxiety may sometimes precede the cancer diagnosis [39,40]. Finally, 11% of all AIDS cases reported annually in the United States are older than 50 years of age [41]. Depression has been directly associated with a decrease in the numbers of natural killer and CD8 cells, which normally inhibit viral activity and are indirectly linked to HIV disease progression because of nonadherence with antiretroviral therapy [19].

In summary, the co-occurrence of depression with medical disorders is common in older adults and frequently affects the course and outcomes of treatment of both the psychiatric and medical disorders. Comorbidity is a cardinal feature of geriatric depression and is relevant to considering variations in the effectiveness of treatment observed in older adults. Hence, any conclusions about the overall efficacy or effectiveness of different treatments should always be considered in the context of the individual patient presentation when making a treatment decision. With this as background for interpreting treatment effectiveness, this review addresses the pharmacologic management of depressive illness in the elderly and the evidence base supporting treatment interventions for geriatric depression.

Methods

Randomized controlled trials, systematic reviews, meta-analyses, and evidence-based reviews were identified by a search of medical literature databases, MEDLINE, EMBASE, and PsychINFO, and selected expert consensus guidelines. A classification scheme was used to categorize the level of evidence for specific treatment recommendations based on a letter grade A, B, C or D (Box 1), summarizing the data supporting the recommendation [42]. This classification approach is used in highlighting the results. Some interventions were assigned a grade C or D recommendation as evidence from meta-analysis of randomized controlled trials (grade A) is not available for all the pharmacologic interventions identified in this review.

In conducting this review, meta-analyses and systematic reviews were identified that summarize the evidence of the comparative efficacy and tolerability of tricyclic antidepressants (TCAs) and SSRIs in geriatric depression. Then, treatment trials restricted to older adults for SSRI and novel non-SSRI antidepressants were identified. Finally, the treatment literature and associated recommendations were reviewed for important clinical issues associated with the pharmacotherapy of geriatric depression, including maintenance treatment and relapse prevention, treatment of psychotic

---

Box 1. Categories of evidence and strength of recommendations

Category of evidence
Ia-evidence from meta-analysis of randomized controlled trials
Ib-evidence from at least one randomized controlled trial
IIa-evidence from at least one controlled study without randomization
IIb-evidence from at least one other type of quasi-experimental study
III-evidence from non-experimental descriptive studies, such as comparative studies, correlation studies, and case-control studies
IV-evidence from expert committee reports or opinions or clinical experience of respected authorities, or both

Strength of recommendation
A-directly based on category I evidence
B-directly based on category II evidence or extrapolated recommendation from category I evidence
C-directly based on category III evidence or extrapolated recommendation from category I or II evidence
D-directly based on category IV evidence or extrapolated recommendation from category I, II or III evidence

---

From Shekelle PG, Woolf SH, Eccles M, et al. Clinical guidelines: developing guidelines. BMJ 1999;318(7183):593–6; with permission.

depression, and the use of electroconvulsive treatment. This review focuses on recent geriatric studies examining the comparative efficacy of SSRIs and serotonin-norepinephrine reuptake inhibitors (SNRIs). The reader is referred elsewhere to recent meta-analyses [43–46] and systematic reviews [47–49] for comprehensive assessments of the effectiveness of TCAs and other agents in the treatment of geriatric depression [46].

Results and meta-analyses

The evidence base supporting different treatment strategies for geriatric depression is illustrated in Table 1. As shown, category I evidence supports the use of antidepressants alone or in combination with psychotherapy in the treatment of geriatric major depressive disorder. The combined use of antidepressants and psychotherapy, antidepressants alone, or psychotherapy alone in the treatment of mild depression is also supported by category I evidence. Table 2 [43,45,46] shows results of meta-analyses comparing the effectiveness of tricyclic antidepressants and selective serotonin reuptake inhibitors in geriatric depression.

As shown, SSRIs and TCAs have comparable efficacy [15,45] and tolerability [45] (see Table 2). Of note, two of the meta-analyses are not restricted to older patients and found different types of side effects and a possible difference in efficacy favoring tricyclic antidepressants in inpatients. However, the most recent meta-analysis conducted by Wilson and Mottram [48] was restricted to studies of older depressed patients and found comparable efficacy and tolerability comparing TCAs with SSRIs.

Geriatric depression and selective serotonin and serotonin-norepinephrine reuptake inhibitor treatment trials

Table 3 [50–56] provides a summary of selected antidepressant trials for older adults consisting of SSRIs and SNRIs. These studies include 5 randomized controlled trials and two open-label studies. Overall, findings from these studies support an evidence base for the efficacy of these agents

Table 1
Treatment strategies in geriatric major depression

Intensity	Treatment strategy (A, D)
Major depression	Antidepressant alone
	Antidepressant and psychotherapy
Mild depression	Antidepressant and psychotherapy
	Antidepressant alone or psychotherapy alone

A, directly based on category I evidence; D, directly based on category IV evidence or extrapolated recommendation from category I, II or III evidence.

Table 2
SSRIs and TCAs have comparable efficacy (A)

Study	Sample size	Type	Comments
Wilson and Mottram 2004 [46]	11 randomized controlled trials; 537 TCA recipients; 554 SSRI recipients	Meta-analysis	TCA-related drugs are comparable to SSRIs in terms of tolerability and may offer an alternative when SSRIs are either contraindicated or clinically unacceptable
Steffens et al 1997 [45]	36 randomized controlled trials; 4076 patients; 995 SSRI recipients; 973 TCA recipients	Meta-analysis	SSRIs resulted in significantly more gastrointestinal problems and sexual dysfunction, whereas treatment with TCAs produced significantly more complaints of sedation, dizziness, and anticholinergic symptoms
Anderson 2000 [43]	102 randomized controlled trials; 10,706 patients	Meta-analysis	Overall efficacy between the two classes is comparable, but SSRIs are not proven to be as effective as TCAs in in-patients and against amitriptyline; SSRIs have a modest advantage in terms of tolerability against most TCAs

A, directly based on category I evidence.

in the treatment of geriatric depression compared with placebo or compared with other SSRI or TCA treatments.

Maintenance treatment and relapse prevention

Treatment outcomes for depression include acute phase outcomes, long-term maintenance, and relapse prevention. As shown in Table 4 [57–59], a variety of different outcomes has been defined to evaluate the treatment effectiveness. The prevention of relapse and recurrence is an important goal in the treatment of geriatric depression because of the potentially chronic and disabling nature of the disorder. The goal of maintenance treatment is to prevent recurrence. This phase begins at the end of the continuation treatment when the patient has entered remission. Executive dysfunction has been associated with relapse and recurrence of geriatric major depression [60]. In a study of treatment for major depression, depressed older adults were randomly assigned to receive nortriptyline, placebo, interpersonal psychotherapy (IPT), or IPT with nortriptyline. In the 3-year follow-up period, the group maintained with combined IPT, and nortriptyline had the lowest recurrence rate (20%) compared with placebo (90%) and was superior in preventing or delaying recurrence [61]. Maintenance treatment is recommended for 12 months after a single episode of depression for older adults and from 1 to 3 years for patients with recurrent depression [62].

Table 3
Selected antidepressant trials (A, B)

Study	Sample size	Age (y)	Dosages (mg)	Type	Scales	Duration (wk)	Comments
Citalopram							
Karlsson et al 2000 [50]	336	≥65	20–40	RCT	MADRS	12	Well tolerated; not sedating for elderly depressed patient with or without dementia
Fluoxetine							
Koran et al 1995 [51]	671	≥60	20	RCT	HAM-D	6	43% response
Paroxetine							
Cassano et al 2002 [52]	242	≥65	20–40	RCT	HAM-D	52	Comparable to fluoxetine
Sertraline							
Bondareff et al 2000 [53]	210	≥60	50–150	RCT	HAM-D	12	Comparable to nortryptiline
Duloxetine							
Wohlreich et al 2004 [54]	101	≥65	80–120	Open label	HAM-D	52	Well tolerated; effective and safe in the long-term treatment of MDD
Nelson et al 2005 [55]	90	≥55	60	RCT	HAM-D	9	30% remission for duloxetine vs 13% for placebo; significant reduction in pain compared with placebo
Venlafaxine							
Dierick 1996 [56]	116	≥65	25–150	Open label	CGI, MADRS	52	67% of patients achieved clinical response by 2 mo

Abbreviations: CGI, Clinical Global Impression; HAM-D, Hamilton Rating Scale for Depression; MADRS, Montgomery-Asberg Depression Rating Scale; RCT, randomized controlled trial.

A, directly based on category I evidence; B, directly based on category II evidence or extrapolated recommendation from category I evidence.

Table 4
Definitions of treatment outcomes

Results	Definition
Improvement	Residual symptoms [57]
Response	50% reduction in symptoms [58]
Remission	Asymptomatic state usually defined as ≤7 on the HAM-D
Relapse	Increase in depressive symptoms to a syndromal level within 6 mo from remission [59]
Recurrence	A new episode of major depression 6 mo after remission
Resistance	No response or partial response to adequate treatment with two or more antidepressants

Abbreviation: HAM-D, Hamilton Rating Scale for Depression.

Treatment of psychotic depression

Psychotic depression occurs in approximately 20% to 45% of hospitalized depressed elderly [63]. One of the earliest treatment studies for psychotic depression (not specific to older adults) resulted in the recommendation that psychotic depression should be treated with amitriptyline and perphenazine [64]. A subsequent randomized study demonstrated that the addition of a moderate dose of perphenazine to nortriptyline was well tolerated but did not improve efficacy [65]. Studies in mixed age adults have found the SSRIs fluvoxamine, paroxetine, and sertraline and the SNRI venlafaxine to be effective in treating psychotic depression [66,67]. Studies of SSRIs alone or in combination with antipsychotic drugs are lacking in the treatment of geriatric psychotic depression. In the absence of empirical data specific to older adults, geriatric expert consensus guidelines suggest the use of a combination of antidepressant and antipsychotic medications or electroconvulsive treatment (ECT) [62]. These guidelines suggest that the SSRIs and venlafaxine are considered first-line agents, with TCAs a high second-line alternative. Atypical antipsychotics were preferred over traditional antipsychotics in these expert consensus guidelines, with risperidone, olanzapine, and quetiapine rated as the first-line choices [62].

Treatment with electroconvulsive therapy

ECT has been found to be highly effective in moderate to severe depression and depression with melancholic features [68]. ECT has been recommended as an initial treatment in patients who have depression with psychotic symptoms or catatonia, severe depressive symptoms and functional impairment, and comorbid medical problems, and when there is an urgent need for response (ie, patients who are acutely suicidal or patients who refuse food and are nutritionally compromised). However, depressed older adults who respond to ECT are at a high risk for relapse unless they receive continuation or maintenance pharmacotherapy or ECT [69]. In a study of patients who underwent ECT because pharmacotherapy failed, patients treated with nortriptyline and lithium had a lower rate of relapse compared with those treated with nortriptyline alone [69].

Discussion

Effective and well-tolerated treatments for late-life depression exist, including antidepressants, psychotherapy, and electroconvulsive therapy. Treatment outcomes include the reduction of depressive symptoms and suicidal ideation, improvement of cognitive and functional status, and prevention of relapse and recurrence. More than half of the elderly patients treated with antidepressants experience treatment response, defined as a 50% reduction in depressive symptoms [45,58]. In intent-to-treat analyses, the response rates to antidepressants are 50% to 65% compared with 25% to 30% on placebo in randomized controlled trials [5,70,71].

Expert consensus recommendations suggest that older adults tolerate SSRIs better than TCAs [59], although empirical studies reveal similar tolerability and rates of side effects. However, the consequences of the side effects may be more serious for TCAs compared with SSRIs. SSRIs are associated with higher rates of nausea, loss of appetite, and sexual dysfunction, but they have less anticholinergic and cardiovascular side effects compared with TCAs [45]. Patients with pre-existing bundle branch block who are treated with TCAs may develop second degree block [72]. The choice among different SSRIs may be guided by the absence of drug interactions, simplicity of dosing, and side-effect profile. The various SSRIs have similar efficacy, and some (escitalopram, citalopram, and sertraline) have a lower potential for drug interactions.

A partial response to treatment is not uncommon in the treatment of geriatric depression, with the result that clinicians prescribe additional agents in the context of augmentation therapies. Augmentation strategies are added early in treatment to accentuate the clinical response, around 4 to 6 weeks of standard antidepressant treatment for patients who have limited improvement [73]. In patients who experience a partial response to treatment, some clinicians combine antidepressants in the hope of realizing synergistic effects. The combination therapy of two antidepressants has not been studied systematically. Hence, there is no empirical evidence base supporting either the effectiveness or lack of effectiveness for augmentation strategies. However, the common occurrence of partial treatment response after several trials of monotherapy has stimulated the development of expert consensus recommendations for partial treatment response in geriatric depression [52]. These expert consensus guidelines suggest that if there is a partial response after the initial antidepressant treatment to (1) SSRI, then add bupropion, lithium, or nortriptyline; to (2) TCA, then add lithium or SSRI;

to (3) bupropion SR, then add SSRI or lithium; or to (4) venlafaxine, then add lithium [62]. Discontinuing the augmentation treatment may put patients at an increased risk of relapse. In one study [74], patients who received brief augmentation during an acute phase had a 52% relapse rate on follow-up. If there is little or no response to an initial SSRI treatment, the experts support switching to venlafaxine or bupropion [62]. Other suggestions are, if there is no response to TCA, then switch to venlafaxine or SSRI; if there is no response to venlafaxine, then switch to SSRI.

Other important clinical issues in the treatment of geriatric depression include the identification and treatment of the older adult with active suicidal ideation or other signs of increased suicide risk. In industrialized countries, men aged 75 years and older have the highest suicide rate among all age groups [75]. Risk factors for suicide in the elderly include physical illness [76], persistent pain [77], mood disorders [78], alcohol abuse [79], anxiety [80], bereavement, and social isolation [81]. More often, among elderly patients, it has been shown that hopelessness best predicts suicidal ideation in the presence of moderate or higher levels of depressive symptoms [82]. Predictors of suicide attempts include previous suicide attempts with serious intent and severity of depression [83]. Elderly patients who have attempted suicide tend to have higher levels of hopelessness even after successful treatment for depression [84]. The use of firearms is the most common method of completed suicide among older adults [85].

Treatment with an antidepressant medication, usually an SSRI or SNRI, is the mainstay of treatment of a depressed suicidal older adult. An examination of double-blind studies does not demonstrate a causal relationship between pharmacotherapy and the emergence of suicidality [86]. In one retrospective analysis [87], depressed patients treated with fluoxetine (n = 1765) were compared with a tricyclic antidepressant (n = 731) or placebo group. There was no increased risk of emergence of suicidal ideation among depressed patients treated with fluoxetine.

Summary

Late-life depression is under-recognized and undertreated in older adults. Depressed older adults who are at an increased risk or undertreatment include patients older than 85 years, those with comorbid medical conditions, and older adults with cognitive impairment receiving home health care or living in nursing homes. Although the existing empirical treatment literature is limited, the available published treatment studies and expert consensus recommendations find that antidepressants are effective. In general the SSRIs and SNRIs pose a low risk for the most serious side effects. Treatment of psychotic depression has not been adequately investigated in older adults, although common practice includes treatment with an SSRI or SNRI in conjunction with an atypical antipsychotic. Treating with antidepressants augmented by psychotherapy can minimize relapse and disability in depressed patients. Continuation and maintenance treatment at an adequate dose and for an adequate length of time is critical in minimizing relapse. Empirical trials are needed that evaluate the selection and effectiveness of pharmacologic combination therapy and other treatment strategies for treatment resistant and partially responsive major depressive disorder in older adults.

References

[1] Reynolds CF III, Lebowitz BD, Schneider LS. The NIH consensus development conference on the diagnosis and treatment of depression in late life: an overview. Psychopharmacol Bull 1993;29(1):83–5.

[2] Jeste DV, Alexopoulos GS, Bartels SJ, et al. Consensus statement on the upcoming crisis in geriatric mental health: research agenda for the next 2 decades. Arch Gen Psychiatry 1999; 56(9):848–53.

[3] Blazer D, Williams CD. Epidemiology of dysphoria and depression in an elderly population. Am J Psychiatry 1980;439–44.

[4] Mulsant BH, Ganguli M. Epidemiology and diagnosis of depression in late life. J Clin Psychiatry 1999;60(Suppl 20):S9–15.

[5] NIH Consensus Conference. Diagnosis and treatment of depression in late life. JAMA 1992; 268(8):1018–24.

[6] Charney DS, Reynolds CF 3rd, Lewis L, et al. Depression and Bipolar Support Alliance consensus statement on the unmet needs in diagnosis and treatment of mood disorders in late life. Arch Gen Psychiatry 2003;60(7):664–72.

[7] Murray CJL, Lopez AD. The global burden of disease: a comprehensive assessment of mortality and disability from diseases, injuries, and risk factors in 1990 and projected to 2020. Cambridge (MA): Harvard University Press; 1996.

[8] Bruce ML, Seeman TE, Merrill SS, et al. The impact of depressive symptomatology on physical disability: MacArthur studies of successful aging. Am J Public Health 1994;84(11): 1796–9.

[9] Penninx BW, et al. Exploring the effect of depression on physical disability: longitudinal evidence from the established populations for epidemiologic studies of the elderly. Am J Public Health 1999;89(9):1346–52.

[10] Alexopoulos GS, Vrontou C, Kakuma T, et al. Disability in geriatric depression. Am J Psychiatry 1996;153(7):877–85.

[11] Lenze EJ, et al. The association of late-life depression and anxiety with physical disability: a review of the literature and prospectus for future research. Am J Geriatr Psychiatry 2001;9(2):113–35.

[12] Bruce ML. Depression and disability in late life: directions for future research. Am J Geriatr Psychiatry 2001;9(2):102–12.

[13] Alexopoulos GS, Young RC, Meyers BS. Geriatric depression: age of onset and dementia. Biol Psychiatry 1993;34(3):141–5.

[14] Lebowitz BD, Pearson JL, Schneider LS, et al. Diagnosis and treatment of depression in late life: consensus statement update. JAMA 1997;278(14):1186–90.

[15] Alexopoulos GS, Kiosses DN, Choi SJ, et al. Frontal white matter microstructure and treatment response of late-life depression: a preliminary study. Am J Psychiatry 2002;1929–32.

[16] Lenze EJ, Mulsant BH, Shear MK, et al. Comorbid anxiety disorders in depressed elderly patients. Am J Psychiatry 2000;157(5):722–8.

[17] Beekman AT, Bremmer MA, Deeg DJ, et al. Anxiety disorders in later life: a report from the Longitudinal Aging Study Amsterdam. Int J Geriatr Psychiatry 1998;13(10):717–26.

[18] Devanand DP. Comorbid psychiatric disorders in late life depression. Biol Psychiatry 2002; 52(3):236–42.

[19] Krishnan KR, Delong M, Kraemer H, et al. Comorbidity of depression with other medical diseases in the elderly. Biol Psychiatry 2002;52(6):559–88.

[20] Mulsant BH, Ganguli M, Seaberg EC. The relationship between self-rated health and depressive symptoms in an epidemiological sample of community-dwelling older adults. J Am Geriatr Soc 1997;45(8):954–8.

[21] Koenig HG, Cohen HJ, Blazer DG, et al. Profile of depressive symptoms in younger and older medical inpatients with major depression. J Am Geriatr Soc 1993;41(11):1169–76.

[22] Ganguli M, Dodge HH, Mulsant BH. Rates and predictors of mortality in an aging, rural, community-based cohort: the role of depression. Arch Gen Psychiatry 2002;59(11):1046–52.

[23] Schulz R, Drayer RA, Rollman BL. Depression as a risk factor for non-suicide mortality in the elderly. Biol Psychiatry 2002;52(3):205–25.

[24] Levine JB, Covino NA, Slack WV, et al. Psychological predictors of subsequent medical care among patients hospitalized with cardiac disease. J Cardiopulm Rehabil 1996;16(2):109–16.

[25] Lesperance F, Frasure-Smith N, Talajic M, et al. Five-year risk of cardiac mortality in relation to initial severity and one-year changes in depression symptoms after myocardial infarction. Circulation 2002;105(9):1049–53.

[26] Kanner AM, Barry JJ. The impact of mood disorders in neurological diseases: should neurologists be concerned? Epilepsy Behav 2003;4(Suppl 3):S3–13.

[27] Robinson RG. Poststroke depression: prevalence, diagnosis, treatment, and disease progression. Biol Psychiatry 2003;54(3):376–87.

[28] Fruehwald S, Gatterbauer E, Rehak P, et al. Early fluoxetine treatment of post-stroke depression: a three-month double-blind placebo-controlled study with an open-label long-term follow up. J Neurol 2003;250(3):347–51.

[29] Anderson RJ, Freedland KE, Clouse RE, et al. The prevalence of comorbid depression in adults with diabetes: a meta-analysis. Diabetes Care 2001;24(6):1069–78.

[30] Ciechanowski PS, Katon WJ, Russo JE. Depression and diabetes: impact of depressive symptoms on adherence, function, and costs. Arch Intern Med 2000;160(21):3278–85.

[31] Laurberg P, et al. Hypothyroidism in the elderly: pathophysiology, diagnosis and treatment. Drugs Aging 2005;22(1):23–38.

[32] Hendrick V, Altshuler L, Whybrow P. Psychoneuroendocrinology of mood disorders: the hypothalamic-pituitary-thyroid axis. Psychiatr Clin North Am 1998;21(2):277–92.

[33] McDonald WM, Richard IH, DeLong MR. Prevalence, etiology, and treatment of depression in Parkinson's disease. Biol Psychiatry 2003;54(3):363–75.

[34] Siegert RJ, Abernethy DA. Depression in multiple sclerosis: a review. J Neurol Neurosurg Psychiatry 2005;76(4):469–75.

[35] Wolfe F, Ross K, Anderson J, et al. The prevalence and characteristics of fibromyalgia in the general population. Arthritis Rheum 1995;38(1):19–28.

[36] Gowin KM. Diffuse pain syndromes in the elderly. Rheum Dis Clin North Am 2000;26(3): 673–82.

[37] Hudson JI, Pope HG Jr. The relationship between fibromyalgia and major depressive disorder. Rheum Dis Clin North Am 1996;22(2):285–303.

[38] Lowenfels AB, Maisonneuve P. Epidemiologic and etiologic factors of pancreatic cancer. Hematol Oncol Clin North Am 2002;16(1):1–16.

[39] Passik SD, Roth AJ. Anxiety symptoms and panic attacks preceding pancreatic cancer diagnosis. Psychooncology 1999;8(3):268–72.

[40] Holland JC, Korzun AH, Tross S, et al. Comparative psychological disturbance in patients with pancreatic and gastric cancer. Am J Psychiatry 1986;143(8):982–6.

[41] Knodel J, Watkins S, VanLandingham M. AIDS and older persons: an international perspective. J Acquir Immun Defic 2003;33(2):1.

[42] Shekelle PG, Woolf SH, Eccles M, et al. Clinical guidelines: developing guidelines. BMJ 1999;318(7183):593–6.

[43] Anderson IM. Selective serotonin reuptake inhibitors versus tricyclic antidepressants: a meta-analysis of efficacy and tolerability. J Affect Disord 2000;58(1):19–36.

[44] Gerson S, Belin TR, Kaufman A, et al. Pharmacological and psychological treatments for depressed older patients: a meta-analysis and overview of recent findings. Harv Rev Psychiatry 1999;7(1):1–28.

[45] Steffens DC, Krishnan KR, Helms MJ. Are SSRIs better than TCAs? Comparison of SSRIs and TCAs: a meta-analysis. Depress Anxiety 1997;6(1):10–8.

[46] Wilson K, Mottram P. A comparison of side effects of selective serotonin reuptake inhibitors and tricyclic antidepressants in older depressed patients: a meta-analysis. Int J Geriatr Psychiatry 2004;19(8):754–62.

[47] Taylor WD, Doraiswamy PM. A systematic review of antidepressant placebo-controlled trials for geriatric depression: limitations of current data and directions for the future. Neuropsychopharmacology 2004;29(12):2285–99.

[48] Wilson K, Mottram P, Sivanranthan A, et al. Antidepressant versus placebo for depressed elderly. Cochrane Database Syst Rev 2005;(3):CD000561.

[49] Bains J, Birks JS, Dening TR. The efficacy of antidepressants in the treatment of depression in dementia. Cochrane Database Syst Rev 2005;(3):CD003944.

[50] Karlsson I, Godderis J, Augusto De Mendonca Lima C, et al. A randomised, double-blind comparison of the efficacy and safety of citalopram compared to mianserin in elderly, depressed patients with or without mild to moderate dementia. Int J Geriatr Psychiatry 2000;15(4):295–305.

[51] Koran LM, Hamilton SH, Hertzman M, et al. Predicting response to fluoxetine in geriatric patients with major depression. J Clin Psychopharmacol 1995;15(6):421–7.

[52] Cassano GB, Puca F, Scapicchio PL, et al. Paroxetine and fluoxetine effects on mood and cognitive functions in depressed nondemented elderly patients. J Clin Psychiatry 2002; 63(5):396–402.

[53] Bondareff W, Alpert M, Friedhoff AJ, et al. Comparison of sertraline and nortriptyline in the treatment of major depressive disorder in late life. Am J Psychiatry 2000;157(5):729–36.

[54] Wohlreich M, Mallinckrodt CH, Watkin JG, et al. Duloxetine for the long-term treatment of major depressive disorder in patients aged 65 and older: an open-label study. BMC Geriatrics 2004;4:11.

[55] Nelson JC, et al. Duloxetine for the treatment of major depressive disorder in older patients. Am J Geriatr Psychiatry 2005;13(3):227–35.

[56] Dierick M. An open-label evaluation of the long-term safety of oral venlafaxine in depressed elderly patients. Ann Clin Psychiatry 1996;8(3):169–78.

[57] Judd LL, Akiskal HS, Maser JD, et al. Major depressive disorder: a prospective study of residual subthreshold depressive symptoms as predictor of rapid relapse. J Affec Disord 1998; 50(2–3):97–108.

[58] Prien RF, Carpenter LL, Kupfer DJ. The definition and operational criteria for treatment outcome of major depressive disorder: a review of the current research literature. Arch Gen Psychiatry 1991;48(9):796–800.

[59] Frank E, Prien RF, Jarrett RB, et al. Conceptualization and rationale for consensus definitions of terms in major depressive disorder: remission, recovery, relapse, and recurrence. Arch Gen Psychiatry 1991;48(9):851–5.

[60] Alexopoulos GS, Meyers BS, Young RC, et al. Executive dysfunction and long-term outcomes of geriatric depression. Arch Gen Psychiatry 2000;57(3):285–90.

[61] Reynolds CF III, Frank E, Perel JM, et al. Nortriptyline and interpersonal psychotherapy as maintenance therapies for recurrent major depression: a randomized controlled trial in patients older than 59 years. JAMA 1999;281(1):39–45.

[62] Alexopoulos G, Katz IR, Reynolds CF, et al. The expert consensus guideline series: pharmacotherapy of depressive disorders in older patients. A Postgraduate Medicine Special Report. October 2001.

[63] Meyers BS. Late-life delusional depression: acute and long-term treatment. Int Psychogeriatr 1995;7(Suppl):113–24.

[64] Spiker DG, Weiss JC, Dealy RS, et al. The pharmacological treatment of delusional depression. Am J Psychiatry 1985;142(4):430–6.

[65] Mulsant BH, Sweet RA, Rosen J, et al. A double-blind randomized comparison of nortriptyline plus perphenazine versus nortriptyline plus placebo in the treatment of psychotic depression in late life. J Clin Psychiatry 2001;62(8):597–604.

[66] Zanardi R, Franchini L, Serretti A, et al. Venlafaxine versus fluvoxamine in the treatment of delusional depression: a pilot double-blind controlled study. J Clin Psychiatry 2000;61(1):26–9.

[67] Zanardi R, Franchini L, Gasperini M, et al. Double-blind controlled trial of sertraline versus paroxetine in the treatment of delusional depression. Am J Psychiatry 1996;153(12):1631–3.

[68] van der Wurff FB, Stek ML, Hoogendijk WJ, et al. The efficacy and safety of ECT in depressed older adults: a literature review. Int J Geriatr Psychiatry 2003;894–904.

[69] Sackeim HA, Haskett RF, Mulsant BH, et al. Continuation pharmacotherapy in the prevention of relapse following electroconvulsive therapy: a randomized controlled trial. JAMA 2001;285(10):1299–307.

[70] Schulberg HC, Katon W, Simon GE, et al. Treating major depression in primary care practice: an update of the Agency for Health Care Policy and Research Practice Guidelines. Arch Gen Psychiatry 1998;55(12):1121–7.

[71] Schulberg HC, Katon WJ, Simon GE, et al. Best clinical practice: guidelines for managing major depression in primary medical care. J Clin Psychiatry 1999;60(suppl 7):19–26; discussion 27–8.

[72] Roose SP, Glassman AH, Giardina EG, et al. Tricyclic antidepressants in depressed patients with cardiac conduction disease. Arch Gen Psychiatry 1987;44(3):273–5.

[73] Nelson JC. Treatment of refractory depression. Depress Anxiety 1997;5(4):165–74.

[74] Reynolds CF III, Frank E, Perel JM, et al. High relapse rate after discontinuation of adjunctive medication for elderly patients with recurrent major depression. Am J Psychiatry 1996; 153(11):1418–22.

[75] Pearson JL, Conwell Y. Suicide in late life: challenges and opportunities for research: introduction. Int Psychogeriatr 1995;7(2):131–6.

[76] Harris EC, Barraclough BM. Suicide as an outcome for medical disorders. Medicine 1994; 73(6):281–96.

[77] Fishbain DA. The association of chronic pain and suicide. Semin Clin Neuropsychiatry 1999;4(3):221–7.

[78] Frierson RL. Suicide attempts by the old and the very old. Arch Intern Med 1991;151(1):141–4.

[79] Murphy GE, Wetzel RD, Robins E, et al. Multiple risk factors predict suicide in alcoholism. Arch Gen Psychiatry 1992;49(6):459–63.

[80] Szanto K, Mulsant BH, Houck PR, et al. Treatment outcome in suicidal vs. non-suicidal elderly patients. Am J Geriatr Psychiatry 2001;9(3):261–8.

[81] Szanto K, Prigerson H, Houck P, et al. Suicidal ideation in elderly bereaved: the role of complicated grief. Suicide Life Threat Behav 1997;27(2):194–207.

[82] Uncapher H, Gallagher-Thompson D, Osgood NJ, et al. Hopelessness and suicidal ideation in older adults. Gerontologist 1998;38(1):62–70.

[83] Alexopoulos GS, Bruce ML, Hull J, et al. Clinical determinants of suicidal ideation and behavior in geriatric depression. Arch Gen Psychiatry 1999;56(11):1048–53.

[84] Szanto K, Reynolds CF 3rd, Conwell Y, et al. High levels of hopelessness persist in geriatric patients with remitted depression and a history of attempted suicide. J Am Geriatr Soc 1998; 46(11):1401–6.

[85] Centers for Disease Control. Suicide among older persons: United States, 1980–1992. JAMA 1996;275(7):509.

[86] Matthews JD, Fava M. Risk of suicidality in depression with serotonergic antidepressants. Ann Clin Psychiatry 2000;12(1):43–50.

[87] Beasley CM Jr, Dornseif BE, Bosomworth JC, et al. Fluoxetine and suicide: a meta-analysis of controlled trials of treatment for depression [erratum appears in BMJ 1991;19;303:968]. BMJ 1991;685–92.

ELSEVIER
SAUNDERS

Psychiatr Clin N Am
28 (2005) 837–869

PSYCHIATRIC
CLINICS
OF NORTH AMERICA

Evidence-Based Pharmacological Treatment of Geriatric Bipolar Disorder

Robert C. Young, MD[a,b,*]

[a]*Payne Whitney Westchester and Institute of Geriatric Psychiatry,
Weill Medical College of Cornell University, White Plains, NY, USA*
[b]*New York Presbyterian Hospital, 21 Bloomingdale Road,
White Plains, NY 10605, USA*

Elderly individuals who have bipolar (BP) disorder present a particular challenge to clinicians, health care services, and caregivers. They are a complex and heterogeneous group of patients who frequently have comorbidities and poor outcomes, including a high mortality rate.

BP elders represent 5% to 19% of patients presenting for acute treatment at geriatric psychiatry services [1,2]. They use health services heavily [3,4]. The psychopathology associated with their illness episodes (ie, mania, mixed mania, hypomania, and depression) can be severe; their signs and symptoms resemble those in younger patients [5]. Elderly BP patients who are treated for manic and mixed episodes often have incomplete response [6,7], further episodes [8–10], and high mortality rate [8,9].

Beyond recognition and careful diagnostic assessment, pharmacotherapy is the cornerstone of their management. This article addresses the current evidence regarding drug treatment of BP disorder in old age. In particular:

- What are the side effects and toxicity of relevant psychotropic agents?
- What is the evidence for their efficacy for acute and continuation/maintenance treatment?
- What age-associated factors may modify these risks and benefits?

The therapeutic armamentarium in BP patients also includes education, other psychosocial interventions, and electroconvulsive therapy. Although these are pertinent to both older and younger BP patients, they will be mentioned only briefly here, because the age-specific literature related to elderly BP individuals is sparse.

---

* New York Presbyterian Hospital, Westchester, 21 Bloomingdale Road, White Plains, NY 10605.

E-mail address: ryoung@med.cornell.edu

The following discussion of the evidence base emphasizes its limitations, as well as its implications for clinical management and public health. This review also suggests strategies and priorities for research.

Methods

Data sources

Articles written in English on the pharmacologic treatment of BP disorder in the elderly between 1966 and May 2005 were identified through a search of the MEDLINE database. Material used in a recent review [11] was updated. Additional data sources included reference lists of the identified articles, other reviews, the author's files, and textbook articles when appropriate.

Selection criteria

"Elderly" was defined as being 60 years of age or older. The keywords "aged" and "geriatric" were combined with words indicating pharmacologic treatments (ie, "pharmacotherapy"), classes of medications (eg, lithium, anti-convulsants, antidepressants), and names of selected individual medications (eg, valproate, divalproex, carbamazepine) with or without names of diagnostic terms (bipolar disorder, mania, hypomania, bipolar depression, depression).

A few articles on "older adults" in which the lower age limits were 50 to 55 years were included for heuristic value and possible extrapolation of their results to the geriatric population. Seminal articles on pharmacotherapy of BP disorder in mixed-age patients were included for evaluation of age effects. All identified original articles were reviewed and reported. Conclusions regarding therapeutics were drawn primarily from studies of more than 10 patients. Case reports and smaller case series were described regarding benefit as appropriate for their heuristic value and when reviewing toxicity issues.

Results

First, the side effects and tolerability in elders of psychotropic agents used in the treatment of BP disorder, and potential modifiers of these effects, are discussed in this article. Thereafter, their efficacy, and potential modifiers of efficacy, are considered. The rationale for this sequence is that tolerability informs drug selection and influences the dose and duration of therapeutic trials. Side effects also determine, in part, adherence to treatment. Side effects and tolerability therefore are important determinants of benefit in these patients.

Overall, the main limitation of the literature is the lack of randomized controlled trials in elderly individuals. The existing evidence is derived mainly from small case series or case reports.

Side effects and toxicity

In the elderly, side effects and toxicity of psychotropics are of particular concern. The medical consequences of specific side effects (eg, falls [12]) may be more severe than the consequences in younger patients. Side effects can also interfere with the quality of remission [13]. The risks of side effects and toxicity of psychotropics may be increased in elders as a result of age-related pharmacokinetic changes. Pharmacodynamic changes that may contribute to increased risks will be outlined separately.

Lithium salts

LI has been widely prescribed in the elderly [14,15]. Among community-based BP patients from Western Pennsylvania in the late 1990s, close to two thirds of those over the age of 65 were treated with LI, and only 31% were receiving anticonvulsants; the proportion of older patients treated with LI was significantly higher than the proportion of younger patients [14].

Table 1 lists 12 studies that include assessment of LI side effects. These reports dealt with more than 10 cases each.

Cognitive and neuromotor impairments. Cognitive and neuromotor impairments range from mild tremor and other "nuisance" effects to life-threatening conditions such as delirium. Neurocognitive side effects were assessed in 9 of these studies [7,16–23]. Although some investigators have suggested that LI can dull cognitive performance [24,25], this has not been examined in the elderly. In aged patients, recovery from LI-induced delirium can be prolonged [26]. However, in a recent study, the incidence of hospitalization for delirium in elderly patients initiated on LI was equivalent to those initiated on valproate [20], and was less than that for benztropine treatment.

Cardiovascular effects. Sick sinus syndrome [27] can occur at moderate LI concentrations in older patients with compromised sinus node function. In a cross-sectional study [28], 58% of elderly BP patients receiving maintenance LI treatment had electrocardiographic abnormalities; interpretation of these findings is limited by the study design.

Other side effects. LI antagonizes thyroid function. In one cross-sectional study, 32% of aged patients treated with LI were prescribed thyroxine replacement or had elevated thyroid stimulating hormone levels [29]. In another study, almost 6% of elderly patients recently initiated on LI treatment received new thyroxine prescriptions, compared with half that rate among elders initiated on VAL [30].

In one report [21], polyuria and polydipsia occurred during LI treatment in approximately 40% of elderly patient visits. Polyuria and polydipsia, weight gain, and edema were categorized as mild side effects in another study, and these occurred at a rate of 46% in patients aged 50 years or older

Table 1
Side effects/toxicity of pharmacotherapy of older adult and eldery BP patients

Agent	Reference	Study design	n	Mean age in years (range)	Dx	Mean dose in mg/d (range)	Mean concentration in mEq/L (range)	Neurocognitive toxicity	Other toxicity	Comment
LI	Hewick et al [22]	R	23 23	NA (50–59) (60–84)	BP, 82%; UP, 9%; other-9%	NA (NA)	NA (NA)	Fine tremor included as "minor"	21/46 (46%) had minor side effects versus 15/36 (42%) of younger patients aged 21–49 yr	Lower concentrations in patients aged ≥60 yr
LI	Roose et al [28]	P	31	67 (60–79)	Primary affective disorder	NA (NA)	NA (0.60–0.70)	NA	4 episodes of toxicity in 18 mo (versus 2/164 younger patients over 18 mo (chi square = 8.32; $P < .01$); 5 had arrhythmias; 14 had conduction abnormality on ECG; hypothyroidism in 1	Concentration in younger group not specified
LI	Himmelhoch et al [7]	R	81	63 (55–)	BP I 74; BP II 7	NA (NA)	NA (NA)	13 (16%)	NA	Predicted by dementiform features and/or extrapyramidal syndrome; not age

LI	Smith and Helms [17]	R	15	70 (65–80)	BP 8; UP 7	NA (NA)	NA (NA)	7 (47%) had moderate to severe side effects – primarily neurotoxicity	NA	LI concentration 1.2–1.5 mEq/L in 5 of those with moderate to severe side effects; in younger group (n = 41) aged 19–61 yr, 12.% had moderate to severe side effects (chi square = 5.84; $P < .02$)
LI	Murray et al [21]	P	37	NA (60–78)	BP 25; UP 12	P (NA)	NA (NA)	Tremor about 40% of visits in BP aged 70–78 (graph)	Graphical presentation	Cross-sectional assessment; no difference in LI concentration with age in BP patients; tremor about 20% of visits in patients aged 20–29 yr, 30% in those aged 30–69 yr; polyuria and polydipsia not greater with age.
LI	Schaffer and Garvey [19]	P	14	67 (65–77)	BP, manic	NA (NA)	NA (0.50–1.10)	3 (21%)	NA	LI discontinued in 2 with toxicity at 0.5–0.8 mEq/L; 1 other when level increased to 1.1 mEq/L

(continued on next page)

Table 1 (*continued*)

Agent	Reference	Study design	n	Mean age in years (range)	Dx	Mean dose in mg/d (range)	Mean concentration in mEq/L (range)	Neurocognitive toxicity	Other toxicity	Comment
LI	Chacko et al [16]	P	19	68 (59–84)	BP	NA (NA)	0.70 (0.30–1.10)	11 (58%) tremor, 8 (42%) sedation	14 (74%) polydipsia, 11 (58%) polyuria; 10 (53%) dry mouth; 6 (32%) weight gain	Only 3 monotherapy; mean duration LI = 3.9 yr; side effects related to number of other psychotropics (r = 0.60, $P < .01$)
LI	Stone 1989 [18]	R	43	NA (65–)	BP, manic	NA (NA)	NA (NA)	11 (26%)	One developed goiter	LI levels in 9 toxic patients were 1.4–2.6 mEq/L; LI discontinued in 2 others with tremor vomiting and ataxia
LI	Head and Dening [29]	R	148	NA (65–85 +)	BP 83; UP 57; other 7	482 (100–1400)	0.64 (0.00–1.50)	NA	47 (32%) were on thyroid replacement or had elevated TSH	Cross sectional
VAL	Puryear et al [141]	R	13	70 (63–77)	BP, manic	1000 (100–1750)	57 (34–82)	1 (8%) delirium; 3 (23%) tremor	2 (15%) weight gain; 5 (38%) dry mouth	VAL discontinued in pt with delirium, also was receiving phenytoin

Drug	Study	Design	N	Age	Diagnosis	Dose		Adverse effects		Comments
VAL	Kando [142]	R	35	71 (63–85)	BP, manic; other	743 (250–2000)	53 (11–102)	2 (6%) sedation; 1 (3%) c/o confusion	2 (6%) nausea; 1 transient leukopenia	VAL was discontinued in 1 pt with nausea
VAL	Ncaguil et al [140]	R	21	71 (60–82)	BP, manic	1405 (500–3000)	72 (31–106)	2 (10%) with sedation	NA	Responded to dose reduction
VAL	Niedermier and Nasrallah [91]	R	39	67 (60–86)	BP	1029 (500–2250)	72 (36–111)	2 (5%) sedation; 1 (3%) slurred speech, 1 confusion; 1 ataxia	1 (3%) nausea; 1 diarrhea; 1 rash;	None required discontinuation; improved with lowering of dose
LI or VAL	Shulman et al [20]	R; population-based cohort study	4,111	73.4 (>65)	NA	NA	NA	NA	Over 18 mo new prescription for thyroxine: 5.65/100 person years in new LI treatment group versus 2.70 in new VAL group	Near 6% treatment in LI group
LI or VAL	Shulman et al [31]	R; as above	5,340	74.7 (>65)	Mood disorder	NA	NA	Over 8 years, hospitalization for delirium at equivalent rates in patients newly treated with LI (2.8 per 100 person years) versus, VAL (4.1 per 100 person years)	NA	Benztropine comparator group had higher rate of delirium than LI group

(continued on next page)

Table 1 (continued)

Agent	Reference	Study design	n	Mean age in years (range)	Dx	Mean dose in mg/d (range)	Mean concentration in mEq/L (range)	Neurocognitive toxicity	Other toxicity	Comment
LI or LTG	Sajatovic et al [23]	P, secondary analysis: following open label phase; randomized, double blind, placebo controlled	98 randomized	61 (55–82)	BP I	LI (n = 34): modal 750 mg/d; LTG (n = 33): modal 240 mg/d (100–400 mg/d); PBO, n = 31	LI (0.8–1.1 mEq/L)	LI adverse events included dypraxia, tremor, amnesia	No cases of serious rash in randomized phase; back pain and headache most common adverse events associated with LTG. Other LI adverse events included xerostomia, headache, infection, dizziness, nausea, fatigue	Adverse events leading to premature withdrawl: LI (29%); LTG (18%); PBO (13%).

Abbreviations: **BP**, bipolar; **ECG**, electrocardiogram; **LI**, lithium; **LTG**, lamotrigine; **NA**, not available; **P**, prospective; **PBO**, placebo; **R**, retrospective; **VAL**, valproate; **UP**, unipolar.

[22]. In another report [17], mild side effects occurred in 27% of elderly patients. In a randomized control trial of stabilized patients, adverse events lead to premature discontinuation in 29% of LI-treated patients compared with 13% for placebo [38].

Dose/concentration and effects. Although case reports in elderly subjects indicate that LI toxicity can occur at moderate blood levels (eg, 0.5–0.8 mEq/L [19]), the relationship of LI concentrations to side effects in the elderly has remained poorly defined. In mixed-age patients, LI concentrations are positively related to side effects, and these increase greatly above 1.0 to 1.5 mEq/L.

Pharmacokinetic distortions in elderly BP patients that lead to increased LI dose/concentration ratios put them at increased risk for side effects. Renal clearance of LI decreases with age, the elimination half-life of LI in the elderly is twice as long as in younger patients [31], and amount of time after which stable concentrations are achieved at a given dose is prolonged. Renal disease and cardiac insufficiency can further reduce LI clearance, and increase in fat/lean body mass ratio may also contribute to higher concentration/dose ratios [31,32]. Finally, medications and special diets for medical disorders, such as thiazide diuretics, nonsteroidal anti-inflammatory agents, angiotension-converting enzyme inhibitors, and sodium restriction, can increase LI dose/concentration ratios, while theophylline can decrease these ratios [33,34].

These pharmacokinetic issues were underscored by Strayhorn and Nash [35]; toxicity in the six elderly subjects in their series occurred in the context of high LI levels (1.58–2.45 mEq/L). In aged patients, brain/peripheral LI concentration ratio can be increased [36], and this may also increase vulnerability to central nervous system toxicity. The relationship of erythrocyte LI concentrations to side effects has not been systematically assessed in elders [37].

Anticonvulsants

Clinicians increasingly prescribe valproate (VAL) for elderly individuals who have BP disorder. Divalproex sodium is more commonly prescribed than valproic acid. In the province of Ontario, VAL has surpassed LI salts as a new prescription for elderly patients with a mood disorder [15].

Table 1 lists six reports concerning VAL in elderly patients that included examination of side effects. Each involves more than 10 patients treated with that agent.

Cognitive and neuromotor impairments. VAL is often well tolerated in elderly individuals [38]. Unimpaired neuropsychologic test performance was reported in geriatric patients with seizure disorder treated with valproate [39]. Neurocognitive side effects including sedation, tremor, and gait disturbance, were noted in a subgroup of patients.

Other anticonvulsants, ie, carbamazepine (CBZ), oxcarbazepine, topiramate, gabapentin and lamotrigine (LTG) have been described in fewer reports as part of the management of geriatric BP disorder. Systematic data on cognitive and other side effects of these agents in nondemented elderly subjects is sparse.

Cardiovascular effects. CBZ can cause bradycardia and atrioventricular conduction delays [40].

Other side effects. VAL and CBZ are associated with blood dyskrasias. VAL is associated with more leukopenia than CBZ. Combined treatment with CBZ in 16 treatment refractory-depressed patients with a mean age of 63 years had to be discontinued in 7 patients due to gastrointestinal complaints, hepatic toxicity, hyponatremia, or rash [41]. Stevens-Johnson syndrome can occur with LTG; it is not known whether advanced aged alters the risk of Stevens-Johnson syndrome, although serious rash did not occur in BP patients aged 55 years of age or older who were randomized to LTG, LI, or placebo [23].

Dose/concentration and effects. The relationship between VAL concentrations and side effects in elderly patients is not well described. In one study, CBZ concentrations in elderly patients presenting with bradyarrythmia or conduction delay were often moderate, while tachyarrythmias in younger patients were often associated with substantially elevated concentrations, including those reflecting intentional overdose [40].

   With increased age, the elimination half-life of VAL can be prolonged [42], and the free fraction of plasma concentrations increases [43]. Aspirin can increase the VAL free fraction [44]. The ratio of total VAL concentration to dose is decreased by phenytoin and CBZ. For example, VAL itself inhibits metabolism of LTG, which may necessitate use of lower LTG doses to minimize its side effects.

   Pharmacokinetic characteristics of CBZ are not well described in aged patients. Drug interactions with phenytoin and barbiturates can decrease CBZ dose/concentration ratios [44]. CBZ itself increases hepatic enzyme activity [45] and decreases levels of VAL and LTG; relatively high doses of those drugs may therefore be necessary to obtain their full benefit when they are used in combination with CBZ.

Antipsychotic agents

   Side effects of antipsychotic agents are probably not specific to BP diagnosis. However, they will be discussed briefly.

   Antipsychotic agents may be used alone or in combination with mood stabilizers in elderly BP patients [46]. Atypical agents have generally supplanted conventional agents as first-line antipsychotics in geriatric clinical practice [47]. They are used as adjuncts or as primary agents.

Cognitive and neuromotor impairments. Conventional antipsychotic drugs can cause sedation and impair cognition, which are particularly problematic when they occur in the elderly. Some atypical agents such as clozapine, olanzapine and quetiapine, also can cause somnolence [48]. On the other hand, atypical antipsychotic treatment may enhance cognition in some elderly patients who are treated for psychosis [49].

Elderly patients are more vulnerable than younger patients to the parkinsonian side effects of antipsychotics, although they may experience acute dystonic reactions less often; their rate of akathisia may be equivalent to that seen in younger patients. The risk of tardive dyskinesia increases with age at first exposure and with cumulative treatment; female patients and patients who have affective disorders may also be at increased risk [50–52]. Atypical antipsychotics, compared with conventional agents, have reduced liability for acute motor side effects [53]; some atypical antipsychotics also may be associated with lower risk for tardive dyskinesia.

Cardiovascular effects. Antipsychotics can prolong QT interval (QTc), which can lead to life-threatening arrhythmia. Pretreatment conduction abnormalities are a risk factor for such changes [54]. Thioridizine and butyrophenones have been particularly implicated in QTc prolongation and arrhythmia [55]; QTc prolongation by ziprasidone is of unknown clinical significance [56].

Both conventional and atypical antipsychotics have anticholinergic effects that can contribute to problematic side effects in the elderly—these include tachycardia, constipation, and urinary hesitancy or obstruction, as well as cognitive toxicity. Lower potency conventional agents and olanzapine, in particular, have such anticholinergic properties. Alpha-1 adrenergic receptor antagonism by antipsychotic drugs, including atypical agents, may contribute to treatment emergent orthostatic hypotension.

Atypical antipsychotics can cause metabolic effects including weight gain, glucose intolerance, and hyperlipidemia in mixed-age populations [57]. Olanzapine and clozapine appear to have the greatest potential for such effects [58]. Although analysis of these effects in geriatric patients is not yet available, preliminary evidence has suggested that advanced age attenuates these effects [59].

Excess mortality has been reported in subgroups of elderly patients treated with atypical antipsychotics [60]. This issue is discussed below under "Neurological and Medical Comorbidities" as modifiers of toxicity.

Doses and effects. Side effects of antipsychotic medications can be dose-dependent. Examples include cognitive toxicity and neuromotor effects such as akathisia.

Antipsychotic dose/concentration ratios can be increased by age-associated factors. This has been reported with risperidone [61] and clozapine [62].

Benzodiazepines

Benzodiazepines have limited, adjunctive use in elderly BP patients.

Cognitive and neuromotor impairments. Benzodiazepines can decrease memory consolidation [63,64]; even short-acting compounds cause memory impairment [64]. There is a pharmacodynamic component to the sensitivity of some elders to diazepam [65]. Benzodiazepines, in particular long-acting drugs such as clonazepam, can also increase disability [66], and risk for falls and fractures [67].

Long-acting benzodiazepines are metabolized to active products by cytochrome P-450-3A4 enzymes, and concentrations of these drugs can accumulate with age [68].

Antidepressants

Antidepressants can be used to treat BP depressed elderly individuals (see below). Their use in unipolar depression in old age, including pharmacokinetics and tolerability, is reviewed elsewhere in this issue. Several types of side effects are only briefly summarized here.

Cognitive and neuromotor impairments. Antidepressants can cause sedation in the elderly. Successful treatment is often associated with improved cognitive performance in elders; however, treatment with selective serotonin reuptake inhibitors (SSRIs) can cause neuromotor side effects.

Cardiovascular effects. Recent practice has favored the use of SSRIs or bupropion in elderly patients, including BP patients. These lack quinidine-like effects and have minimal orthostatic hypotensive effects. SSRIs can, however, cause bradycardia. Dose-related hypertension can occur with venlafaxine. Nonspecific monoamine oxidase inhibitors require dietary restriction to avoid tyramine reaction; phenelzine is associated with delayed orthostatic hypotension [69].

Other side effects. SSRI treatment can cause hyponatremia in elderly individuals.

Pharmacodynamic modifiers of toxicity

In addition to pharmacokinetic changes with age, pharmacodynamic differences may contribute to vulnerability to side effects. To assess pharmacodynamic factors requires accounting for pharmacokinetic differences, when appropriate, using therapeutic drug monitoring. It is difficult to interpret studies of agents where this information is relevant, but is lacking, or in which there are differences in concentrations between patient groups of interest.

Age

Evidence regarding the influence of age on side effects of medications used in the management of BP disorders is sparse. Such influences have been examined in some studies of LI treatment. Although they did not find greater overall side effects in elderly patients compared with younger patients, Smith and Helms [17] did find greater moderate to severe LI side effects in aged patients. Murray and colleagues [21] reported greater tremor but not greater polydipsia/polyuria in aged compared with younger patients. Although Roose and colleagues [28] observed that overall LI toxicity was greater in older patients, no age effect was found in two other studies [7,22]. Himmelhoch and colleagues [7] included only patients aged more than 55 years, and differences in LI concentration limit interpretation of findings from another study [22].

Patterns of carbamazepine cardiotoxicity may differ by age and sex [40]. In that study, young men with cardiotoxicity often have tachyarrythmias and high drug concentrations and overdose; elderly women more often have bradyarrythmias and conduction delay without excessive drug exposure.

Neurological and medical comorbidity

As illustrated by the following reports, comorbid dementia in pariticular may increase vulnerability to side effects of psychotropics. Thus, the central nervous system side effects of LI may be greater in aged patients with dementia. Himmelhoch [7] reported, for example, that among elderly patients, LI was poorly tolerated in those with dementia and in those with parkinsonian features. Anticonvulsant side effects may also be greater in elders with dementia, but, as is the case for LI [7], available reports have not included nondemented patients [70,71]. In a randomized double blind, placebo-controlled study of VAL, elderly patients with dementia and manic features had a discontinuation rate due to adverse events, primarily sedation, of 22% during initiation of treatment at doses greater than 15 mg/kg [70]; this suggests that demented patients tolerate lower doses than do nondemented patients. Also, CBZ caused diplopia or ataxia in 23% of elders with dementia [71].

Excess mortality associated with atypical antipsychotic agents has been reported in a subgroup of geriatric patients. Excess cerebrovascular accidents and deaths have been reported in patients with dementia; other risk factors appear to include advanced age and vascular disease [60].

Cardiovascular disorders are a potential modifier of side effects of other psychotropics in the elderly. Thus, they can increase vulnerability to orthostatic hypotensive, and quinidine-like effects [72].

Pharmacodynamic drug–drug interactions

Polypharmacy is liable to be associated with high side effect burden as a result of pharmacodynamic as well as pharmacokinetic interactions. Examples of pharmacodynamic effects include the potentiation of extrapyramidal side effects of antipsychotic agents used in conjunction with LI [73], and the potentiation of anticholinergic effects by combining agents with that property [74]. However, such interactions can also be used for clinical benefit—for example, potentiation of sedative effects.

What is the evidence for efficacy in the elderly?

Treatment of manic states

Lithium. The efficacy of lithium (LI) in mania has been demonstrated in placebo-controlled studies of mixed-age patients [75]. Cade [76] reported efficacy of LI in ten patients; of these three were elderly and they responded. However, there have been no placebo-controlled acute efficacy trials of LI in the geriatric population. Studies of efficacy in purely geriatric samples have been primarily retrospective; they have described outcomes of naturalistic treatment of differing duration. Table 2 includes five studies that involved more than 10 elders treated with LI. LI dose and levels were not reported in all of these.

In addition, Wylie and colleagues [77] included 39 manic patients in a group of 62 elderly BP patients assessed for outcome of naturalistic treatment; 37 of these patients were treated with LI. Although the patients fared well overall, the authors did not evaluate the outcomes of treatment with LI separately. Gildengers and colleagues [78] reported the feasibility of protocol-based treatment, primarily with LI or VAL, of BP elderly subjects in various clinical states; they noted that most patients did not experience sustained recovery. In another study, LI was more efficacious than chlorpromazine in a sample of manic patients with a mean age of 56 years [79].

The relationship between plasma LI concentrations and acute antimanic response has not been defined in elderly patients. Case series [19,28] have suggested that geriatric patients may respond to levels of LI that are lower ($0.5-0.8$ mEq/L) than those considered optimal ($0.8-1.2$ mEq/L) in mixed-age adults [80]. However, other reports have suggested that geriatric patients benefit best from conventional LI levels when tolerated [81,82]. Studies that can identify subgroups of elderly individuals who benefit from low concentration of LI and other psychotropic drugs are needed; concentration-dependent side effects could be avoided in these patients.

Monotherapy with mood stabilizers, together with elimination of other unnecessary psychotropics, is considered an optimal first step in the management of elderly patients. Monotherapy, if efficacious, can avoid the additional side effect burden of combined treatment. Nevertheless, the time course of antimanic response to LI or other monotherapy, under particular dosing conditions, has not been described in aged manic patients. Defining adequate trials of antimanic agents such as LI in elderly patients requires considering both treatment duration and dose.

Anticonvulsants. Whereas placebo-controlled studies of VAL (divalproex) in mixed-age patients support its efficacy in mania [83], there are no published data comparing VAL to placebo or to LI in the elderly. Nevertheless, retrospective and open studies indicate that VAL can have antimanic effects in geriatric patients [38,84–86]. Table 2 includes five studies that included more than 10 elders treated with VAL. A total of 137 elderly patients were studied. The doses ranged between 250 and 2250 mg/d. The total VAL concentrations were 25 to 120 µg/mL. Overall, 59% of patients met various improvement criteria. Other reports regarding VAL treatment were consistent with these findings [38,84–87].

One retrospective report [88] compared VAL with LI treatment in manic BP elders; the therapeutic benefits of the two agents were comparable. In another report, although either VAL or LI were mainly prescribed, the limited number of manic patients precluded such comparison [71].

The relationship between blood levels of VAL and antimanic response is not established in the elderly. Bowden [89] recommended total concentrations between 50 and 120 µg/mL based on data from a mixed-age sample with an average age of 39 years. Findings from retrospective naturalistic series are difficult to interpret [88,90]. However, Chen and colleagues [88] found that manic elders with VAL concentrations of 65 to 90 µg/mL improved more than patients who had levels of 45 to 65 µg/mL. Recently, VAL administered intravenously reduced psychopathology in three geriatric patients with concentrates between 44 and 87 µg/mL [91]. While the proportion of VAL not bound to proteins is higher with increased age [43]; the clinical significance of these differences in protein binding is not known.

Information is limited regarding therapeutic benefit of VAL in combination with LI in aged BP patients. This combination was reportedly beneficial for elderly patients who were only partially responsive to LI [92,93], and it can also be useful in rapid cycling BP elders [93,94].

The antimanic effect of CBZ has not been a focus of controlled trials in the elderly [95]. Okuma and colleagues [96], in their double-blind comparison of the efficacy of CBZ and LI, included 7 elderly manic patients out of 50 in the CBZ arm, treated with a mean level of 8 µg/mL, and 6 out of 51 patients in the LI arm. Overall, both drugs were efficacious.

With regard to other anticonvulsants (eg, oxcarbazepine, gabapentin, and topiramate) in elderly manic patients, information is limited to case reports and case series. For example, gabapentin in combination with an antipsychotic or VAL was associated with reduction in manic symptoms in 7 elderly patients [97]. Thus, the role of these agents in geriatric practice is not established.

Antipsychotic agents. There is little data regarding the efficacy of atypical antipsychotic medications in aged BP patients. Although newer agents such as aripiprazole may have particular advantages in elders, the broadest experience for mixed-age BP patients relates to risperidone and olanzapine as adjunct therapy [98,99] or as monotherapy [100]. Risperidone, olanzapine, quetiapine, aripiprazole, and ziprasidone have US Food and Drug

Table 2
Acute efficacy of pharmacotherapy in older adult and elderly BP patients

Agent	Reference	Study design	n	Mean age in years (range)	Dx	Mean dose in mg/d (range)	Mean concentration in mEq/L (range)	Outcome measures	Duration (wk)	Benefit	Comments
LI	van der Velde [6]	R	12	67 (60–74)	BP, manic	NA (700–2100)	NA (0.60–2.00)	Global improvement (–4 severe depression, +4 severe mania)	2	4 (33%) improved	51/63 (81%) of younger (age 17–59 yr) BP manic patients responded
LI	Himmelhoch et al [7]	R	81	63 (55–88)	BP I 74; BP II 7	NA (NA)	(NA)	Global efficacy/improvement scale: 1–6 (1 = optimum, 6 = none)	3–8	56 (69%) improved	23/25 of the poor responders had dementia, intermittent confusion, and/or extrapyramidal syndromes; drug abuse also was a negative predictor
LI	Schaffer and Garvey [19]	P	14	69 (65–77)	BP, manic	NA (NA)	NA (0.50–0.90)	Discharge	>2	11 (71%) improved	
VAL	Puryear et al [141]	R	13	70 (63–77)	7 BP, manic, mixed; 6 other	1000 (100–1750)	57 (34–82)	BPRS, Cohen Mansfield Agitation Inventory	NA (inpatient)	Reduction in BPRS in 12 (92%)	

VAL	Kando et al [142]	R	35 71 (63–85)	24 BP I, manic, 11 other affective disorder	743 (250–2000)	53 (11–102)	Global McElroy scale 0-3 (0 no improvement, 3 complete remission)	0.5–21	18/29 (62%) improved with adequate trial	No data for inadequate trial group; 27 patients had past trial with LI, 19% did not respond
VAL	Noaguil et al [140]	R	21 71 (60–82)	BP, manic	1405 (500–3000)	72 (31–106)	Improvement of CGI (responders: CGI 1 and 2)	1–7	19 (90%) improved	20 patients received neuroleptics
VAL	Niedermier and Nasrallah [91]	R	39 67 (60–86)	16 BP, 7 BP and dementia	1029 (500–2250)	72 (36–111)	CGI	≥1	14/16 (88%) BP responded; 7 (100%) BP and dementia responded	
LI or VAL	Chen et al [89]	R	59 69 (NA)	BP, manic	NA	LI (n = 30): 0.30–1.30 mEq/L; VAL (n = 29): 25–116 µg/mL	Improvement of CGI (score of 1 and 2)	Mean 2.3	LI: 20 (67%) improved overall; 9/11 (82%) improved with ≥ 0.8 mEq/L (CGI = 2 ± 0.6). VAL: 11 (38%) improved overall; 6/8 (75%) with 65-90 µg/mL (CGI = 2.1 ± 0.6)	Response rates to LI better than VAL for classic mania; similar efficacy for mixed mania

Abbreviations: BP, bipolar; BPRS, Brief Psychiatric Rating Scale; CGI, clinical global impression; LI, lithium; NA, not available; P, prospective; PBO, placebo; R, retrospective; VAL, valproate.

Administration–approved indications for use in BP disorder. A preliminary analysis of manic patients aged 50 years or more suggests efficacy of olanzapine monotherapy [101]. Also, preliminary experience has suggested a role for quetiapine in management of BP elders [102,103]. In addition, Shulman and colleagues [104] and Frye [105] noted response to clozapine in geriatric manic patients.

Relationships between antipsychotic dose or serum/plasma concentrations to efficacy in the elderly are not defined.

Benzodiazepines. The benefits of benzodiazepines, such as lorazepam, as adjuncts in elderly manic patients have not been studied. Clinicians must weigh their potential benefits against associated risks.

Treatment of BP depression

There is no systematic literature focused on the treatment of elderly patients who have BP depression [106]. Indeed, the pharmacotherapy of acute BP depression has not been adequately studied in mixed-age populations. The pharmacologic strategies used in BP depression differ from those used in unipolar depression in their focus on mood stabilizers and on combination treatments [107]. In a series of five elderly BP depressed patients, LTG (75–100 mg/d) augmentation of LI or VAL led to remission [106].

The efficacy of antidepressant pharmacotherapy in aged BP patients has not been tested. Nemeroff and colleagues [108] found that the combination of paroxetine and LI, at a concentration of 0.8 mEq/L or less, was more efficacious than LI alone in patients aged 21 to 71 years. No age dependence of response was reported.

In elderly patients, "switching" to mania during pharmacotherapy with tricyclic and other antidepressant agents can occur [109,110]. Comparisons of treatment-emergent mania related to alternative antidepressants in the elderly are needed.

Monoamine oxidase inhibitors can benefit younger BP depressed patients [111], and they are effective in geriatric unipolar depression [69]. They have not been studied in elderly individuals who have BP.

What factors may modify acute efficacy?

Age-associated factors may modify benefit from pharmacotherapy in elderly individuals who have BP. The evidence for such effects is summarized as follows:

Age. There are limited findings regarding the influence of age on acute treatment outcomes in BP disorders. Van der Velde [6] noted poorer acute benefit of LI in elderly BP patients compared with younger patients (Table 2). One study of naturalistic LI treatment in mixed-age manic patients suggested that benefit was attenuated by increased age [112]; however, only four patients in this study were elderly. No age effect was reported in a placebo-controlled study of the efficacy of LI in mixed-age manic patients, 18% of whom were 60 years of age or older [113]. Apparently, no analyses address age effects on VAL or CBZ efficacy in mania. Cycling into a depressive episode may occur more often during treatment of mania in elders than in younger patients [114]. The effects of age on treatment outcomes in BP depression are not known.

Age at onset. There is little information regarding the relationship of age at onset and treatment outcome in geriatric BP patients [115]. No effect of age at onset on outcome at end point was found in one naturalistic study [116], or in one retrospective report [117]. In BP patients, both age at first affective episode and at first manic episode may be pertinent. The reliability of course assessment in geriatric patients is a limiting factor in research, and multiple sources of information must be used.

Neurological comorbidity/cognitive impairment. Elderly manic patients with neurological compromise may have relatively poor therapeutic outcomes. Berrios and Bakshi [118] reported an association between higher Hachinski scores, indicating cerebrovascular disease, and worse acute outcome. Himmelhoch [7] observed chronic mania in 19 elderly subjects despite treatment with LI; 12 of these subjects had extrapyramidal syndromes, and 5 had dementia.

Cognitive impairments may be associated with attenuated acute treatment outcomes in older BP patients. Executive impairments, for example, are prevalent in BP disorders, particularly in late life [119–121]; these are often associated with frontostriatal pathology. These impairments were associated with limited acute response to LI pharmacotherapy in a preliminary study of elderly manic patients [122]. Comorbid dementia may also be associated with worse antimanic outcomes of LI treatment [7]. In a randomized, placebo-controlled trial in demented patients with manic symptoms, VAL reduced agitation but not mania ratings [70].

Acute treatment can improve cognitive performance in geriatric BP patients [77]; however, one mechanism for such improvement is alleviation of affective psychopathology, sometimes referred to as "reversible dementia." In addition, mood stabilizers may have neuroprotective effects [123,124], and may promote regeneration of cortical gray matter [125]. However, cognitive impairments may also persist despite successful treatment of BP patients [126], and these impairments may have implications for long-term management.

Comorbid medical conditions. Comorbid medical conditions are prevalent among elderly BP patients [7] and may also predict poor LI response. In a mixed-age sample, patients with medical comorbidity had higher age (mean 51 yr) and poorer response to naturalistic LI treatment compared with patients without such comorbidity [127]. Studies focusing on the implications of specific medical disorders in the elderly are needed.

Substance abuse. Substance abuse may be relatively prevalent in aged BP patients. It was associated with poor antimanic response to LI in elderly manic patients in one report [7].

Symptom profile. The relationship between symptom profile and treatment outcome in geriatric mania has received little study. For example, the presence of mixed features or psychosis and outcomes await investigation in the elderly. In a retrospective report, LI treatment was associated with better therapeutic effect than VAL treatment in patients with classic mania compared with those with mixed mania; drug levels were not provided in this comparison. Treatments for hypomania and rapid cycling also have not been systematically studied in late life.

Continuation/maintenance treatment

Because BP patients, including the elderly, are at risk for repeated episodes requiring treatment, continuation and maintenance pharmacotherapy is critical to their care. The literature regarding the long-term treatment of elderly BP patients is even more limited than for acute management.

Information concerning long-term treatment of elderly BP patients is primarily derived from naturalistic treatment in mixed-age samples. Table 3 presents five studies that each included at least 10 elderly BP patients. All of these studies included LI treatment. Stone [18] did not find fewer psychiatric rehospitalizations in patients naturalistically maintained on LI compared with those who were not. These studies do not allow assessment of the efficacy of LI.

In a secondary analysis of BP I patients 55 years of age or older treated in randomized double-blind studies after open-label stabilization, LTG delayed time to intervention for any mood episode and for depressive episode, while LI delayed time to intervention for manic, hypomanic, and mixed episodes [23].

Clinical experience suggests that many elders with BP disorder receive combined psychotropic regimens [77,103]. The optimal duration of adjunctive agents, ie, antidepressants or antipsychotic agents, after successful treatment is not defined in elderly BP patients.

There is no adequate information to guide mood stabilizer dosing in the context of continuation and maintenance treatment in BP elders. The patients followed by Stone [18] were treated with LI at concentrations of 0.5 to 1.00 mEq/L, and those of Sajatovic and colleagues [23] at 0.8 to 1.1 mEq/L.

Studies in mixed-age patients have suggested that LI treatment can have an antisuicide effect [128]. Although BP patients are at risk for suicide [129], BP elderly indivuduals have yet to be studied from this perspective.

Nonsuicide mortality rates on follow-up of manic elders are greater than those of same-age patients who have major depression [8]. The effect of psychiatric interventions on mortality in BP elderly individuals is not known.

What factors may modify efficacy of continuation-maintenance treatment?

Age. There has been conflicting evidence whether advanced age has adverse implications for long-term affective outcomes, and this evidence is limited to LI treatment. Three of the studies listed in Table 3 included younger patients treated with LI. While one of these studies indicated more recurrent affective episodes in elderly subjects [6], another [21] found only trends for greater manic psychopathology but not more frequent hospitalizations. Interpretation of the third report [22] was confounded by differing LI concentrations with age. Other studies of LI maintenance treatment in mixed-age populations that have examined age as a predictor have included few elderly subjects, or, despite a wide age range, did not indicate the number of elderly subjects; these reported no age effect on various outcome measures [130–133].

Course of illness. In the naturalistic follow-up of geriatric mania by Stone [18], patients with prior episodes had a greater rate of recurrence. Schurhoff and colleagues [133] did find differences in outcome of LI treatment in mixed-age BP patients with illness onset after age 40 years compared with those with earlier age at onset.

Neurological status/cognitive impairment. Elderly BP patients with neurologic comorbidity had higher risk of psychiatric rehospitalization and institutionalization in one study. Also, enduring cognitive impairments, despite acute control of affective symptoms, may have adverse implications for long-term treatment outcomes. In geriatric BP patients, cognitive deficits have been limited to poor community living skills and deficits in performing activities of daily living, as well as with nursing home placement [134], but not greater relapse with hospitalization [9].

Thus, factors that alter acute treatment outcomes in elderly BP patients may also influence outcomes of long-term management information. However, controlled treatment trials are needed.

Discussion

The results noted in this article provide limited direction for clinical practice and have implications for health care delivery. They also highlight the need for clinical investigation and suggest directions for such research.

Limitations of the search strategy need to be kept in mind in considering the literature reviewed. Few articles published before 1966 were identified, only English language literature was searched, and abstracts and reports at research meetings are not identified by MEDLINE. The challenges of using unfiltered databases such as MEDLINE have been emphasized by Bartels and colleagues [135].

Table 3
Efficacy of continuation-maintenance treatment in older adult and elderly BP patients

Agent	Reference	Study design	n	Mean age in years (range)	Dx	Mean dose in mg/d (range)	Mean concentration in mEq/L (range)	Outcome measures	Duration (yr)	Results	Comments
LI	Van der Velde [6]	R	12	67 (60–74)	BP, manic	NA (900–2100)	NA (0.60–2.00)	Recurrence of affective episodes	3 years after acute inpatient phase	2/12 (17%) had no recurrence in 1 year, 1 (8%) in 2 and 3 years	Younger patients (n = 63; age 17 -59) remained better during follow-up.
LI	Hewick et al [22]	R	23 23	NA (50–59) (60–84)	BP 82%; UP 9%; other 9%	NA (NA)	NA (NA)	Global (0–3) after > 3 mo of treatment	NA	13/46 (28%) not optimally controlled (rating > 0) versus 6/36 (17%) of younger patients	Lower concentrations in elders
LI	Murray et al [21]	P	37	NA (60–78)	BP 25; UP 12	NA (NA)	NA (NA)	Global (0–3)	2	Trend for more severe and prolonged mania in elders	Similar LI levels in elderly and younger patients (n = 129; range 25-59 yr); 69% of patients on LI for at least 12 mo
LI	Stone [18]	R	43	NA (65–)	BP, manic	NA (NA)	NA (0.50–1.00)	No. of readmissions	Mean 3.2	1.1 on LI versus 1.6 not on LI (n = 44)	

| LI or LTG | Sajatovic et al [23] | P; secondary analysis: following open label phase; randomized, double-blind, placebo-controlled | 98 randomized | 61 (55–82) | BP I; stabilization criteria after 8–16 weeks open label phase | LI (n = 34), modal 750 mg/d; LTG (n = 33), modal 240 mg/d (100–400 mg/day); PBO, n = 31 | LI (0.8–1.1 mEq/L) | Time to intervention | Up to 18 mo | LTG delayed time to intervention for any mood episode (median 201 d) and for depressive but not mania/hypomania/mixed episode; LI delayed time to intervention for mania/hypomania/mixed episode, but not depression or any episode (median 138 d); for PBO the median was 98 d for any episode. |

Abbreviations: **BP**, bipolar; **LI**, lithium; **LTG**, lamotrigine; **NA**, not available; **P**, prospective; **PBO**, placebo; **R**, retrospective; **UP**, unipolar.

Implications for clinical practice and health care delivery

The tolerability of specific agents is a major determinant guiding treatment selection and dosing in elderly BP patients. Central clinical tasks are to obtain and critically review history of adverse response, benefit, and drug levels where appropriate. The initial clinical and laboratory evaluation needs to focus not only on excluding aggravating or causative factors, but also on identification of conditions that can influence drug selection. Lying and standing blood pressure and pulse, an electrocardiogram, neurologic examination, and cognitive assessment are important in management of aged patients. In considering acute treatment, clinicians should be sensitive to the potential role of nonadherence in patients with limited benefit, relapse, or recurrence. Geropsychiatrists, while choosing from among alternatives based on side effect profile and treatment history, should avoid unnecessary abandonment of previously effective agents—for example, when side effect history is given without corroboration or when associated drug concentrations were documented as excessive.

LI remains one of the treatments of choice for BP manic episodes. Clinicians should target concentration ranges from 0.4 to 1.0 mEq/L and expect that concentrations at the upper end may be necessary. LI dose should be titrated gradually because of the higher dose/concentration ratio and longer time to steady state levels compared with younger patients. Diseases and treatments that increase dose/concentration ratio require more conservative dosing. In the presence of brain pathology, more conservative LI concentrations may be warranted. Worsening of cognitive status, coarse tremor, and hypothyroidism are important side effects to avoid.

VAL is a rational alternative to LI in elderly manic patients. It can be used as a first-line mood stabilizer in most cases. It may replace LI in patients who develop adverse effects of LI. Given the state of the evidence, clinicians should expect to use concentrations in the range of 40 to 100 μg/mL. The most clinically important side effects are sedation, gait disturbance, and thrombocytopenia.

CBZ can be considered a second-line agent for the treatment of mania in the elderly. The role of other anticonvulsants as antimanic agents in elderly individuals is unclear. In using CBZ, the preinitiation workup should place particular emphasis on the electrocardiogram, liver function tests and hematology. Adverse reactions include cardiovascular effects and hematologic effects.

Monotherapy with mood stabilizer, together with elimination of unnecessary psychotropic agents, is considered a reasonable first approach.

The optimal timing of treatment changes for manic elders with partial response or nonresponse—that is, augmentation or change to alternative treatment, respectively—remains to be clarified. In the absence of evidence-based guidelines, clinical experience suggests a a duration of several weeks to assess the initial strategy.

Partial response to initial monotherapy suggests addition of atypical antipsychotic or another mood stabilizer. Clinicians have virtually no age-specific systematic information to guide atypical antipsychotic use. The greatest amount of experience has come with olanzapine and risperidone as adjunctive agents for manic and mixed states in late life. The potential metabolic effects of atypical agents mean that laboratory monitoring is needed.

The treatment of BP depression in the elderly is guided only by sporadic age-specific reports and extrapolation from other age and diagnostic groups. Initial mood stabilizer treatment has potential advantages, and LI may be used when feasible, in anticipation of its use either as a primary agent or in later combination with antidepressants. LTG is a promising medication for BP depression, especially because the risk of Stevens-Johnson syndrome appears to be low in older patients. The dosing schedule for LTG should follow the same guidelines as in younger patients.

When an antidepressant is needed in addition to a mood stabilizer, the treatment history and toxicity profile of particular agents should guide treatment selection. Electroconvulsive therapy (ECT) is effective in BP depression and should be considered in refractory elderly patients in addition to elderly patients who exhibit suicidality or inadequate nutritional intake. ECT should also be considered in patients with mania or mood states refractory to pharmacotherapy. However, there are no systematic data comparing ECT and pharmacotherapy in elderly BP patients.

Pharmacotherapy that has proved to be efficacious for acute treatment of mania or BP depression should be continued for 6 to 12 months. After that period of continuation treatment, if remission is sustained, slow discontinuation of adjunctive antidepressants, antipsychotics, or antianxiety agents can be attempted under close monitoring.

Clinicians should expect to provide maintenance pharmacologic management despite the absence of clear guidelines for this in BP elders; mood stabilizers should in general be continued indefinitely. Although acute and long-term treatment benefits may be attenuated in some elders, in particular those with comorbid brain disease, this should not preclude attempts to provide adequate treatment trials in these patients.

Directions for research

The development of evidence-based treatment of late-life BP disorders has been limited by several factors. First, a relatively small numbers of patients can be studied prospectively at individual academic centers, as is reflected by the fact that the existing literature consists primarily of small sample case series. Additional challenges include the rigors of working with these patients, and the complex design issues that must be faced in such research.

Recently, these challenges are being met through new strategies, including analysis of clinical administrative databases, and collaborative multicenter studies in which investigators with expertise in studying young BP patients are participating. The elderly BP population was recognized as a priority for funding at the National Institute of Mental Health Depression and BP Support Alliance Consensus Conference 2001 and its report [136].

The existing literature in elderly patients can help formulate further hypotheses for systematic and controlled efficacy and safety trials. Randomized controlled trials comparing available agents are needed. Initial studies of acute treatment can provide a basis for designing continuation and maintenance treatment studies. Research should focus on defining those dosing and duration conditions for first-line drugs (eg, LI and VAL) that provide the best balance between benefit and side effects. New agents (eg, LTG and atypical antipsychotic medications) also need to be studied systematically in these patients.

Given the significance of side effects in elders, one important agenda for research in this population is the identification of patients who respond adequately to monotherapy to minimize side effects. For the same reason, characterization of patients who respond to low exposure (ie, relatively low drug blood levels) is an important aim. Further, such research provides a focus for examination of the utility of experimental measures related to drug distribution—for example, VAL not bound to peripheral protein, and central or erythrocyte LI concentrations.

Another major research need is to define rationale alternative approaches in patients who receive limited benefit from initial treatments and to explore the heuristic opportunities presented by such patients. In partially responsive elderly patients, the efficacies of standard augmentation regimens need to be tested. Dementia, cognitive impairments, and other neurologic dysfunction may characterize patients who require such augmentation. Specific features such as these can provide a framework for selection from among innovative augmentation approaches that are particularly relevant to particular elderly BP patients and may be adequately tolerated. One example is the use of cholinesterase inhibitors [137].

Given the prevalence of various comorbid conditions in BP elders, patients who have stable comorbid medical conditions or mild cognitive impairment need to be included in initial studies so that their findings can influence practice. In addition to symptom measures, the assessment of outcome in geriatric BP treatment studies should include other dimensions, including measures of side effects, behavioral and cognitive function, and medical status.

The management of type II BP disorder and of schizoaffective BP disorder [138] needs to be studied separately in the elderly.

Effectiveness studies become a higher priority as information regarding efficacy becomes available. For example, nonadherence is a particularly important issue in the elderly; laboratory monitoring of treatment can be improved by nurse intervention programs [139].

Summary

In BP elders, there is a clear disparity between the sparse age-specific evidence base that can contribute to rational treatment approaches and their illness severity, high mortality, vulnerability to side effects, chronicity and relapse/recurrence, high services use, and potential caregiver burden. Pressure from managed care providers to minimize inpatient management increases the need for timely symptom reduction and the prevention of relapse and recurrence. Yet extrapolations regarding the efficacy of medications used in younger BP patients are not yet supported by data from aged patients.

Case series suggest differences in side effect profile between lithium salts and anticonvulsants, and between atypical compared with conventional antipsychotics. Dementia and other comorbidities may exacerbate side effects. Case series also indicate that lithium and valproate both can have efficacy in manic states. Age-associated factors including dementia and cognitive impairment may attenuate benefit.

Research priorities include the need for randomized controlled trials of both acute and continuation/maintenance treatments. Elderly BP patients highlight the issues of monotherapy and timing of augmentation strategies and offer opportunities for investigation of the mechanisms of attenuation of response and testing innovative interventions.

Acknowledgments

Supported by National Institute of Mental Health grants K02 MH067028 and U01MH074511.

References

[1] Dunn KL, Rabins PV. Mania in old age. In: Shulman KI, Tohen M, Kutcher SP, editors. mood disorders across the life span. New York: John Wiley & Sons; 1996. p. 399–406.

[2] Yassa R, Nair V, Nastase C. Prevalence of bipolar disorder in a psychogeriatric population. J Affect Disord 1988;14:197–201.

[3] Sajatovic M, Vernon L, Semple W. Clinical characteristics and health resource use of men and women veterans with serious mental illness. Psych Serv 1997;48:1461–3.

[4] Bartels SJ, Forester B, Miles KM, et al. Mental health service use by elderly patients with bipolar disorder and unipolar major depression. Am J Ger Psychiatry 2000;8:160–6.

[5] Young RC. Bipolar disorders. In: Roose S, Sackeim HA, editors. Phenomenology of late life depression in affective disorders. Oxford: Oxford University Press; 2004.

[6] van der Velde CD. Effectiveness of lithium carbonate in the treatment of manic-depressive illness. Am J Psychiatry 1970;123:345–51.

[7] Himmelhoch J, Neil JR, Ray SJ, et al. Age, dementia, dyskinesias, and lithium response. Am J Psychiatry 1980;137:941–5.

[8] Shulman KI, Tohen M, Satlin A, et al. Mania compared with unipolar depression in old age. Am J Psychiatry 1993;149:341–5.

[9] Dhingra U, Rabins PV. Mania in the elderly: a five-to-seven year follow-up. J Am Ger Soc 1991;39:581–3.

[10] Tohen M, Shulman KI, Satlin A. First-episode mania in late life. Am J Psychiatry 1994;151: 130–2.

[11] Young RC, Gyulai L, Mulsant BH, et al. Pharmacotherapy of bipolar disorder in old age. Am J Ger Psychiatry 2004;12:342–57.

[12] Tinetti ME, Speechley M, Ginter SF. Risk factors for falls among elderly persons living in the community. N Engl J Med 1988;319:1701–7.

[13] Krishnan KRR. Biological risk factors in late life depression. Biol Psychiatry 2002;52:185–92.

[14] Umapathy C, Mulsant BH, Pollock BG. Bipolar disorder in the elderly. Psychiatr Ann 2000;30:473–80.

[15] Shulman KI, Rochon P, Sykora K, et al. Changing prescription patterns for lithium and divalproex in old age: shifting without evidence. BMJ 2003;326:960–1.

[16] Chacko RC, Marsh B, Marmion J, et al. Lithium side effects in elderly bipolar outpatients. J Clin Psychiatry 1987;9:79–88.

[17] Smith RE, Helms PM. Adverse effects of lithium therapy in the acutely ill elderly patient. J Clin Psychiatry 1982;43:94–9.

[18] Stone K. Mania in the elderly. Br J Psychiatry 1989;155:220–4.

[19] Schaffer CB, Garvey MJ. Use of lithium in acutely manic elderly patients. Clin Gerontologist 1984;3:58–60.

[20] Shulman KI, Sykora K, Gill SS, et al. New thyroxine treatment in older adults beginning lithium therapy: implications for clinical practice. Am J Geriatric Psychiatry 2005;13:299–304.

[21] Murray E, Hopwood S, Balfour JK. The influence of age on lithium efficacy and side-effects in out-patients. Psychol Med 1983;13:53–60.

[22] Hewick DS, Newburg P, Hopwood S, et al. Age as a factor affecting lithium therapy. Br K Clin Pharmacol 1977;4:201–5.

[23] Sajatovic M, Gyulai L, Calabrese JR, et al. Maintenance treatment outcomes in older patients with bipolar I disorder. Am J Geriatr Psychiatry 2005;13:305–11.

[24] Judd LL, Hubbard B, Janowsky DS, et al. The effect of lithium carbonate on the cognitive functions of normal subjects. Arch Gen Psychiatry 1977;34:355–7.

[25] Judd LL, Hubbard B, Janowsky DS, et al. The effect of lithium carbonate on the affect, mood, and personality of normal subjects. Arch Gen Psychiatry 1977;34:346–51.

[26] Nambudiri DE, Meyers BS, Young RC. Delayed recovery from lithium neurotoxicity. J Ger Psychiat Neurol 1991;4:40–3.

[27] Roose SP, Nurnberger J, Dunner D, et al. Cardiac sinus mode dysfunction during lithium treatment. Am J Psychiatry 1979;136:804–6.

[28] Roose SP, Bone S, Haidorfer C, et al. Lithium treatment in older patients. Am J Psychiatry 1979;136:843–4.

[29] Head L, Dening T. Lithium in the over-65s: who is taking it and who is monitoring it? A survey of older adults on lithium in the Cambridge Mental Health Services catchment area. Int J Geriatr Psychiatry 1998;13:164–71.

[30] Shulman KI, Sykora K, Gill S, et al. Incidence of delirium in older adults newly prescribed lithium or valproate: a population-based study. J Clin Psychiatry 2005;66:424–7.

[31] Hardy BG, Shulman KI, Mackenzie SE. Pharmacokinetics of lithium therapy. J Clin Psychopharmacol 1987;4:201–5.

[32] MacKinnon DF, Jamison KR, DePaulo JR. Genetics of manic depressive illness. Annu Rev Neurosci 1997;20:355–73.

[33] Satlin A, Lipzin B, Young RC. Diagnosis and treatment of mania. In: Salzman C, editor. Clinical geriatric psychopharmacology. 4th edition. New York: Williams and Wilkins; 2005. p. 353–84.

[34] Sarid-Segal O, Creelman WL, Ciraulo DA, et al, editors. Drug interactions in psychiatry. 2nd edition. Baltimore: Williams and Wilkins; 1995. p. 175–213.

[35] Strayhorn JM, Nash JL. Severe neurotoxicity despite therapeutic serum lithium levels. Dis Nerv Syst 1977;38:107–11.

[36] Moore CM, Demopoulos CM, Henry ME, et al. Brain-to-serum lithium ratio and age: an in vivo magnetic resonance spectroscopy study. Am J Psychiatry 2002;159:1240–2.

[37] Foster JR, Silver M, Boksay IJ. The potential use of adjunctive intra-erythrocyte (RBC) lithium levels in detecting serious impending neurotoxicity in the elderly: two case reports. Int J Ger Psychiatry 1990;5:9–14.

[38] McFarland BH, Miller MR, Strumfjord AA. Valproate use in the older manic patient. J Clin Psychiatry 1990;51:479–81.

[39] Craig I, Tallis R. Impact of valproate and phenytoin on cognitive function in elderly patients: results of a single-blind randomized comparative study. Epilepsia. New York: Raven Press, Ltd.; 1994. p. 381–90.

[40] Kasarskis EJ, Kuo CS, Berger R, et al. Carbamazepine-induced cardiac dysfunction. Arch Intern Med 1992;152:186–91.

[41] Cullen M, Mitchell P, Brodaty H, et al. Carbamazepine for treatment-resistant melancholia. J Clin Psychiatry 1991;52:11:472–6.

[42] Bryson SM, Verma N, Scott PJW, et al. Pharmacokinetics of valproic acid in young and elderly subjects. Br J Clin Psychiatry 1983;16:104–5.

[43] Bauer LA, Davis R, Wilensky A, et al. Valproic acid clearance: unbound fraction and dirunal variations in young and elderly adults. Clin Pharmacol Ther 1985;37:697–700.

[44] Patel J, Salzman C. Drug interactions wtih psychotropic medications. In: Salzman C, editor. Clinical geriatric psychopharmacology. New York: Williams and Wilkins; 1998. p. 553–78.

[45] Pollock B. Drug interactions. In: Nelson JC, editor. Geriatric psychopharmacology. New York: Marcel Dekker, Inc.; 1998. p. 43–60.

[46] Beyer J, Siegal A, Kennedy J, et al. Olanzapine, divalproex and placebo treatment non-head-to-head comparisons of older adult acute mania. International Psychogeriatric Association; Nice, France. September 9–14, 2001. p. 203.

[47] Jeste DV, Rockwell E, Harris MJ, et al. Conventional vs. newer antipsychotics in elderly patients. Am J Geriatr Psychiatry 1999;7:70–6.

[48] Jeste DV, Sable JA, Salzman C. Treatment of late-life disordered behavior, agitation, and psychosis. In: Salzman C, editor. Clinical geriatric psychopharmacology. 4th edition. Philadelphia: Williams and Wilkins; 2005. p. 129–95.

[49] Harvey PD, Napolitano JA, Mao L, et al. Comparative effects of risperidone and olanzapine on cognition in elderly patients with schizophrenia or schizoaffective disorder. Int J Geriatr Psychiatry 2003;18:820–9.

[50] Yassa R, Nastase C. Dupont Dea. Tardive dyskinesia in elderly psychiatric patients: a 5 year study. Am J Psychiatry 1992;149:1206–11.

[51] Woerner MG, Kane JM, Lieerman JA, et al. The prevalence of tardive dyskinesia. J Clin Psychopharmacol 1991;11:34–42.

[52] Jeste DV, Wyatt RJ. Aging and tardive dyskinesia. In: Miller NE, Cohen GD, editors. Schizophrenia and aging. New York: Guilford; 1987. p. 275–86.

[53] Caligiuri MF, Jeste DV, Lacro JP. Antipsychotic induced movement disorders in the elderly: epidemiology and treatment recommendations. Drug Aging 2000;17:363–84.

[54] Glassman AH, Bigger JT. Antipsychotic drugs: prolonged QTc interval, torsade de pointes, and sudden death. Am J Psychiatry 2001;158:1774–82.

[55] Reilly JG, Ayis SA, Ferrier IN, et al. QT-interval abnormalities and psychotropic drug therapy in psychiatric patients. Lancet 2000;355:1048–52.

[56] Haverkamp W, Breithardt G, Camm AJ, et al. The potential for t prolongation and proarrhythmia by non-antiarrhythmic drugs: clinical and regulatory implications. Eur Heart J 2000;21:1216–31.

[57] Meltzer HY. Putting metabolic side effects into perspective:risks versus benefits of atypical antipsychotics. J Clin Psychiatry 2001;62:39.

[58] Kane JM, Barrett EJ, Casey DE, et al. Metabolic effects of treatment with atypical antipsychotics. J Clin Psychiatry 2004;65:1447–55.

[59] Meyer JM. A retrospective comparison of weight, lipid, and glucose changes between risperidone and olanzapine treated inpatients: metabolic outcomes after one year. J Clin Psychiatry 2002;63:425–33.

[60] Brodaty H, Ames D, Snowdon J, et al. A randomized placebo-controlled trial of risperidone for the treatment of aggression, agitation, and psychosis of dementia. J Clin Psychiatry 2003;64:134–43.

[61] Balant-Gorgia AE, Gex-Febry M, Genet C, et al. Therapeutic drug monitoring of risperidone using a new, rapid HPLC method: reappraisal of interindividual variability factors. Ther Drug Monit 1999;21:105–15.

[62] Haring C, Meise U, Humpel C, et al. Influence of patient-related variables on clozapine plasma levels. Am J Psychiatry 1990;147:1471–5.

[63] Rickels K, Schweizer E, Lucki I. Benzodiazepine side effects. Washington, DC: American Psychiatric Association; Vol. 6, 1987

[64] Pomara N, Tun H, DaSilva D, et al. The acute and chronic performance effects of alprazolam and lorazepam in the elderly: relationship to duration of treatment and self-rated sedation. Psychopharmacol Bull 1998;34:139–53.

[65] Reidenberg MM, Levy M, Warner H, et al. Relationship between diazepam dose, plasma level, age, and central nervous system depression. Clin Pharm Ther 1978;23:371–4.

[66] Sarkisian CA, Liu H, Gutierrez PR, et al. Modifiable risk factors predict functional decline among older women: a prospectively validated clinical prediction tool. The stufy of osteoporotic fractures research group. J Am Geriatr Soc 2000;48:170–8.

[67] Sgadari A, Lapane KL, Mor V, et al. Oxidative and nonoxidative benzodiazepines and the risk of femur fracture. The Systematic Assessment of Geriatric Drug Use Via Epidemiology Study Group. J Clin Psychopharmacol 2000;20:234–9.

[68] von Moltke LL, Abernathy DR, Greenblatt DJ. Kinetics and dynamics of psychotropic drugs in the elderly. In: Salzman C, editor. Clinical geriatric psychopharmacology. 3rd edition. Baltimore (MD): Williams & Wilkins; 1998. p. 70–93.

[69] Georgotas A, McCue RE, Hapworth W, et al. Comparative efficacy and safety of MAOIs versus TCAs in treating depression in the elderly. Biol Psychiatry 1986;21:1155–66.

[70] Tariot PN, Schneider LS, Mintzer JE, et al. Safety and tolerability of divalproex sodium in the treatment of signs and symptoms of mania in elderly patients with dementia: results of a double-blind, placebo-controlled trial. Curr Ther Res Clin Exp 2001;62:51–67.

[71] Smith DA, Perry PJ. Nonneuroleptic treatment of disruptive behavior in organic mental syndromes. Ann Pharmacother 1992;26:1400–8.

[72] Meyers BS, Young RC. Psychopharmacology. In: Sadavoy, et al, editors. Comprehensive review of geriatric psychiatry. 3rd edition. New York: Norton; 2003.

[73] Miller F, Menninger J, Whitchup SM. Lithium neuroleptic neurotoxicity in the elderly bipolar patient. J Clin Psychopharmacol 1986;6:176–8.

[74] Mulsant BH, Pollock BG, Kirshner M, et al. Seurm anticholinergic activity in a community sample of older adults. Arch Gen Psychiatry 2003;60:198–203.

[75] Goodwin FK, Jamison KR. Manic depressive illness. New York: Oxford University Press; 1990.

[76] Cade JFJ. Lithium salts in the treatment of psychotic excitement. Med J Aust 1949;36: 349–52.

[77] Wylie ME, Mulsant BH, Pollock B, et al. Age at onset in geriatric bipolar disorder. Am J Geriatr Psychiatry 1999;7:77–83.

[78] Gildengers AG, Mulsant BH, Begley AE, et al. A pilot study of standardized treatment in geriatric bipolar disorder. Am J Geriatr Psychiatry 2005;13:319–23.

[79] Platman SR. A comparison of lithium carbonate and chlorpromazine in mania. Am J Psychiatry 1970;127:351–3.

[80] Prien RF, Caffey EM, Klett CJ. Relationship between serum lithium level and clinical response in acute mania treated with lithium. Br J Psychiatry 1972;120:409–14.

[81] Young RC, Kalayam B, Tsuboyama G, et al. Mania: response to lithium across the age spectrum. Abstr Soc Neurosci 1992;18:669.

[82] DeBattista C, Schatzberg AF. Current psychotropic dosing and monitoring guidelines. Primary Psychiatry 1999;65-6.

[83] Pope HG, McElroy SL, Keck PE, et al. Valproate in the treatment of acute mania: a placebo controlled study. Arch Gen Psychiatry 1991;48:62-8.

[84] Gnam W, Flint AJ. New onset rapid cycling bipolar disorder in an 87 year old woman. Can J Psychiatry 1993;38:324-6.

[85] Risinger RC, Risby ED, Risch SC. Safety and efficacy of divalproex sodium in elderly bipolar patients. J Clin Psychiatry 1994;55:215.

[86] Mordecai DJ, Sheik JI, Glick ID. Divalproex for the treatment of geriatric bipolar disorder. Int J Geriatr Psychiatry 1998;14:494-6.

[87] Yassa R, Cvejic J. Valproate in the treatment of posttraumatic bipolar disorder in a psychogeriatric patient. J Geriatr Psychiatry Neurol 1994;7:55-7.

[88] Chen ST, Altshuler LL, Melnyk KA, et al. Efficacy of lithium vs valproate in the treatment of mania in the elderly: a retrospective study. J Clin Psychiatry 1999;60:181-5.

[89] Bowden C. Anticonvulsants in bipolar elderly. In: Nelson JC, editor. Geriatric psychopharmacology. New York: Marcel Dekker; 1998. p. 285-99.

[90] Niedermier JA, Nasrallah HA. Clinical correlates of response to valproate in geriatric inpatients. Ann Clin Psychiatry 1998;10:165-8.

[91] Regenold WT, Prasad M. Use of intravenous valproate in geriatric psychiatry. Am J Ger Psychiatry 2001;9:306-8.

[92] Goldberg JF, Sachs MH, Kocsis JH. Low-dose lithium augmentation of divalproex in geriatric mania. J Clin Psychiatry 2000;61:304.

[93] Schneider AL, Wilcox CS. Divalproate augmentation in lithium-resistant rapid cycling mania in four geriatric patients. J Affect Dis 1998;47:201-5.

[94] Sharma V, Prasad E, Mazmanian D, et al. Treatment of rapid cycling bipolar disorder with combination therapy of valproate and lithium. Can J Psychiatry 1993;38:137-9.

[95] Kellner MB, Neher F. A first episode of mania after age 80. Can J Psychiatry 1991;36: 607-8.

[96] Okuma T, Yamashita I, Takahashi R, et al. Comparison of the antimanic efficacy of carbamazepine and lithium carbonate by double-blind controlled study. Pharmacopsychiatry 1990;23:143-50.

[97] Sethi MA, Mehta R, Devenand DP. Gabapentin in geriatric mania. J Geriatr Psychiatry Neurol 2003;16:117-20.

[98] Tohen M, Zarate CA, Centorrino F, et al. Risperidone in the treatment of mania. J Clin Psychiatry 1996;57:249-53.

[99] Tohen M, Chengappa KN, Suppes T, et al. Efficacy of olanzapine in combination with valproate or lithium in the treatment of mania in patients partially nonresponsive to valproate or lithium monotherapy. Arch Gen Psychiatry 2002;59:62-9.

[100] Tohen M, Jacobs RG, Grundy SL, et al. Efficacy of olanzapine in acute bipolar mania: a double-blind placebo-controlled study. The Olanzapine HGGW Study Group. Arch Gen Psychiatry 2000;57:841-9.

[101] Beyer JL, Shulman K, Young R, et al. Olanzapine, divalproex, and placebo. Treatment comparison of older adults with acute mania. 2003.

[102] Yeung PP, Tariot PN, Schneider LS, et al. Quetiapine for elderly patients with psychotic disorders. Psychiatr Ann 1999;30:197-201.

[103] Sajatovic M. Treatment of bipolar disorder in older adults. Int J Geriatr Psychiatry 2002; 17:865-73.

[104] Shulman RW, Singh A, Shulman KI. Treatment of elderly institutionalized bipolar patients with clozapine. Psychopharmacol Bull 1997;33:113-8.

[105] Frye MA, Altshuler LL, Bitran JA. Clozapine in rapid cycling bipolar disorder [letter]. Clin Psychopharmacol 1996;16:87-90.

[106] Robillard M, Conn DK. Lamotrigine use in geriatric patients with bipolar depression. Can J Psychiatry 2002;47(8):767–70.

[107] American Psychiatric Association. Practice guidelines for the treatment of patients with bipolar disorder (revision). Am J Psychiatry 2002;159:1–50.

[108] Nemeroff CB, Evans DL, Gyulai L, et al. Double-blind, placebo-controlled comparison of imipramine and paroxetine in the treatment of bipolar depression. Am J Psychiatry 2001; 158:906–12.

[109] Bittman B, Young RC. Mania in an elderly man treated with bupropion. Am J Psychiatry 1991;148:541.

[110] Young RC, Jain H, Kiosses D, et al. Antidepressant-associated mania in late life. Int J Geriatr Psychiatry.

[111] Himmelhoch J, Fuchs CZ, Symons BJ. Double-blind study of tranylcypromine treatment of major anergic depression. J Nerv Ment Dis 1982;170:628–34.

[112] Young RC, Falk JR. Age, manic psychopathology and treatment response. Int J Geriatr Psychiatry 1989;4:73–8.

[113] Stokes PE, Stoll PM, Shamoian CA, et al. Efficacy of lithium as acute treatment of manic-depressive illness. Lancet 1971;1:1319–25.

[114] Broadhead J, Jacoby R. Mania in old age: a first prospective study. Int J Geriatr Psychiatry 1990;5:215–22.

[115] Young RC, Klerman GL. Mania in latelife: focus on age at onset. Am J Psychiatry 1992; 149:867–76.

[116] Young RC, Moline M, Kleyman F. Hormone replacement therapy and late life mania. Am J Geriatr Psychiatry 1997;5:179–81.

[117] Lehman S, Rabins P. Factors influencing treatment outcomes in geriatrid mania. Biol Psychiatry 2001.

[118] Berrios GE, Bakshi N. Manic and depressive symptoms in the elderly: their relationships to treatment outcome, cognition and motor symptoms. Psychopathology 1991;24:31–8.

[119] Bearden CE, Hoffman KM, Kannon TD. The neuropsychology of neuroanatomy of bipolar affective disorder. Bipolar Disord 2001;3:106–50.

[120] Gildengers A, Butters MA, Seligman K, et al. Cognitive impairment in late life bipolar disorder. Am J Psychiatry 2004;161:731–8.

[121] Young RC, Murphy CF, Heo M. Cognitive impairment in bipolar disorder in old age: literature review and findings in manic patients. J Affect Disord, in press.

[122] Young RC, Murphy CF, DeAsis JM, et al. Executive function and treatment outcome in geriatric mania. Presented and the American Psychiatric Association Annual Meeting. New Orleans, LA; May 5–10, 2001.

[123] Moore GJ, Bebchuk JM, Wilds IB, et al. Lithium-induced increase in human brain grey matter. Lancet 2000;356:1241–2.

[124] Manji HK, Moore GJ, Chen G. Lithium at 50: have the neuroprotective effects of this unique cation been overlooked? Biol Psychiatry 1999;46:929–40.

[125] Moore GJ, Bebchuk JM, Hasanat K, et al. In vivo evidence in support of bcl-2's neurotrophic effects? Biol Psychiatry 2000;48:1–8.

[126] Ferrier IN, Thompson JM. Cognitive impairment in bipolar affective disorder: implications for the bipolar diathesis. Br J Psychiatry 2002;180:293–5.

[127] Black DW, Winokur G, Bell S, et al. Complicated mania. Arch Gen Psychiatry 1988;45: 232–6.

[128] Tondo L, Hennen J, Baldessarini RJ. Lower suicide risk with long-term lithium treatment in major affective illness: a meta-analysis. Acta Psychiatr Scand 2001;104:163–72.

[129] Muller-Oerlinghausen B, Berghofer A, Bauer M. Bipolar disorder. Lancet 2002;359:241–7.

[130] Angst J, Weis P, Grof P, et al. Lithium propylaxis in recurrent affective disorders. Br J Psychiatry 1970;116:604–14.

[131] O'Connell RA, Mayo JA, Flatow L, et al. Outcome of bipolar disorder on long-term treatment with lithium. Br J Psychiatry 1991;159:123–9.

[132] Abou-Saleh MT, Coppen A. Prognosis of depression in old age: the case for lithium therapy. Br J Psychiatry 1983;143:527–8.

[133] Schurhoff F, Bellivier F, Jouvent R, et al. Early and late onset bipolar disorders: two different forms of manic-depressive illness? J Affect Disord 2000;58:215–21.

[134] Bartels SJ, Meuser KT, Miles KM. A comparative study of elderly patients with schizophrenia and bipolar disorder in nursing homes and the community. Schiz Res 1997;27: 181–90.

[135] Bartels SJ, Dums AR, Oxman TE, et al. The practice of evidence-based geriatric psychiatry. In: Sadavoy J, Jarvik LF, Grossberg GT, editors. Comprehensive textbook of geriatric psychiatry. 3rd edition. New York: American Association for Geriatric Psychiatry; 2004. p. 817–44.

[136] Charney DS, Reynolds CF, Lewis L, et al. Depression and bipolar support alliance consensus statement on the unmet needs in diagnosis and treatment of mood disorders in late life. Arch Gen Psychiatry 2003;60:664–72.

[137] Burt T, Sachs G, Demopoulos C. Donepezil in the treatment-resistant bipolar disorder. Biol Psychiatry 1999;45:959–64.

[138] Yu XL, Young RC. Geriatric schizoaffective disorders [abstract]. Biol Psychiatry 2001;49: 125.

[139] Fielding S, Kerr S, Godber C. Lithium in the over-65s: a dedicated monitoring service leads to a better quality of treatment supervision. Int J Geriatr Psychiatry 1999;14:985–7.

[140] Noagiul S, Narayan M, Nelson CJ. Divalproex treatment of mania in elderly patients. Am J Geriatr Psychiatry 1998;6:257–62.

[141] Puryear LJ, Kunik ME, Workman R. Tolerability of divalproex solium in elderly psychiatric patients with mixed diagnoses. J Geriatr Psychiatry Neurol 1995;8:234–7.

[142] Kando JC, Tohen M, Castillo J, et al. The use of valproate in an elderly population with affective symptoms. J Clin Psychiatry 1996;57:238–40.

ELSEVIER
SAUNDERS

Psychiatr Clin N Am
28 (2005) 871–896

PSYCHIATRIC
CLINICS
OF NORTH AMERICA

Evidence-Based Treatment of Geriatric Anxiety Disorders

Julie Loebach Wetherell, PhD[a], Eric J. Lenze, MD[b], Melinda A. Stanley, PhD[c],*

[a]*Department of Psychiatry, University of California San Diego, VA San Diego Healthcare System, 3350 La Jolla Village Drive (116B), San Diego, CA 92161, USA*
[b]*Western Psychiatric Institute and Clinic, Room E1124, 3811 O'Hara Street, Pittsburgh, PA 15213, USA*
[c]*Menninger Department of Psychiatry and Behavioral Sciences, Baylor College of Medicine, 2002 Holcombe Boulevard (152), Houston, TX 77030, USA*

Until the last decade, anxiety disorders were a relatively unrecognized public health problem among older adults. Recent emerging data have suggested a high prevalence and significant impact of anxiety in later life. A growing body of literature provides evidence-based guidelines for care, although the data still lag far behind what is known about the treatment of depression in later life. Treatment studies of late-life anxiety and clinical standards of care in this arena have focused largely on the impact of pharmacologic and cognitive behavioral approaches, following the large body of work in younger adults with anxiety. This article presents an overview of what is known about the prevalence and impact of late-life anxiety, followed by a more detailed, critical review of the available treatment outcome literature.

Community prevalence rates for anxiety disorders in older adults range from 3.5% [1] to 10.2% [2], suggesting a higher prevalence than late-life depression. The prevalence of late-life anxiety disorders is even higher among homebound elderly [3], nursing homes residents [4], older medical patients [5], and patients who have chronic medical illness [6,7]. Of all the anxiety disorders in later life, generalized anxiety disorder (GAD) is one of the most frequently diagnosed, with community prevalence ranging from 1.9% [8] to 7.3% [2]. GAD also seems to be the most frequently diagnosed anxiety disorder in primary care, where older adults most often present

This work was supported by National Institute of Mental Health grants MH53932, MH067643, and MH064196.

* Corresponding author.
E-mail address: mstanley@bcm.tmc.edu (M.A. Stanley).

doi:10.1016/j.psc.2005.09.006
psych.theclinics.com

for assistance, with rates ranging from 3.1% [9] to 11.2% [5]. Anxiety symptoms that do not necessarily meet criteria for a psychiatric diagnosis occur even more often, with rates as high as 15% to 20% in general community and primary care samples [9–11] and over 40% in patients who have disability or chronic medical illnesses [6,12]. Many available prevalence rates, however, are likely serious underestimates, given the tendencies of older adults to underreport or deny psychologic symptoms [13] and difficulties with recognition of anxiety in older medical patients [8].

Among older people, anxiety symptoms and disorders are associated with decreased physical activity and functional status, poorer self-perceptions of health, decreased life satisfaction, and increased loneliness, even with adjustments for demographic variables and severity of chronic disease [14,15]. Anxiety in later life also is associated with increased physical disability [16,17], decreased quality of life [18–20], and increased service use [21]. Rates of coexistent depressive disorders are high [22,23], and anxiety has been associated with increased mortality in men [24,25].

Despite the relatively high prevalence and significant impact, however, anxiety symptoms and disorders frequently remain unrecognized and undertreated among older adults. Although anxiety disorders are particularly prevalent in medical settings, naturalistic data from ambulatory medical care settings suggest that anxiety disorders are diagnosed during only a small percentage of office visits made by older adults (1.3%) [21]. The recognition of anxiety in older patients is complicated by the presence of coexistent medical illness and treatments as well as a symptom presentation characterized more often by a somatic picture and the reluctance to acknowledge psychologic difficulties [8]. Nevertheless, anxiety is clearly a serious public health problem for older adults.

Anxiety in older adults has traditionally been treated pharmacologically, often with benzodiazepines [26]. However, the clinical recommendations for pharmacologic treatment actually have been much broader, including suggestions to consider serotonergic antidepressants, buspirone, and venlafaxine, given efficacy data from younger adults and a small body of emerging studies with older anxious patients [27,28]. Another growing body of literature has examined the impact of cognitive-behavioral therapy (CBT) treatments for late-life anxiety [29]. These studies follow from the body of efficacy data resulting from studies conducted with younger adults [30], the increased risk of adverse drug reactions in older patients [28], data suggesting the acceptability or preference for nonmedication interventions among older adults [31,32], and the time-limited, directive, and collaborative nature of a CBT approach [33].

Method

MEDLINE and PsychINFO searches were conducted using the population term "aged" and keywords "anxiety disorders," "treatment," and "therapy." The citation index in PsychINFO also was used to locate articles that cited relevant articles on the topic of treatment of anxiety in older adults. Reference lists from review articles and chapters on the treatment of geriatric anxiety also were examined, and investigators working in the field were contacted to solicit unpublished or in-press manuscripts.

Inclusion criteria consisted of reports in which (1) participants were at least 55 years old, with a principal or co-principal diagnosis of any anxiety disorder diagnosed according to criteria of the Diagnostic and Statistical Manual of Mental Disorders III-R or IV; (2) the study design was either a randomized controlled trial in which the intervention was compared with a waiting list, usual care, or a pill or attention placebo, or it was an open-label trial or a case series of more than five participants; and (3) data were reported on at least one outcome measure, either self-reported or interviewer-rated. Studies focusing on open trials with fewer than five participants or on patients who had anxiety symptoms rather than disorders were excluded.

The studies included and the associated statistically significant findings are reported in Tables 1 and 2 [34–54]. To compare clinical significance across studies, effect sizes were calculated where possible for each outcome measure within each study using the formula for Cohen's $d = (\text{mean}_{\text{treatment}} - \text{mean}_{\text{control}})/\text{standard deviation}_{\text{pooled}}$. For reports of case series, the pretreatment mean for the control group mean was substituted.

Results

Cognitive behavioral interventions

Generalized anxiety disorder

Most psychotherapy studies of late-life anxiety have focused on GAD. The first such study [34] compared 14 weeks of group-administered CBT with supportive psychotherapy (SP) in a sample of 48 GAD patients who were at least 55 years of age. Participants were required to discontinue psychotropic medications before enrolling in the study. CBT consisted of education about anxiety, its symptoms, and its triggers; symptom monitoring; progressive, passive, and cue-controlled relaxation training; cognitive restructuring, in which participants were taught to challenge their thoughts about the likelihood of negative events and catastrophic consequences; and imaginal and in vivo exposure to anxiety cues and triggers using systematic desensitization. SP emphasized empathic listening. In this investigation, CBT and SP were equally effective in decreasing symptoms of anxiety and depression. Effect sizes for CBT immediately after treatment ranged from −.06 to .62, with a mean of .20. Post-treatment response rates, defined by an improvement of at least 20% on three of four measures of anxiety and worry, were 28% in CBT and 54% in SP. Gains were maintained or enhanced in both conditions at 6-month follow-up, and response rates at

Table 1
Summary of cognitive behavioral interventions for geriatric anxiety disorders

Study	Study design	Model/conditions	Sample (size, setting, diagnosis, age, gender, other)	Follow-up (duration and completion rate)	Outcome measures and results	Limitations/comments
Barrowclough et al [45] 2001	RCT	8–12 sessions of individual, home-delivered (1) CBT; (2) SC	55 patients (27 CBT, 28 SC) with panic disorder, social phobia, GAD, or anxiety NOS; mean age 72y; 77% women. All patients stabilized on psychotropic medications for at least 3 mo before enrollment in study (58% on anxiolytics, 51% on antidepressants, 9% on both) Exclusions: certain medical conditions and cognitive impairment	43 patients completed treatment (19 CBT, 24 SC); 39 completed 12-month follow-up (16 CBT, 23 SC)	BAI, GDS: CBT > SC at post, 12 mo BDI: CBT = SC at post, 12 mo HAMA, STAI-T: CBT = SC at post, CBT > SC at 12 mo	Attrition; results not reported separately by diagnosis.
Carmin et al [42] 1998	Case series based on chart review	Inpatient multidisciplinary treatment including at least 2 h/d of exposure and response prevention; education about OCD, anxiety management skills training, family therapy, group CBT	11 patients with OCD from inpatient psychiatric unit; mean age 69y; gender not reported; some patients received concurrent pharmacotherapy Exclusions: psychosis, mental retardation, gross neurological impairment	Information not reported	Patient-rated improvement: mean 7/10 Staff-rated responder (50% reduction in symptoms): 72%	No standard objective outcome measures; multifaceted inpatient intervention; retrospective case series design.

Study	Design	Intervention	Sample	Completers/follow-up	Results	Comments
Gorenstein et al [46] 2005	RCT	13 individual sessions of (1) CBT plus MM; (2) MM alone	42 patients (23 CBT + MM, 19 MM) with GAD, panic disorder, or anxiety NOS, and on anxiolytic medication for at least 8 wk; mean age 68y; 50% women. Exclusions: major depression, history of bipolar disorder or psychosis, substance abuse, recent suicidality, serious medical condition, and cognitive impairment	28 patients completed treatment (14 CBT + MM, 14 MM); 11 CBT patients completed 6 monthly booster sessions and 6-mo follow-up	Medication use, CGI, STAI-T, PSWQ, BDI, SCL-Anxiety: CBT + MM = MM. SCL Phobia, OC, Som, GS: CBT + MM > MM. Gains in medication use, CGI, SCL Anxiety, and SCL Phobia maintained at follow-up	Attrition, results not reported separately by diagnosis.
King and Barrowclough [44] 1991	Case series	3–12 individual sessions of CBT; 6 patients were seen in their own homes	10 patients with panic disorder, GAD, or agoraphobia; mean age 73y; 80% women; 7 patients on psychotropic medications. Exclusions: organic impairment and psychosis	10 patients completed treatment; 9 patients completed 3–6-mo follow-up	Self-reported panic, dizziness, headaches, agoraphobic avoidance, hypochondriacal beliefs: 7/10 patients showed no symptoms and 9/10 decreased symptoms at post, 8/9 showed no symptoms, 9/9 showed decrease at follow-up. BAI: 6/8 improved at post, 5/7 maintained gains at follow-up. BDI: 6/7 improved at post, 3/7 maintained gains at follow-up	No comparison group, variability of treatment

(continued on next page)

Table 1 (*continued*)

Study	Study design	Model/conditions	Sample (size, setting, diagnosis, age, gender, other)	Follow-up (duration and completion rate)	Outcome measures and results	Limitations/ comments
Ladouceur et al [40] 2004	Case series	14 individual sessions CBT.	8 GAD patients; mean age 64y; 7 women, 1 man; 5 patients stabilized on psychotropic medications for at least 8 wk Exclusions: suicidal intent, substance dependence, history of schizophrenia, bipolar disorder, or organic mental disorder	8 patients completed treatment, 6-and 12-mo follow-ups	PSWQ d = 2.4; WAQ d = 1.6; WDQ d = 1.6; BAI d = 1.0; BDI d = 1.1 Gains maintained at follow-up	No comparison group, young sample (oldest patient was 71y).
Mohlman et al [37] 2003	RCT	Study 1: (1) 13 individual sessions of CBT; (2) WL Study 2: (1) 13 individual sessions of enhanced CBT (ECBT); (2) WL	Study 1: 27 GAD patients (14 CBT, 13 WL); mean age 66y; 70% women Study 2: 15 GAD patients (8 ECBT; 7 WL); mean age 68y; 60% women Exclusions, both studies: use of psychotropic medications, active suicidality, major depression, psychosis, organic brain disease, use of medications with anxiety-like effects, cognitive impairment	Study 1: 21 patients completed treatment, 6 monthly booster sessions, and 6-mo follow-up (11 CBT, 10 WL) Study 2: 15 patients completed treatment, booster sessions, and follow-up (8 ECBT, 7 WL)	Study 1: BAI, BDI, PSWQ, STAI-T, SCL Anxiety, SCI GS: CBT = WL Study 2: BAI, PSWQ, SCL Anxiety, SCI GS: ECBT > WL BDI, STAI-T: ECBT = WL Gains maintained at follow-up	Small sample; no direct comparison between CBT and ECBT; WL rather than alternative treatment.

Study	Design	Treatment	Patients	Completion	Outcomes	Comments
Mohlman and Gorman [38] 2005	RCT	(1) 13 individual sessions of CBT for patients with intact EF, improved EF, and impaired EF; (2) WL	32 GAD patients (10 intact EF, 5 improved EF, 7 impaired EF, 10 WL); mean age 69y; 53% women. Exclusions: current major depression, recent suicidality, history of psychotic symptoms, use of anxiolytic or antidepressant medications	30 patients completed treatment (8 intact EF, 5 improved EF, 7 impaired EF, 10 WL); 15 CBT patients (5 intact EF, 5 improved EF, 5 impaired EF) completed 12-mo follow-up	BAI: intact EF = improved; EF = impaired; EF = WL. BDI: improved EF > WL. PSWQ: intact EF = improved; EF > WL. STAI-T: Improved EF > impaired; EF = WL. SCL-GSI: improved; EF > WL = impaired EF. Improved EF group maintained gains at follow-up	Small group sizes.
Radley et al [43] 1997	Multiple baseline design	4-wk no-treatment control period followed by 8 group sessions of CBT	9 patients with specific phobia, agoraphobia, social phobia, or GAD; mean age 71y; 7 women, 2 men; 1 on psychotropic medication for 4 wk prior to enrollment	6 patients completed treatment	HADS-A $d = .37$; HAMA $d = .88$; GAS $d = 1.1$; STAI-T $d = 1.0$; STAI-S $d = .39$; FI $d = 0$; PSI $d = .51$; CAQ $d = .26$; ELI $d = -.17$	Attrition; no comparison group; no follow-up.
Stanley et al [34] 1996	RCT	14 group sessions of (1) CBT; (2) SP	48 GAD patients (26 CBT, 20 SP; 2 dropped before randomization); mean age 68y; 71% women; patients required to discontinue psychotropic medications. Exclusions: current psychotherapy, serious medical conditions, substance abuse, psychosis, and cognitive impairment	31 patients completed treatment and 6-mo follow-up (18 CBT, 13 SP)	GAD severity, percent worry, PSWQ, WS, STAI-T, HAMA, DBI, HAMD, FQ: CBT = SP. Gains maintained at follow-up	Attrition; assessors not blind to treatment condition.

(continued on next page)

Table 1 (*continued*)

Study	Study design	Model/conditions	Sample (size, setting, diagnosis, age, gender, other)	Follow-up (duration and completion rate)	Outcome measures and results	Limitations/comments
Stanley et al [35] 2003	RCT	(1) 15 group sessions of CBT; (2) MCC	85 GAD patients (39 CBT, 41 MCC); 5 dropped before randomization; mean age 66y; 75% women; patients required to discontinue psychotropic medications Exclusions: current psychotherapy, substance abuse, serious medical conditions, psychotic symptoms, and cognitive impairment	66 patients completed treatment (29 CBT, 35 MCC); 27 CBT patients completed 12-mo follow-up	GAD severity, PSWQ, STAI-T, HAMA, BDI, GDS, HAMD, QOLI, LSI-Z: CBT > MCC WS: CBT = MCC Gains maintained at follow-up	Attrition; MCC rather than alternative treatment.
Stanley et al [39] 2003	RCT	(1) 8 individual sessions of CBT; (2) usual care (UC)	12 medical patients with GAD (6 CBT, 6 UC); mean age 71y; 83% women; 50% on psychotropic medications Exclusions: suicidality, psychosis or bipolar disorder, substance abuse, and cognitive impairment excluded	9 patients completed treatment (5 CBT, 4 UC)	GAD severity, PSWQ, BDI, SF-36 VT: CBT > UC BAI, QOLI, SF-36 MH, RE, GH, PF, RP, BP, SF: CBT = UC	Small sample; no follow-up; UC rather than alternative treatment.

Study	Design	Treatment	Sample	Completers	Results	Comments
Swales et al [41] 1996	Open-label trial	10 individual sessions of CBT	20 panic disorder patients, mean age 63y; 80% women. Exclusions: bipolar disorder, psychosis, borderline personality disorder, OCD, substance abuse within past 6 mo, current use of anxiolytics or other anxiety treatment, cognitive impairment, and unstable cardiopulmonary conditions	15 patients completed treatment and 3-mo follow-up	$ACQ\ d = 1.5$; BSQ $d = 1.1$; $TPRPS\ d = .7$; $MI\ d = .6$; $FQ\ d = .9$; $BAI\ d = 1.6$; Panic attacks $d = 1.0$ Gains maintained at follow-up	No comparison group.
Wetherell et al [36] 2003	RCT	12 group sessions of (1) CBT; (2) DG focused on common topics of worry among older adults; (3) WL	75 GAD patients (26 CBT, 26 DG, 23 WL); mean age 67y; 80% women; 40% on psychotropic medications. Exclusions: history of mania or psychosis, cognitive impairment, current psychotherapy, substance abuse, and lack of recent medical check-up	57 patients completed treatment (18 CBT, 18 DG, 21 WL); 18 CBT patients and 17 DG patients completed 6-mo follow-up	GAD severity: CBT = DG > WL; DG = WL Percent worry: CBT > DG; CBT = WL; DG = WL PSWQ: CBT = DG > WL HAMA, BAI, HAMD, SF-36 SF: CBT = DG = WL BDI, SF-36 RE, VT: CBT > WL; DG = WL, CBT = DG CBT = DG on all measures at 6 mo	Attrition; attention placebo rather than alternative treatment.

Abbreviations: ACQ, Agoraphobia Cognitions Questionnaire; BAI, Beck Anxiety Inventory; BDI, Beck Depression Inventory; BP, SF-36 Bodily Pain; BSQ, Body Symptoms Questionnaire; CAQ, Cognitive Anxiety Questionnaire; CGI, Clinical Global Impression; ECBT, enhanced CBT; ELI, Effects on Life Inventory; FI, Fear Inventory; FQ, Fear Questionnaire; GDS, Geriatric Depression Scale; GH, SF-36 General Health; GSI, Global Severity Index; HADS-A, Hospital Anxiety and Depression Scale-Anxiety; HAMA, Hamilton Anxiety Scale; LSI-Z, Life Satisfaction Index; MH, SF-36 Mental Health; MI, Mobility Inventory for Agoraphobia; NOS, not otherwise specified; PF, SF-36 Physical Functioning; PSI, Physical Symptom Inventory; PSWQ, Penn State Worry Questionnaire; QOLI, Quality of Life Index; RE, SF-36 Role Functioning - Emotional; RP, SF-36 Role Functioning - Physical; SCL, Hopkins Symptom Checklist; SF, SF-36 Social Functioning; SF-36, Medical Outcomes Study 36-item Short Form Health Survey; STAI-T, Spielberger State-Trait Anxiety Inventory-Trait; TPRPS, Texas Panic-Related Phobia Scale; TPRPS, Texas Panic-Related Phobia Scale; WAQ, Worry and Anxiety Questionnaire; WDQ, Worry Domains Questionnaire.

Table 2
Summary of psychopharmacological interventions for geriatric anxiety disorders

Study	Study design	Model/ conditions	Sample (size, setting, diagnosis, age, gender, other)	Follow-up (duration and completion rate)	Outcome measures and results	Limitations/comments
Bresolin et al [52] 1988	Prospective randomized controlled trial	Ketazolam vs placebo	63 outpatients; multicenter; aged 66–85 (mean 74y) with GAD for at least 1 mo and HAMA ≥ 18	15 d of placebo or ketazolam for 15 d Nonresponders in both conditions received an additional dose of ketazolam Responders continued with the same treatment 60 completed first phase, 59 completed the study	At 15 days: HAMA: ketazolam > placebo Response rates: HAMA ≥ 25%; 83% ketazolam vs 43% placebo ($P \leq 0.01$)	Short trial with unusual study design making second phase results hard to characterize. Ketazolam is not available in the US. 25% reduction in HAMA is not usually considered response. Current GAD criteria are 6 mo not 1 mo. Nevertheless, these data support acute efficacy of benzodiazepines for late-life GAD.
Frattola et al [53] 1992	Prospective randomized controlled trial	Alpidem vs placebo	40 outpatients at two sites; aged 65–80 (mean 70y), with GAD (n = 33) or adjustment disorder with anxious mood (n = 7) of at least 1 mo duration	3 wk; 37 completed	HAMA, STAI, VAS: alpidem > placebo Response rates: HAMA ≥ 25%; 55% alpidem vs 15% placebo ($P = .02$)	Alpidem is not available in the US. Short trial. 25% reduction in HAMA is not usually considered response.

Study	Design	Intervention	Sample	Duration	Results	Comments
Katz et al [55] 2002	Pooled secondary analysis of 5 phase III randomized controlled trials	Venlafaxine XR vs placebo	184 outpatients; multisite; aged 60+ (mean 66y) with GAD	8 wk (2 studies provided 24-wk data), 134 completed 8 wk	Completer analysis: HAMA, CGI, HAD: venlafaxine > placebo Response rates: HAMA ≥ 50%; 65% venlafaxine vs 39% placebo ($P \leq .05$); CGI 1 or 2: 77% venlafaxine vs 48% placebo ($P \leq .01$) ITT analysis: HAD: venlafaxine > placebo; HAMA, CGI: venlafaxine = placebo Response rates: HAMA ≥ 50%: 53% venlafaxine vs 38% placebo (ns); CGI 1 or 2: 66% venlafaxine vs 41% placebo ($P < .01$) Response rates and tolerability were comparable to younger adults.	Limited by retrospective nature of data and industry sample. Nevertheless, this study provides evidence that venlafaxine is efficacious for late-life GAD.

(continued on next page)

Table 2 (*continued*)

Study	Study design	Model/ conditions	Sample (size, setting, diagnosis, age, gender, other)	Follow-up (duration and completion rate)	Outcome measures and results	Limitations/comments
Koepke et al [54] 1982	Prospective randomized controlled trial	Oxazepam vs placebo	220 outpatients; multicenter; "all but one" aged ≥60 (mean age 67.5y) with anxiety neurosis (n = 201); adjustment reaction with anxiety (n = 7) or anxiety reaction with depression (n = 12)	4 wk; 182 completed (roughly equivalent dropouts in drug and placebo groups)	Completer analysis: HAMA, Physician's Target Symptom Scale, Hopkins 35-item Symptom Checklist, and Global Improvement Scale: oxazepam > placebo	Completer-only analysis (although roughly equivalent dropouts); short trial. "Anxiety neurosis" is non-specific diagnosis. Nevertheless this trial demonstrates benzodiazepine efficacy for late-life anxiety disorders.
Lenze et al [56] 2005[a]	Prospective randomized controlled trial	Citalopram vs placebo	34 outpatients; single site; aged 60+ (mean 69y) with GAD (n = 31), panic disorder (n = 2), or PTSD (n = 1) and HAMA ≥ 17	8 wk; 29/34 completed	HAMA: citalopram > placebo ($d = .52$) Response rates: (HAMA ≥ 50% reduction or CGI = 1 or 2) 65% citalopram compared with 24% placebo ($P < .02$)	Small study with some diagnostic heterogeneity (though mainly GAD). This study provides preliminary evidence that SSRIs are efficacious for geriatric anxiety disorders, particularly GAD.
Sheikh et al [57] 2004	Open-label trial	Sertraline	10 outpatients; single site; mean age 72.5, with panic disorder	12 wk; Completion rate unknown	90% panic-free in week before last visit HAMA $d = .96$ CGI $d = 3.17$	Small open-label study. Nevertheless, data are promising for SSRIs in late-life panic disorder.

Sheikh and Swales [58] 1999	Pilot randomized controlled trial	Imipramine vs alprazolam vs placebo	25 outpatients; single site; age 55–73 (mean 61y) with panic disorder	8 wk; 18/25 completed (dropout = 0% in alprazolam; 10% in imipramine; 86% in placebo)	No group comparisons conducted due to small sample sizes HAMA: imipramine $d = 1.6$; alprazolam $d = 1.5$; placebo $d = .5$ HAMD: imipramine $d = 1.6$; alprazolam $d = 1.4$; placebo $d = .6$	Study was terminated early because of concerns that imipramine was causing adverse events. On unblinding, this concern was not substantiated.
Wylie et al [59] 2000	Open-label trial	Fluvoxamine	19 outpatients; single site; aged 50+ (mean 67y), with GAD (n = 11), panic disorder (n = 3), GAD and panic (n = 3), or OCD (n = 2)	21 wk; 12/19 completed	Completer analysis: HAMA $d = 1.02$ Response rates: HAMA $\geq 50\%$, 67%; CGI 1 or 2: 58% ITT analyses: response rates: HAMA $\geq 50\%$: 42%; CBI 1 or 2: 37%	Small open-label study with diagnostic heterogeneity. Large dropout rate limits efficacy.

Abbreviations: CGI, Clinical Global Impression; HAD, Hospital Anxiety and Depression; HAMA, Hamilton Anxiety Scale; ITT, Intent-to-treat; ns, not significant; SSRI, selective serotonin reuptake inhibitor; STAI, Spielberger State-Trait Anxiety Inventory; VAS, Visual Analogue Scale.

[a] Lenze et al [51] reported an effect size of .79.

this time were 50% (CBT) and 77% (SP), a difference that was not significant. Although this study was the first randomized controlled psychotherapy trial among older adults with a diagnosed anxiety disorder, a number of serious limitations warrant caution in the interpretation of results, namely, the absence of an inactive control condition, the relatively young age and demographic homogeneity of the sample, the use of nonblind raters to assess outcomes, and the relatively brief follow-up interval.

In a follow-up study designed to address some of these limitations, 85 adults with GAD who were at least 60 years old were withdrawn from psychotropic medications (when appropriate) and offered 15 weeks of group-administered CBT or a minimal contact control (MCC) condition [35]. The CBT protocol in this investigation was similar to the one described earlier. The effects of CBT on measures of worry, anxiety, depression, and quality of life were superior by comparison with MCC, with effect sizes ranging from −.05 to 1.1 (mean, .71). Gains were maintained over a 1-year follow-up period. Post-treatment response rates, defined as in the previous trial, were 45% (CBT) and 8% (MCC). By the 12-month follow-up, the response to CBT was 63%. Strengths of the study included the relatively large sample size, the attention to quality of life outcomes, and 12-month follow-up. However, the study sample was still relatively young and demographically restricted. The absence of an alternative active treatment condition also limited conclusions about the specific benefits of CBT.

Another team of investigators [36] compared interventions consisting of 12 weeks of group-administered CBT, an attention placebo consisting of a discussion group (DG) focused on worry-provoking topics, and a waiting list (WL), using a sample of 75 older adults with GAD, 40% of whom were taking psychotropic medications. This CBT protocol was similar to the one described earlier. CBT participants did better than WL participants on five measures of anxiety, depression, and quality of life. DG was superior to WL on two measures of anxiety. However, CBT was superior to DG only on one measure of anxiety, and this difference was no longer significant at the 6-month follow-up. Effect sizes for CBT relative to WL ranged from .39 to 1.4, with a mean of .71. Effect sizes for CBT relative to DG ranged from −.11 to .45, with a mean of .24. In both active treatment groups, patients tended to n.aintain or enhance their gains over time. Post-treatment response rates, defined as in earlier studies, were 33% in CBT, 33% in DG, and 5% in WL. By the 6-month follow-up, response rates were 50% in CBT and 53% in DG. This study is the only one to date that has compared CBT simultaneously with active and inactive control conditions. However, as in the previous studies, patients included in this trial were relatively young, healthy, well educated, and mainly white, and thus were not representative of more heterogeneous groups of older adults.

Another independent investigation [37] compared standard, individually administered CBT with WL in a sample of 27 older adults with GAD and also compared an enhanced form of individually administered CBT with

WL in a sample of 15 older adults with GAD. None of the patients in any condition was taking psychotropic medications. Enhanced CBT included the standard CBT elements of relaxation training, cognitive therapy, prevention of overly cautious behaviors, problem-solving skills training, daily structure, and sleep hygiene, as well as additional attention to at-home practice assignments, reminder telephone calls, and weekly reviews of concepts and techniques. No significant group differences were found between standard CBT and WL on any outcome measure. Effect sizes ranged from .09 to 1.0, with a mean of .43. However, enhanced CBT participants did significantly better than WL participants on two outcome measures, and significantly fewer enhanced CBT participants than WL participants met GAD criteria after the intervention. Effect sizes ranged from .04 to 1.6, with a mean of .81. The response rate to enhanced CBT (defined as in previous trials) was 75%, relative to 40% in standard CBT, and 9% to 14% in WL. Gains were maintained in the enhanced CBT condition at 6-month follow-up after monthly booster sessions. Overall, results suggest that CBT enhancements to counteract cognitive changes associated with aging may help to improve the response of anxious older adults. Unfortunately, enhanced and standard CBT were not directly compared in this study, and sample sizes were small. As in other studies, patients also were relatively young, largely white, and high functioning.

A follow-up investigation compared CBT with a WL among 32 older GAD patients who had intact executive function (EF), impaired EF, and those who initially showed impaired EF but also demonstrated improvement in cognitive function along with anxiety symptoms [38]. CBT in this study followed the enhanced format described above, with reminder telephone calls and feedback on at-home practice assignments. Results suggest that individuals with impaired EF did not respond to CBT (mean effect size .31 relative to WL, and no patients classified as responders), whereas those with intact and improved EF were more likely to respond (mean effect sizes of .78 and 1.3 and response rates of 50% and 67%, respectively, compared with WL). This study makes a unique contribution in exploring predictors of response to CBT in older adults with GAD and the possible impact of cognitive limitations, although samples were quite small and replication of study findings is necessary.

In an effort to examine the value of CBT for a broader and more representative sample of older adults, a small sample of 12 primary care patients who had GAD, half of whom were taking psychotropic medication, were assigned to receive eight sessions of individually administered CBT or usual care (UC). The response to CBT was superior to UC on measures of anxiety and depression [39]. CBT in this protocol included psychoeducation, symptom monitoring, relaxation training, cognitive therapy, exposure, problem-solving skills training, and guidelines for good sleep. Effect sizes ranged from .41 to 3.7, with a mean of 1.3, and all five patients who completed CBT (100%) were classified as responders. In the UC group, 25% of patients were classified similarly. However, sample sizes were very small, and conclusions await completion of a larger clinical trial. Nevertheless, this investigation was an important initial effort to disseminate anxiety treatment to the primary care setting, where most older adults with GAD present for treatment. Patients in this trial also were somewhat older, less well educated, and more ethnically diverse than in previous studies.

A recent promising case series presented data on a form of CBT based on intolerance of uncertainty as a key feature of GAD [40]. In this study, eight older adults with GAD received 14 weekly sessions of individual CBT consisting of awareness training, increasing tolerance of uncertainty using behavioral experiments (eg, driving to an event at an unknown location without taking the route the day before), reevaluating beliefs about the usefulness of worry, problem-solving skills training, exposure to worrisome thoughts using a looped tape, prevention of behaviors used to distract attention or neutralize the worry, and relapse prevention by reviewing skills learned and distinguishing between normal and pathologic worry. Seven of the eight participants no longer met diagnostic criteria for GAD after treatment, and these gains were maintained at 6- and 12-month followups. The mean effect size was 1.7. Future investigations will need to compare this protocol with an alternative condition in a randomized trial.

Panic disorder

To date, no randomized controlled psychosocial intervention trials have been conducted exclusively among older adults with panic disorder. In an open-label trial, 20 older adults whose symptoms met criteria for panic disorder with or without agoraphobia, none of whom was taking anxiolytic medication, received 10 individual 90-minute sessions of CBT consisting of education, challenging inappropriate or maladaptive thoughts, muscle relaxation, breathing, and exposure to panic cues and triggers. Results showed large and clinically significant gains on measures of panic, anxiety, and depression [41]. Effect sizes ranged from .6 to 1.6, with a mean of 1.0. Although this study suggests that older adults can be treated successfully for panic disorder using exposure to internal sensations and external triggers without adverse cardiac or other consequences, the lack of any control condition seriously limits the conclusions that can be drawn.

Obsessive-compulsive disorder

The only report [42] on the treatment of geriatric obsessive-compulsive disorder (OCD) that met criteria for inclusion in this review was a retrospective chart review of 11 older patients who received treatment in an inpatient behavioral medicine unit. Treatment was multidisciplinary and included at least 2 hours per day of exposure to obsessional thoughts and situations combined with the prevention of ritualized, compulsive responses. Additional treatment components included education about OCD, anxiety management training, family therapy, and group CBT. Some patients also received adjunctive pharmacotherapy, but no details were reported. Information on the duration of treatment also was not reported. Outcomes included self-reported improvement on 11-point scales (0 to 10) for the frequency of obsessions and time spent engaging in compulsive rituals. Patients were classified as treatment responders if they experienced a 50% reduction in targeted OCD symptoms, as rated by staff. Self-reported improvement and staff-rated response rates were both high. No long-term follow-up data were reported. Weaknesses of this investigation include the retrospective chart review methodology, lack of a comparison condition, and lack of follow-up.

Mixed anxiety disorders

In a small open trial, nine patients who had specific phobias, agoraphobia, social phobia, or generalized anxiety symptoms were evaluated before and after a 4-week baseline control period and then received 8 weeks of group-administered CBT, consisting of relaxation and breathing training, avoidance reduction, increasing self-confidence, strategies for coping with anxiety, and cognitive therapy [43]. Patients also received booster sessions 4 and 12 weeks after treatment. There was a significant increase in a measure of cognitive anxiety during the baseline control period. After treatment, patients improved significantly on several measures of anxiety symptoms, with a mean effect size of .56. The use of a baseline no-treatment period in this study was a creative method for controlling for the effects of time passage without resorting to a WL condition. However, the small sample size and lack of longer-term follow-up restrict the ability to generalize the findings.

In a case series of 10 patients who had panic disorder, GAD, or agoraphobia, individual CBT was offered over 3 to 12 sessions [44]. CBT in this trial included self-monitoring, reinterpretation of physical sensations as nonthreatening, controlled breathing, and behavioral experiments. Some patients had comorbid conditions such as depression and hypochondriasis. Most patients improved, and most maintained their gains at 3- to 6-month follow-up. Because of differences in outcome measures, however, it was not possible to calculate effect sizes. Limitations included diagnostic heterogeneity and the lack of a comparison condition.

A randomized trial with 55 anxious older adults compared 8 to 12 sessions of individual, home-delivered CBT to supportive counseling (SC) [45]. Most of the sample (51%) had panic disorder, whereas 2% had social phobia, 19% had GAD, and 28% had anxiety disorder not otherwise specified (NOS). Specific CBT elements varied by disorder but included education, cognitive restructuring, and, for the panic patients, exposure to bodily sensations associated with panic attacks as well as to external triggers. The SC condition focused on empathic listening. One of the strengths of this investigation was that all participants had failed at least one 3-month trial of psychotropic medication before enrollment in the study and also failed to recover after an additional 6-week baseline period following enrollment but before the initiation of psychotherapy. Results provided some evidence for the superiority of CBT on self-ratings of anxiety and depression immediately after treatment, with better performance for CBT on most measures across a 12-month follow-up period. Effect sizes for CBT immediately after treatment ranged from 0.1 to .74, with a mean of .38. Response rates, defined by a 20% reduction on two measures of anxiety, were 71% in CBT and 39% in SC. One major limitation of this study was the failure to report results separately by diagnosis, at least for the panic disorder patients.

Another recently completed study investigated the efficacy of CBT plus medication management (MM) versus MM alone in 42 older adults who wished to discontinue their use of anxiolytic medication [46]. At enrollment, patients had been taking medications, including benzodiazepines (62%), meprobamate (12%), antidepressants (17%), opiates (5%), valerian (2%), and diphenhydramine (2%), for at least 8 weeks. Patients had GAD (55%), panic disorder (17%), comorbid panic disorder and GAD (9%), or anxiety disorder NOS (19%). CBT was conducted in 13 individual 50-minute sessions, with components that included education about anxiety, monitoring anxiety symptoms, diaphragmatic breathing, progressive muscle relaxation, cognitive restructuring, prevention of overly cautious behaviors, exposure to internal and external anxiety cues, problem-solving skills training, daily structure, guidelines for managing medication withdrawal, and sleep hygiene. MM involved 13 weekly 15-minute sessions and included medication taper, discussing symptoms, and monitoring efficacy and side effects. Results indicated that CBT plus MM was more effective than MM alone in reducing scores on several Hopkins Symptom Checklist-90 subscales, with equivalent efficacy in reducing dependence on anxiolytic medications. However, there was no differential efficacy on worry, state or trait anxiety, or depression. CBT effect sizes ranged from −0.3 to .95, with a mean of .40. Gains tended to erode by the 6-month follow-up, despite the fact that patients received monthly booster sessions. However, response rates at post-treatment, defined according to global clinician rating, were 64% in CBT and MM and 36% in MM alone. The greatest strength of this investigation was the focus on patients wishing to discontinue psychotropic medications, particularly benzodiazepines, the long-term use of which is often contraindicated in older adults because of adverse effects on cognition and balance. Limitations included an attrition rate of 39% from CBT and the failure to report results separately by diagnostic group.

Pharmacologic intervention

Given that older adults with anxiety disorders present most often for care to medical settings, it is no surprise that pharmacologic intervention is the most frequently used avenue of care. Naturalistic data, in fact, demonstrate that approximately half of the patients assigned an anxiety disorder diagnosis in primary care were prescribed an anxiolytic or antidepressant [21]. However, very few treatment trials have addressed the impact of pharmacologic treatment for anxiety disorders in older patients. Consequently, clinical recommendations are often derived from clinical trials with younger adults, even though outcome data from these studies may not generalize to older samples, given the differential pharmacokinetic properties of medications, the greater potential impact of adverse events among older patients, and the increased frequency of coexistent medical problems that complicate treatment. The literature in this area that met inclusion criteria for this report has focused largely on the use of benzodiazepines and antidepressant medications. Other medications with potential benefit (eg, buspirone, a typical antipsychotic) warrant further investigation [47,48].

Benzodiazepines

Benzodiazepines continue to be the medications most frequently prescribed for anxiety in later life, with epidemiologic data suggesting general prevalence rates of 10% [49] to 12% [50] and as high as 43% for individuals with persistent anxiety [51]. However, only three randomized controlled trials have investigated the impact of benzodiazepines for anxiety disorders in later life [52–54]. Two of these trials have focused on GAD [52,53], and one trial has studied an earlier, potentially comparable category of anxiety neurosis [54]. In all of these studies, medication was efficacious relative to placebo, with treatment effects evident within as early as 7 days [53]. Only one study [53] provided sufficient data for the calculation of effect size, with *d* ranging from 0.79 to 0.95 (mean *d*, .85). Response rates to medication ranged from 57% to 83% [52,53], but the definition of response in these trials was more liberal than in more recent studies [55,56]. Attrition rates were generally low ($\leq 17\%$). Overall, the data from these trials suggest the value of benzodiazepines for treating anxiety disorders in older adults, although only one of the medications investigated (oxazepam) is commonly used or even available in the United States [54].

The treatment duration across all benzodiazepine trials was brief, ranging from 3 to 6 weeks. Although this treatment interval is typical and expected for acute pharmacologic trials with these types of medications, studies with longer treatment intervals are of value given the chronic nature and serious impact of anxiety disorders, particularly GAD, in later life. However, longer-term treatment with benzodiazepines generally is not recommended, particularly for older adults, given the potential for more serious adverse events. Benzodiazepines can affect cognitive functioning and psychomotor performance, leading to an increased risk of hip fractures caused by falls, a decreased ability to drive, and an increase in memory problems. As such, clinical recommendations for the use of benzodiazepines with older adults suggest that lower doses of compounds with shorter half-lives be used over a briefer interval than might be the case for younger patients [28].

Antidepressant medications

Five pharmacotherapy studies of late-life anxiety disorders have examined the value of antidepressant medications. Two of these studies focused on patients who had panic disorder [57,58], one study focused on a mixed group of patients who had GAD, panic disorder, or OCD [59], and two studies focused on GAD [55,56].

Panic disorder. Sheikh and Swales [58] compared the effects of imipramine, alprazolam, and placebo for the treatment of panic disorder in 25 older patients. This study was stopped prematurely because of concerns about adverse events and high attrition, resulting in sample sizes that were too small to generate solid conclusions regarding the efficacy of either medication. Nevertheless, the calculation of effect sizes suggests equivalent effects of imipramine and alprazolam relative to placebo for anxiety and depressive symptoms. In a subsequent small open-label trial of sertraline [57], 10 patients who had panic disorder were treated over the course of 12 weeks. Results at post-treatment suggest significant improvement in anxiety symptoms according to the Hamilton anxiety scale and ratings of global severity. Of course, the small sample size and lack of controlled design seriously limit the conclusions that can be drawn from this report. Nevertheless, the data from these two preliminary studies are encouraging with regard to the potential pharmacologic treatment of late-life panic disorder.

Mixed anxiety disorders. In an open trial with 19 patients whose symptoms met criteria for GAD, panic disorder, or OCD, Wylie and colleagues [59] demonstrated some potential value of fluvoxamine. Response rates ranged from 37% to 67%, with variation based on the measure used and the evaluation of completer or intent-to-treat samples. Response rate among the GAD subgroup was 57%, but interestingly, none of the three patients who had panic disorder responded. These data highlight the need for attention to diagnostic heterogeneity. Although the cut-off age for study inclusion was only 50 years, data analyses suggest comparable response for patients who are 50 to 64 years and those who are 65 years or older. Nevertheless, the mean age of the study sample was still relatively young. The small sample size, high attrition rate (37%), and uncontrolled nature of the trial also limit conclusions that can be drawn.

Generalized anxiety disorder. Katz and colleagues [55] conducted a secondary analysis of data from patients aged 60 years and older who participated in five randomized clinical trials of venlafaxine for the treatment of GAD. Results suggest a significant impact of treatment relative to placebo for older adults, although findings were less robust in intent-to-treat analyses. Response rates were generally comparable across older and younger samples. Attrition rates from venlafaxine (older adults, 23% and younger adults, 27%) and placebo (older adults, 31% and younger adults, 28%)

also were equivalent across age subgroups. As such, these data support the potential value of venlafaxine for the treatment of late-life GAD. However, little attention was given to the maintenance of gains over long-term follow-up. The power to detect significant age effects also was limited, and the replication of these findings is necessary in a prospective study with a larger sample of older adults. Older patients in these studies also were relatively young and likely more healthy and functional than older patients seen in primary care.

In the only prospective, randomized clinical trial of a serotonergic antidepressant conducted to date, Lenze and colleagues [56] examined the effect of citalopram versus placebo in a sample of 34 patients, 31 of whom were diagnosed with GAD. Results demonstrate significant improvement in Hamilton anxiety ratings, with an effect size of 0.52, calculated according to the formula used in this review. Response rates were 65% after citalopram and 27% after placebo. Again, however, no data addressed long-term maintenance of gains, and patients were recruited largely through the media, limiting generalizability to more representative samples of older adults with mental health needs.

Discussion

Overall, the available data suggest the potential value of both CBT and pharmacologic treatments for late-life anxiety disorders, most notably GAD. The CBT literature consistently documents a positive response relative to no treatment, although response rates are lower than is evident for younger adults and there is no consistent evidence of a significant CBT benefit relative to other psychosocial treatment options (eg, supportive therapy). The response to pharmacologic treatment may be more robust [60], although differential definitions of response across psychologic and pharmacologic studies and the lack of direct comparisons of these two forms of treatment make this kind of comparison very difficult. However, there remains room for significant future advances in both treatment arenas.

Across the majority of clinical trials conducted to date, samples of patients are relatively homogeneous and often are not representative of older adults in general with regard to age, functional status, ethnicity, education, or medical health. For the most part, treatment trials also have been conducted in academic mental health settings where older patients do not present routinely for clinical care. Relatively few data have addressed the value of treatment in more real-world settings, with patients who represent a broad range of demographic and clinical characteristics. Future research will need to examine more closely the outcomes of treatment for late-life anxiety in primary care and other community-based settings where older adults typically often receive services. A number of efforts are ongoing in this domain and data from these trials will provide more evidence related to the translational value of available efficacy data.

Another serious limitation of the research literature in both psychologic and pharmacologic domains is the predominant focus on late-life GAD. Although GAD is one of the most prevalent anxiety disorders among older adults, other common and potentially more disabling anxiety conditions, including agoraphobia and post-traumatic stress disorder (PTSD), have largely been neglected. The lack of attention to PTSD is particularly striking given the high prevalence among war veterans, Holocaust survivors, and disaster victims [61]. Specific phobias that interfere with necessary medical procedures, such as fear of injections and claustrophobia, also merit research and clinical attention.

In the psychologic research literature, the rates of attrition in many trials are higher among older adults (21%–39%) than among younger adults (approximate average of 10%) [62]. Attention needs to be given to this issue, perhaps with improved treatment strategies that better meet the needs of individual patients. In pharmacologic treatment studies, attrition is somewhat lower (15%–23%) [23,55] and comparable to what is seen in trials of younger adults with anxiety disorders.

One clear limitation of the CBT literature to date, particularly with regard to studies of GAD, is the focus on group interventions. A group intervention was selected for early trials in this area given the hypothesized importance of social support and reduced cost for older patients. However, meta-analytic work with data from younger adults has documented reduced outcomes for group versus individual interventions [62], which may explain some of the relatively modest response rates in early trials of CBT for late-life GAD. More recent work [39,46] and ongoing studies are focused on the use of individual treatments that allow for greater idiosyncratic tailoring of treatment to the clinical and personal needs of patients, with the goal of creating an intervention that is better suited to more heterogeneous populations seen in typical care settings.

Another limitation specific to CBT trials includes the emphasis of primary analyses on outcome data from completers. Pharmacologic trials, on the other hand, more often analyze data on an intent-to-treat basis. Completer analyses tend to inflate treatment effects. Furthermore, psychotherapy studies typically use a large number of outcome measures, often assessing the same construct, which complicates the interpretation of results when significant effects are found on some but not all measures. Finally, there is no psychotherapeutic comparison condition equivalent to a pill placebo. It is impossible to craft a double-blind psychotherapy study. So-called nonspecific therapeutic effects are associated with almost any credible intervention, making it difficult to find a significant effect for a comparison of a CBT with an alternative treatment or attention placebo. The comparison with wait list control conditions or usual care, however, not only raise ethical issues, they sometimes fail to deliver the critical component of equal expectancies for each condition.

Studies of both psychologic and pharmacologic treatment will need to focus further on the long-term maintenance of treatment gains. In studies of

CBT to date, follow-up is limited to 12 months or less, and no attention has been given to comparisons of methods for increasing response further over follow-up or to extension of gains beyond this time interval. Pharmacologic trials also have not yet attended to the nature and efficacy of various maintenance options. These issues are of critical importance given the enduring nature and significant impact of anxiety disorders in later life.

Summary

Available data point to the potential value of pharmacologic and cognitive-behavioral interventions for the treatment of late-life anxiety disorders, with modest improvement and response rates in most cases. Further efficacy work is needed to investigate the impact of improved psychosocial approaches that allow for more idiosyncratic attention to the needs of older patients and outcomes following a broader range of pharmacologic treatments. Attention in this work needs to be given to long-term outcomes and generalizability of findings to broader and more representative samples of older patients. Additional effectiveness work also is needed to address the value of various treatment options in the settings where older adults typically receive care (eg, primary care, community-based programs) and to the methods for optimal dissemination of evidence-based interventions.

References

[1] Bland RC, Newman SC, Orn H. Prevalence of psychiatric disorders in the elderly in Edmonton. Acta Psychiatr Scand Suppl 1988;338:57–63.
[2] Beekman AT, Bremmer MA, Deeg DJ, et al. Anxiety disorders in later life: a report from the Longitudinal Aging Study Amsterdam. Int J Geriatr Psychiatry 1998;13(10):717–26.
[3] Bruce ML, McNamara R. Psychiatric status among the homebound elderly: an epidemiologic perspective. J Am Geriatr Soc 1992;40(6):561–6.
[4] Junginger J, Phelan E, Cherry K, et al. Prevalence of psychopathology in elderly persons in nursing homes and in the community. Hosp Community Psychiatry 1993;44(4):381–3.
[5] Tolin DF, Robison JT, Gaztambide S, et al. Anxiety disorders in older Puerto Rican primary care patients. Am J Geriatr Psychiatry 2005;13(2):150–6.
[6] Kunik ME, Roundy K, Veazey C, et al. Surprisingly high prevalence of anxiety and depression in chronic breathing disorders. Chest 2005;127(4):1205–11.
[7] Stein MB, Heuser IJ, Juncos JL, et al. Anxiety disorders in patients with Parkinson's disease. Am J Psychiatry 1990;147(2):217–20.
[8] Blazer D, George LK, Hughes D. Anxiety in the elderly: treatment and research. In: Salzman C, Lebowitz BD, editors. The epidemiology of anxiety disorders: an age comparison. New York: Springer Publishing Company; 1991. p. 17–30.
[9] Wittchen HU, Kessler RC, Beesdo K, et al. Generalized anxiety and depression in primary care: prevalence, recognition, and management. J Clin Psychiatry 2002;63(Suppl 8):24–34.
[10] Himmelfarb S, Murrell SA. The prevalence and correlates of anxiety symptoms in older adults [part 2]. J Psychol 1984;116:159–67.
[11] Mehta KM, Simonsick EM, Penninx BW, et al. Prevalence and correlates of anxiety symptoms in well-functioning older adults: findings from the health aging and body composition study. J Am Geriatr Soc 2003;51(4):499–504.

[12] Brenes GA, Guralnik JM, Williamson J, et al. Correlates of anxiety symptoms in physically disabled older women. Am J Geriatr Psychiatry 2005;13(1):15–22.

[13] Gurian BS, Minor JH. Anxiety in the elderly: treatment and research. In: Salzman C, Lebowitz BD, editors. Clinical presentation of anxiety in the elderly. New York: Springer; 1991. p. 31–44.

[14] de Beurs E, Beekman AT, van Balkom AJ, Deeg DJ, et al. Consequences of anxiety in older persons: its effect on disability, well-being and use of health services. Psychol Med 1999; 29(3):583–93.

[15] Kim HF, Kunik ME, Molinari VA, et al. Functional impairment in COPD patients: the impact of anxiety and depression. Psychosomatics 2000;41(6):465–71.

[16] Brenes GA, Guralnik JM, Williamson JD, et al. The influence of anxiety on the progression of disability. J Am Geriatr Soc 2005;53(1):34–9.

[17] Lenze EJ, Rogers JC, Martire LM, et al. The association of late-life depression and anxiety with physical disability: a review of the literature and prospectus for future research. Am J Geriatr Psychiatry 2001;9(2):113–35.

[18] Bourland SL, Stanley MA, Snyder AG, et al. Quality of life in older adults with generalized anxiety disorder. Aging Ment Health 2000;4(4):315–23.

[19] Stanley MA, Diefenbach GJ, Hopko DR, et al. The nature of generalized anxiety in older primary care patients: preliminary findings. Journal of Psychopathology and Behavioral Assessment 2003;25(4):273–80.

[20] Wetherell JL, Thorp SR, Patterson TL, et al. Quality of life in geriatric generalized anxiety disorder: a preliminary investigation. J Psychiatr Res 2004;38(3):305–12.

[21] Stanley MA, Roberts RE, Bourland SL, et al. Anxiety disorders among older primary care patients. Journal of Clinical Geropsychology 2001;7105–16.

[22] Beekman AT, de Beurs E, van Balkom AJ, Deeg DJ, et al. Anxiety and depression in later life: co-occurrence and communality of risk factors. Am J Psychiatry 2000;157(1):89–95.

[23] Lenze EJ, Mulsant BH, Shear MK, et al. Comorbid anxiety disorders in depressed elderly patients. Am J Psychiatry 2000;157(5):722–8.

[24] Kawachi I, Sparrow D, Vokonas PS, et al. Symptoms of anxiety and risk of coronary heart disease: the Normative Aging Study. Circulation 1994;90(5):2225–9.

[25] van Hout HP, Beekman AT, de Beurs E, Comijs H, et al. Anxiety and the risk of death in older men and women. Br J Psychiatry 2004;185:399–404.

[26] van Balkom AJ, Beekman AT, de Beurs E, Deeg DJ, et al. Comorbidity of the anxiety disorders in a community-based older population in The Netherlands. Acta Psychiatr Scand 2000;101(1):37–45.

[27] Dada F, Sethi S, Grossberg GT. Generalized anxiety disorder in the elderly. Psychiatr Clin North Am 2001;24(1):155–64.

[28] Sheikh JI, Cassidy EL. Treatment of anxiety disorders in the elderly: issues and strategies. J Anxiety Disord 2000;14(2):173–90.

[29] Nordhus IH, Pallesen S. Psychological treatment of late-life anxiety: an empirical review. J Consult Clin Psychol 2003;71(4):643–51.

[30] Barlow DH. Anxiety and its disorders: the nature and treatment of anxiety and panic. 2nd edition. New York: Guilford Publications; 2002.

[31] Landreville P, Landry J, Baillargeon L, et al. Older adults' acceptance of psychological and pharmacological treatments for depression. J Gerontol B Psychol Sci Soc Sci 2001;56(5): 285–91.

[32] Unützer J, Katon W, Callahan CM, et al. Collaborative care management of late-life depression in the primary care setting: a randomized controlled trial. JAMA 2002;288(22): 2836–45.

[33] Zeiss AM, Steffan A. Behavioral and cognitive-behavioral treatments: an overview of social learning. In: Zarit SH, Knight BG, editors. A guide to psychotherapy and aging: effective clinical interventions in a life-stage context. Washington (DC): American Psychological Association; 1996. p. 35–60.

[34] Stanley MA, Beck JG, Glassco JD. Treatment of generalized anxiety in older adults: a preliminary comparison of cognitive-behavioral and supportive approaches. Behav Ther 1996; 27(4):565–81.

[35] Stanley MA, Beck JG, Novy DM, et al. Cognitive-behavioral treatment of late-life generalized anxiety disorder. J Consult Clin Psychol 2003;71(2):309–19.

[36] Wetherell JL, Gatz M, Craske MG. Treatment of generalized anxiety disorder in older adults. J Consult Clin Psychol 2003;71(1):31–40.

[37] Mohlman J, Gorenstein EE, Kleber M, et al. Standard and enhanced cognitive-behavior therapy for late-life generalized anxiety disorder: two pilot investigations. Am J Geriatr Psychiatry 2003;11(1):24–32.

[38] Mohlman J, Gorman JM. The role of executive functioning in CBT: a pilot study with anxious older adults. Behav Res Ther 2005;43(4):447–65.

[39] Stanley MA, Hopko DR, Diefenbach GJ, et al. Cognitive-behavior therapy for late-life generalized anxiety disorder in primary care: preliminary findings. Am J Geriatr Psychiatry 2003;11(1):92–6.

[40] Ladouceur R, Leger E, Dugas M, et al. Cognitive-behavioral treatment of generalized anxiety disorder (GAD) for older adults. Int Psychogeriatr 2004;16(2):195–207.

[41] Swales PJ, Solfvin JF, Sheikh JI. Cognitive-behavioral therapy in older panic disorder patients. Am J Geriatr Psychiatry 1996;4(1):46–60.

[42] Carmin CN, Pollard CA, Ownby RL. Obsessive-compulsive disorder: Cognitive behavioral treatment of older versus younger adults. Clin Gerontol 1998;19:1977–81.

[43] Radley M, Redston C, Bates F, et al. Effectiveness of group anxiety management with elderly clients of a community psychogeriatric team. Int J Geriatr Psychiatry 1997;12(1): 79–84.

[44] King P, Barrowclough C. A clinical pilot-study of cognitive-behavioral therapy for anxiety disorders in the elderly. Behavioural Psychotherapy 1991;19(4):337–45.

[45] Barrowclough C, King P, Colville J, et al. A randomized trial of the effectiveness of cognitive-behavioral therapy and supportive counseling for anxiety symptoms in older adults. J Consult Clin Psychol 2001;69(5):756–62.

[46] Gorenstein EE, Kleber MS, Mohlman J, et al. Cognitive-behavioral therapy for management of anxiety and medication taper in older adults. Am J Geriatr Psychiatry 2005; 13(10):901–9.

[47] Bohm C, Robinson DS, Gammans RE. Buspirone therapy for elderly patients with anxiety or depressive neurosis. J Clin Psychiatry 1990;51(7):309.

[48] Morinigo A, Blanco M, Labrador J, et al. Risperidone for resistant anxiety in elderly persons. Am J Geriatr Psychiatry 2005;13(1):81–2.

[49] Gleason PP, Schulz R, Smith NL, et al. Correlates and prevalence of benzodiazepine use in community-dwelling elderly. J Gen Intern Med 1998;13(4):243–50.

[50] Gray SL, Eggen AE, Blough D, et al. Benzodiazepine use in older adults enrolled in a health maintenance organization. Am J Geriatr Psychiatry 2003;11(5):568–76.

[51] Schuurmans J, Comijs HC, Beekman AT, et al. The outcome of anxiety disorders in older people at 6-year follow-up: results from the Longitudinal Aging Study Amsterdam. Acta Psychiatr Scand 2005;111(6):420–8.

[52] Bresolin N, Monza G, Scarpini E, et al. Treatment of anxiety with ketazolam in elderly patients. Clin Ther 1988;10(5):536–42.

[53] Frattola L, Piolti R, Bassi S, et al. Effects of alpidem in anxious elderly outpatients: a double-blind, placebo-controlled trial. Clin Neuropharmacol 1992;15(6):477–87.

[54] Koepke HH, Gold RL, Linden ME, et al. Multicenter controlled study of oxazepam in anxious elderly outpatients. Psychosomatics 1982;23(6):641–5.

[55] Katz IR, Reynolds CF III, Alexopoulos GS, et al. Venlafaxine ER as a treatment for generalized anxiety disorder in older adults: pooled analysis of five randomized placebo-controlled clinical trials. J Am Geriatr Soc 2002;50(1):18–25.

[56] Lenze EJ, Mulsant BH, Shear MK, et al. Efficacy and tolerability of citalopram in the treatment of late-life anxiety disorders: results from an 8-week randomized, placebo-controlled trial. Am J Psychiatry 2005;162(1):146–50.

[57] Sheikh JI, Lauderdale SA, Cassidy EL. Efficacy of sertraline for panic disorder in older adults: a preliminary open-label trial. Am J Geriatr Psychiatry 2004;12(2):230.

[58] Sheikh JI, Swales PJ. Treatment of panic disorder in older adults: a pilot study comparison of alprazolam, imipramine, and placebo. Int J Psychiatry Med 1999;29(1):107–17.

[59] Wylie ME, Miller MD, Shear MK, et al. Fluvoxamine pharmacotherapy of anxiety disorders in later life: preliminary open-trial data. J Geriatr Psychiatry Neurol 2000;13(1):43–8.

[60] Wetherell JL, Sorrel JT, Stanley MA, et al. Comparison of cognitive-behavioral therapy and citalopram for late-life generalized anxiety disorder [abstract]. Presented at the 25th Annual Meeting of the Anxiety Disorder Association of America. Seattle (WA), March 17–20, 2005.

[61] Averill PM, Beck JG. Posttraumatic stress disorder in older adults: a conceptual review. J Anxiety Disord 2000;14(2):133–56.

[62] Gould RA, Safren SA, Washington DO, et al. A meta-analytic review of cognitive-behavioral treatments: generalized anxiety disorder: advances in research and practice. New York: Guilford; 2004. p. 248–64.

ELSEVIER
SAUNDERS

Psychiatr Clin N Am
28 (2005) 897–911

PSYCHIATRIC
CLINICS
OF NORTH AMERICA

Evidence-Based Treatment of Geriatric Substance Abuse

David W. Oslin, MD

*Section of Geriatric Psychiatry, Department of Psychiatry, University of Pennsylvania,
3535 Market Street, Room 3002 Philadelphia, PA 19104, USA*

Alcohol and drug dependence are two of the leading causes of disability worldwide. However, substance use is often not appreciated as relevant to the care of older adults [1]. As the number of older adults increases, the magnitude of mental health disorders also will increase [2]. The public health impact of alcohol and other substance abuse disorders will likely follow this trend. In addition to increases that follow from the growth of the elderly population, the prevalence of late-life addiction is predicted to increase because of cohort changes. The current cohort of 30- to 50-year-old people represents a group who were raised during the 1950s and 1960s and, as such, participated in the increased use of and addiction to heroin, cocaine, tobacco, and alcohol. Both a history of and continued substance dependence will have physical and mental health consequences for this cohort as it ages.

Research on the treatment of late-life addictions has developed slowly. However, recent epidemiologic data underscore the anticipated cohort changes and provide the background for future development of interventions targeted to older adults. This article outlines the current state of knowledge regarding the magnitude of late-life addictions and considers interventions that target prevention, early intervention, or treatment. The focus is on late-life alcohol misuse and introduces concepts regarding medication misuse and the potential emergence of problems related to illicit substance misuse and nicotine.

Before describing the methods and review, it is important to define concepts used in this review, including recommended drinking limits, at-risk

This work was supported in part by National Institute of Mental Health Grants 5R01AA014851 and P30 MH66270 and by the Mental Illness Research, Education, and Clinical Center at the Philadelphia Veterans Affairs Medical Center.

E-mail address: oslin@mail.med.upenn.edu

drinking, and alcohol dependence. Drinking limits have been established and endorsed by a number of agencies. The National Institute on Alcohol Abuse and Alcoholism and the Center for Substance Abuse Treatment, Treatment Improvement Protocol on older adults recommend that persons age 65 and older consume no more than on standard drink per day or seven standard drinks per week [3,4]. In addition, older adults should consume no more than four standard drinks on any drinking day. These drinking limit recommendations are consistent with data regarding the relationship between heavy consumption and alcohol-related problems within this age group [5]. These recommendations are also consistent with the current evidence for a beneficial health effect of low-risk drinking [6,7].

Providers may be confused by drinking limits because alcohol use can lead to benefits (at low to moderate intake) as well as to increased morbidity and mortality. Prescription medications pose a similar dilemma in that, when they are used properly, they can reduce morbidity and mortality but can also lead to marked disability and economic burden. Illicit substances and nicotine do not share these characteristics; currently any use is considered to have greater risk than benefit. Adding to the confusion about drinking limits, the limits are lower for older adults compared with younger adults. The reason for the different limits is related to increased sensitivity to alcohol as well as over-the-counter and prescription medications. There is an age-related decrease in lean body mass and total body water content in relation to total fat volume, and the resultant decrease in total body volume increases the serum concentration of alcohol and other mood-altering chemicals in the body. Central nervous system sensitivity to alcohol also increases with age, and the interactions between medication and alcohol are a particular concern in this age group. Indeed, for some patients, any alcohol use coupled with the use of specific over-the-counter or prescription medications can be problematic.

Drinking guidelines also highlight an important distinction between problem or at-risk drinking and alcohol dependence. Alcohol dependence refers to a medical illness characterized by the loss of control, preoccupation with alcohol, continued alcohol use despite adverse consequences, and physiologic symptoms such as tolerance and withdrawal [8]. Older adults engaging in problem, abusive, or at-risk use are drinking at a level that either already has resulted in adverse medical, psychologic, or social consequences or substantially increases the likelihood of such problems but not to a level that meets the criteria of dependence. Because some of the classic symptoms of dependence, such as employment or legal problems, are not present, individuals and practitioners may underestimate the risks of this level of consumption. However, because of the risks associated with this level of drinking, problem and at-risk drinking do represent an appropriate target for interventions, particularly those interventions that are focused on a prevention model as opposed to a disease model.

Methods

Articles for consideration were obtained using online searching (MEDLINE), first for articles focused on randomized trials of treatment, either focused on older adults or including older adults as a reported subgroup. A secondary list of articles was obtained by reviewing the bibliographies of several recent reviews for additional articles focused on interventions. It is inevitable that some important reports were missed, especially non-English publications, articles reporting on treatment outcomes in which older adults are mentioned, or recently published works.

Both randomized controlled trials and well-designed descriptive treatment studies of either psychopharmacologic or psychotherapeutic interventions were included. In weighting the support of the current literature, a distinction was made between these two lines of evidence, giving more weight to the randomized trials. Given the small number of trials, other considerations such as sample sizes, relevance of comparison groups, and availability of manual-based approaches received less attention.

Results

Epidemiology

Current estimates from community-based epidemiologic studies suggest that the 1-year prevalence rate for alcohol abuse and dependence is 2.75% for elderly men and 0.51% for elderly women [9]. Despite the common occurrence and disability associated with alcohol misuse in older patients, these problems are more often unrecognized in older adults [10]. In other settings, prevalence rates will be higher. For instance, in primary care, at-risk drinking has been estimated to occur in 5% to 15% of the population [4–7]. Behavioral health care settings also have higher prevalence rates than are seen in the community (8.6%) [11–13]. There is also consistent evidence throughout these studies indicating that men drink more and have a greater prevalence of at-risk use or dependence than women have. These studies are less clear on the differences between ethnic groups, although in certain ethnic minorities such as elderly Asian populations, drinking is very uncommon [14].

Little is known about the epidemiology of substance use disorders other than alcoholism in the elderly. The general belief is that older drug addicts represent only younger addicts who have grown old. The Epidemiologic Catchment Area Study [15] has found the lifetime prevalence rates of drug abuse and dependence to be 0.12% for elderly men and 0.06% for elderly women. The lifetime history of illicit drug use was 2.88% and 0.66%, respectively. There were no active cases reported in either gender. In contrast, there are a few more recent reports suggesting that illicit substance abuse is becoming more common in treatment-seeking adults. In a study of 684 persons over the age of 50 who had a lifetime history of intravenous cocaine and heroin use, McBride and colleagues [16] have found that 13% were actively using cocaine more than once per day. Schonfeld and colleagues [17] note relatively high rates of recent illicit substance use (38%) in a Veterans Affairs (VA) older adult treatment program. Although smoking rates decrease with age (primarily because of differential mortality among smokers and nonsmokers), one of every five smokers is age 50 or older [18,19]. Approximately 15.2% of community-dwelling individuals age 65 to 74 and 8.4% of those age 75 and older are smokers.

Perhaps a unique problem with the elderly is the misuse of prescription and over-the-counter medications. This includes the misuse of substances such as sedatives and hypnotics, narcotic and non-narcotic analgesics, diet aids, decongestants, and a wide variety of other over-the-counter medications. Although dependence on these substances exists, a more common problem with medications is the inappropriate and indiscriminant use of products with limited documentation of demonstrated effectiveness in an individual and the use of multiple medications. Although not considered a disorder by the Diagnostic and Statistical Manual of Mental Disorders, revised 4th edition, there is a growing body of literature on the increase in morbidity and mortality associated with misusing prescription and nonprescription medications. To highlight the issue, 32% of community-dwelling elderly are taking an analgesic, 8.9% are taking an antidepressant, and 10.4% are taking a benzodiazepine [20]. Many medications used by the elderly have the potential for inducing tolerance, withdrawal syndromes, and harmful medical consequences such as cognitive changes and renal and hepatic diseases.

Defining an evidence base for screening and diagnosis

Based on a host of studies demonstrating the decreased drinking and objective benefits associated with early interventions, including decreased systolic blood pressure, liver function tests, and health care use, the US Preventive Services Task Force recommends routine alcohol screening followed by assessment and brief alcohol counseling (BAC) with appropriate patients [21–23]. Screening can be performed as part of routine mental and physical health care and should be updated annually, before the older adult begins taking any new medications or in response to problems that may be alcohol- or medication-related. Screening questions can be asked by a verbal interview, by a paper-and-pencil questionnaire, or by a computerized questionnaire. All three methods have equivalent reliability and validity [24,25]. Any positive responses can lead to further assessment. To successfully incorporate alcohol (and other drug) screening into clinical practice with older adults, it should be simple and consistent with other screening procedures already in place [26–28].

In addition to quantity and frequency questions to ascertain the patient's use, the Short Michigan Alcoholism Screening Test-Geriatric version (SMAST-G), the Cutdown, Annoyed, Feeling Guilty, and use of an Eye-opener (CAGE), and the Alcohol Use Disorders Identification Test (AUDIT) or a shorter version, the AUDIT-C, are often used with older adults. Of these assessments, the SMAST-G was developed specifically for older adults. The choice of screening instruments really depends on the purpose of the screening. For instance, if the goal is to identify those patients with alcohol dependence only, then a questionnaire such as the CAGE provides high specificity for the most severe cases. On the other hand, if the goal is to reduce the disability from the broader spectrum of alcohol misuse, then the CAGE is of minimal value and the SMAST-G or AUDIT-C are of great value.

Although screening is important, it is also insufficient in providing care. Within the Department of Veterans Affairs, the majority of veterans are screened annually for alcohol misuse using the AUDIT-C. However, a recent World Health Organization multinational trial has indicated such low rates of alcohol screening and implementation of BAC that providers who screened over 20% of their patients and offered counseling to over 10% of screen-positive patients were considered to have "high" rates of implementation [29]. The VA's Large Health Study and the multisite VA Ambulatory Care Quality Improvement (ACQUIP) study has found similar low rates of alcohol-related advice even after routine screening [30,31], despite patient reports of readiness for change [32].

Toward an evidence base for treatment

Prevention and early intervention approaches

Over the last two decades, there have been multiple controlled clinical trials to evaluate the effectiveness of early identification and secondary prevention using BAC to address alcohol misuse [33–37]. Strategies have ranged from relatively unstructured counseling and feedback to more formal structured therapy [38–40] and have relied heavily on concepts and techniques from the behavioral self-control literature [41,42]. The interventions generally include an expression of concern, feedback to patients linking their drinking and health, and explicit advice to cut down. The US Preventive Services Task Force and other educational programs [21,43] recommend the "Five A's" approach (ask, assess, advise, agree, assist). A number of large randomized controlled trials of BAC with both younger and older adults have found significantly reduced alcohol use at follow-up in patients who were offered the intervention, compared with those in the control groups. These trials have been summarized in six meta-analyses [33–37], including one for the US Preventive Services Task Force [44], which resulted in the 2004 recommendation that routine alcohol screening should be followed by BAC [21].

An example of BAC research is the Trial for Early Alcohol Treatment (ie, Project TrEAT), which was the first United States randomized clinical trial to test the effectiveness of two 15-minute counseling sessions and two follow-up telephone calls for patients who screened positive for alcohol misuse in primary care settings [40,45]. At the 12-month follow-up, there was a significant reduction in alcohol use and binge drinking in the intervention group compared with the control group. At the 2-year follow-up, drinking, health care costs, and medical care use were all decreased [46]. To date, there have been two brief alcohol intervention trials with older adults. Fleming and colleagues [45] and Blow [47] conducted randomized clinical brief intervention trials to reduce hazardous drinking with older adults in primary care settings. These studies have shown that older adults can be engaged in brief intervention protocols, that the protocols are acceptable in this population, and that there is a substantial reduction in drinking among the at-risk drinkers receiving interventions compared with a control group.

The first study, Project GOAL [45], was a randomized, controlled clinical trial (sample size, 158) conducted in Wisconsin with 24 community-based primary care practices (43 practitioners). The intervention consisted of two 10- to 15-minute physician-delivered counseling visits and two follow-up telephone calls by clinic staff, which included advice, education, and contracting using a scripted workbook. At the 12-month follow-up, the intervention group drank significantly less than the control group ($P \leq .001$). The second elder-specific study, the Health Profile Project [47], randomized a total of 452 subjects to usual care or to a single brief intervention session. At the 12-month follow-up, there were significant reductions in alcohol consumption among those receiving the BAC compared with usual care. Although these trials were conducted in primary care settings, brief interventions for older adults are likely to be effective in other settings, including mental health settings. The evidence base of BAC for prevention and early intervention is robust across the lifespan and should be considered standard practice for patients with at-risk and problem drinking. There is no literature on the use of early intervention and brief counseling for older adults with illicit substance use or medication misuse, although theoretically these approaches may have value.

Formal treatment for patients with abuse or dependence

Despite a growing evidence base demonstrating effective treatments for younger adults, relatively little formal research has been conducted on the comparative efficacy of various approaches to addiction treatment in older adults. Because traditional alcohol treatment programs generally provide services to few older adults, sample size issues have been a barrier to studying treatment outcomes for elderly alcoholics in most settings. However, several naturalistic studies suggest that older adults who do engage in treatment can have as good or substantially better outcomes compared with younger adults [48–51]. Thus in contrast to popular beliefs, older adults are quite amenable to treatment, especially in programs that offer age-appropriate care with providers who are knowledgeable about aging issues.

There is a small evidence base demonstrating that age-specific programming can improve treatment completion and result in higher rates of attendance at group meetings compared with mixed age treatment [52]. Oslin and colleagues [50] have reported that older adults are more compliant with addiction treatment than younger adults are, as measured by treatment attendance. This is consistent with other published reports on older versus middle-aged adults [22,23]. Previous literature has suggested that compliance with addiction treatment is directly related to a better outcome [53]. If this relationship holds for older adults, the expectation would be that treatment outcome would be better in the elderly. Although the age of onset of alcohol problems has been suggested as a risk factor for poor treatment outcomes, this has not been demonstrated in clinical trials. It is important to remark on traditional 12-step peer support as a model treatment. Self-help programs have been the central focus of most community-based programs for many years and have clearly been successful for a number of people. There is some concern that group-based approaches, including 12-step programs, are not effective for all patients. This may be particularly true if the group is composed of only a few older adults and mostly younger adults. In support of this, Oslin and colleagues [54] have found that older adults leaving a traditional 12-step rehabilitation program were less likely to engage in formal treatment than middle-aged adults were. This effect was seen as early as 1 month after discharge and may be related to issues of stigma as well as practical issues such as transportation or health problems.

There are almost no randomized treatment outcome studies reported in the literature that are focused on older adults, in part because of the complexity of studying older adults in treatment and in part because of difficulties in following them after completion of treatment. Thus, sample sizes tend to be too small to provide definitive results. An exception is a study of 137 male veterans (age 45–59, n = 64; age 60–69, n = 62; and age ≥ 70, n = 11) who had alcohol problems, who were randomly assigned after detoxification to age-specific treatment or standard mixed-age treatment [55]. Outcomes at 6 months and 1 year showed that elder-specific-program patients were 2.9 times more likely at 6 months and 2.1 times more likely at 1 year to report abstinence compared with mixed-age group patients. Treatment groups, however, could not be compared at baseline because baseline alcohol consumption and alcohol severity data were not included in the study.

Pharmacotherapy of addiction

Pharmacologic treatments have not traditionally played a major role in the long-term treatment of older alcohol dependent adults. Until recently, disulfiram was the only medication approved for the treatment of alcohol dependence but was seldom used in older patients because of concerns related to adverse effects. In 1995, the opioid antagonist naltrexone was approved by the US Food and Drug Administration (FDA) for the treatment of alcohol dependence. The FDA approval of naltrexone was based on studies demonstrating the efficacy of naltrexone for the treatment of middle-aged patients with alcohol dependence [56,57]. In both studies, naltrexone was found to be safe and effective in preventing relapse and reducing the craving for alcohol. The use of naltrexone is based on the interaction between endogenous endorphin activity and alcohol intake and reward.

Oslin and colleagues [58] have extended this line of research by studying a group of older veterans, age 50 to 70. The study was designed as a double-blind placebo-controlled randomized trial with naltrexone, 50 mg/d. The results were similar to the other clinical trials with half as many subjects treated with naltrexone who relapsed to significant drinking compared with those treated with placebo. It is important to note that there was no improvement in total abstinence but there was a decrease in the rate of relapse to heavy drinking among those who had any drinking. Thus, the failure to achieve abstinence should not be seen as a failure of treatment.

Recently, acamprosate was approved for the treatment of alcohol dependence. Although the exact action of acamprosate is still unknown, it is believed to reduce glutamate release and thus effect the rewarding properties of alcohol [59]. Although there are no studies focused on older adults, the clinical evidence favoring acamprosate is impressive. For instance, Sass and colleagues [60] studied 272 alcohol-dependent subjects in Europe for up to 48 weeks using a randomized placebo-controlled study of acamprosate. Forty-three percent of the acamprosate-treated group was abstinent at the conclusion of the study, compared with 21% in the placebo group.

Detoxification and withdrawal

Alcohol withdrawal symptoms occur commonly in patients who stop drinking or markedly cut down their drinking after regular heavy use. During hospitalizations, patients may be particularly vulnerable to alcohol or benzodiazepine withdrawal if the clinical team is unaware of the use of these substances. Alcohol withdrawal can range from mild and almost unnoticeable symptoms to severe and life-threatening ones. The classical set of symptoms associated with alcohol withdrawal includes autonomic hyperactivity (increased pulse rate, increased blood pressure, and increased temperature), restlessness, disturbed sleep, anxiety, nausea, and tremor. More severe withdrawal can be manifested by auditory, visual, or tactile hallucinations, delirium, seizures, and coma. Other substances of abuse such as benzodiazepines, opioids and cocaine have distinct withdrawal symptoms that are also potentially life threatening. Elderly patients have been shown to have a longer duration of withdrawal symptoms, and withdrawal has the potential for complicating other medical and psychiatric illnesses. However, there is no evidence to suggest that older patients are more prone to alcohol withdrawal or need longer treatment for withdrawal symptoms [61].

Treatment studies for other substance disorders are lacking among the elderly. Although smoking is clearly linked to increased disability and mortality in late life, there have been relatively few studies of smoking cessation focused on the elderly. Orleans and colleagues [62] have found that the use of transdermal nicotine replacement resulted in a 29% self-reported quit rate and greater success in patients who received professional (physician or pharmacist) encouragement to stop. This study was an open-label descriptive study of lower income smokers. The antidepressants bupropion and nortriptyline have both been shown to be effective in improving quit rates among middle-aged smokers [63,64]. Future studies should include more elderly subjects because there are clearly defined benefits from smoking cessation, including among the elderly [65,66]. Finally, although Rickels and colleagues [67] have demonstrated that the elderly could successfully be withdrawn from chronic benzodiazepine use, they also demonstrated that the elderly are more likely to return to benzodiazepine use within 3 years of discontinuation [67,68].

Future research directions for treatment

Traditionally, treatment studies in addiction have excluded patients over the age of 65. This bias has left a tremendous gap in knowledge regarding treatment outcomes and understanding of the neurobiology of addiction in older adults. Table 1 [45,47,52,58,69] summarizes the existing knowledge base, with important priorities listed for the future. With the substantial cohort effects already leading to increases in the prevalence of substance misuse, it is vital that new research begin to unravel the complexities of treating late-life addiction.

Summary

Over the past several years there has been a growing awareness that addictive disorders among the elderly are a common public health problem. Epidemiologic studies suggest that alcohol dependence is present in up to 4% of community-dwelling elderly, and evidence indicates that the prevalence of alcohol abuse or dependence among older adults is on the rise [70,71]. Moreover, problem or hazardous drinking is estimated to be even more common than alcohol dependence among the elderly [71–73]. However, there continues to be a gap in the number of older adults who are referred for treatment or who receive treatment for addictive disorders. This gap in treatment is likely to become broader as geriatric care providers venture into unfamiliar dialogues with patients about illicit substance use. The evidence base for formal treatments is strong for younger adults, particularly those with alcohol, opioid, or nicotine dependence. However, it is not clear whether these treatments can be applied with equal success to older adults. The one exception to the lack of an evidence base is in the early intervention work on brief alcohol interventions. Clearly, brief alcohol interventions should be learned by the broad array of clinicians working with older adults, both as a mechanism for dialogue between patient and

Table 1
Summary of evidence-based research on late-life alcoholism

	Evidence base from randomized trials	General effect	Other evidence base	Future needs
Problem and at-risk drinking				
Brief interventions	2 randomized trials [45,47]	50%–75% of patients reduced drinking to moderate levels	None	Randomized trials in other high-risk settings such as behavioral health, home care, and the emergency room
Alcohol dependence				
Psychotherapy	1 randomized trial [52]	2-fold improvement with age-appropriate treatment	Several naturalistic trials demonstrating increased adherence to treatment and generally better outcomes for older adults compared to middle aged adults	Randomized trials designed to better understand age-dependent adherence and treatment outcomes
Naltrexone	1 randomized trial [58]	Medication was well tolerated and showed some evidence for efficacy in post hoc analyses	None	Clinical pharmacology trials need to begin enrolling older adults rather than excluding them, which is the general practice; greater advocacy from the geriatrics field should be focused on this issue in the addiction field; there are specific needs for safety studies as well as efficacy studies
Antabuse	No trials specifically in older adults		Antabuse reaction may be particularly harmful for older adults with pre-existing medical problems	

Other agents	No trials			Antidepressants, mood stabilizing agents, and acamprosate are all used clinically but with no evidence base in older adults
Comorbidity	1 randomized trial for depressed alcohol-dependent patients [69]	There was no evidence for efficacy of naltrexone when added to sertraline and psychosocial support	One trial in alcohol related dementia shows stabilization of dementia with abstinence; some evidence that a history of at-risk drinking or dependence results in higher rates of treatment-resistant depression	This is a critical area of need both for patients with current alcohol dependence or at-risk drinking and for those with histories of alcohol dependence or at-risk drinking

Adapted from Oslin DW. Late-life alcoholism: issues relevant to the geriatric psychiatrist. Am J Geriatr Psychiatry 2004;12(6):571–83; with permission.

provider and as an intervention that can be effective. Clearly, more research from basic neuroscience to implementation and policy work are warranted.

References

[1] Murray C, Lopez A, editors. The global burden of disease: a comprehensive assessment of mortality and disability from diseases, injuries, and risk factors in 1990 and projected to 2020. In: The global burden of disease and injury series, vol. 1. Boston: Harvard University Press; 1996. p. 23–26 and 31–9.

[2] Jeste DV, Alexopoulos GS, Bartels SJ, et al. Consensus statement on the upcoming crisis in geriatric mental health: research agenda for the next 2 decades. Arch Gen Psychiatry 1999; 56(9):848–53.

[3] Blow F. Substance abuse among older Americans. In: Treatment Improvement Protocol, #26. Washington DC: Center for Substance Abuse Prevention, DHHS No. (SMA) 98–3179. US Government Printing Office, Bethesda, MD; 1998.

[4] National Institute on Alcohol Abuse and Alcoholism. Diagnostic criteria for alcohol abuse. Alcohol Alert 1995;30(PH 359):1–6.

[5] Chermack ST, Blow FC, Hill EM, et al. The relationship between alcohol symptoms and consumption among older drinkers. Alcohol Clin Exp Res 1996;20:1153–8.

[6] Klatsky AL, Armstrong A. Alcohol use, other traits and risk of unnatural death: a prospective study. Alcohol Clin Exp Res 1993;17:1156–62.

[7] Poikolainen K. Epidemiologic assessment of population risks and benefits of alcohol use. Alcohol Alcohol 1991;(Suppl 1):S27–34.

[8] American Psychiatric Association. Diagnostic and statistical manual of mental disorders. 4th edition. Washington (DC): American Psychiatric Press; 1994.

[9] Grant BF, Dawson DA, Stinson FS, et al. The 12-month prevalence and trends in DSM-IV alcohol abuse and dependence: United States, 1991–1992 and 2001–2002. Drug Alcohol Depend 2004;74(3):223–34.

[10] Curtis J, Geller G, Stokes E, et al. Characteristics, diagnosis, and treatment of alcoholism in elderly patients. J Am Geriatr Soc 1989;37:310–6.

[11] Holroyd S, Duryee J. Substance use disorders in a geriatric psychiatry outpatient clinic: prevalence and epidemiologic characteristics. J Nerv Ment Dis 1997;185(10):627–32.

[12] Joseph CL, Ganzini L, Atkinson R. Screening for alcohol use disorders in the nursing home. J Am Geriatr Soc 1995;43:368–73.

[13] Oslin DW, Streim JE, Parmelee P, et al. Alcohol abuse: a source of reversible functional disability among residents of a VA nursing home. Int J Geriatr Psychiatry 1997;12(8):825–32.

[14] Kirchner J, Zubritsky C, Cody M, et al. Alcohol consumption among older adults in primary care. JAMA, in press.

[15] Anthony JC, Helzer JE. Syndromes of drug abuse and dependence. In: Robins LN, Regier DA, editors. Psychiatric disorders in America: the Epidemiologic Catchment Area Study. New York: The Free Press; 1991. p. 116–54.

[16] McBride DC, Inciardi JA, Chitwood DD, et al. Consortium TNAR: crack use and correlates of use in a national population of street heroin users. J Psychoactive Drugs 1992;24(4):411–6.

[17] Schonfeld L, Dupree LW, Dickson-Fuhrmann E, et al. Cognitive-behavioral treatment of older veterans with substance abuse problems. J Geriatr Psychiatry Neurol 2000;13:124–9.

[18] Gourlay S, Benowitz N. The benefits of stopping smoking and the role of nicotine replacement therapy in older patients. Drugs Aging 1996;9:8–23.

[19] Orleans C, Rimer B, Salmon M, et al. Psychological and behavioral consequences and correlates of smoking cessation. In: The health benefits of smoking cessation: a report of the Surgeon General; 1990. US Department of Health and Human Services Services, US Government Printing Office: Rockville, MD. pp. 521–78.

[20] Moxey E, O'Connor J, Novielli K, et al. Prescription drug use in the elderly: a descriptive analysis. Health Care Financ Rev 2003;24(4):127–44.

[21] US Preventive Services Task Force. Screening and behavioral counseling interventions in primary care to reduce alcohol misuse: recommendation statement. Ann Intern Med 2004; 140:554–6.

[22] Schuckit M, Pastor P. The elderly as a unique population. Alcohol Clin Exp Res 1978;2: 31–8.

[23] Wiens AN, Menustik CE, Miller SI, et al. Medical-behavioral treatment for the older alcoholic patient. Am J Drug Alcohol Abuse 1982;9:461–75.

[24] Barry K, Fleming M. Computerized administration of alcoholism screening tests in a primary care setting. J Am Board Fam Pract 1990;3:93–8.

[25] Greist J, Klein M, Erdman H, Bires J. Comparison of computer- and interviewer-administered versions of the Diagnostic Interview Schedule. Hosp Community Psychiatry 1987; 38:1304–11.

[26] Barry KL, Oslin DW, Blow FC. Prevention and management of alcohol problems in older adults. New York: Springer Publishing; 2001.

[27] Bradley K, Epler A, Bush K, et al. Alcohol-related discussions during general medicine appointments of patients who screen positive for at-risk drinking. J Gen Intern Med 2002;17(5): 315–27.

[28] McCormick K, Bradley K, Cochran N, et al. How primary care providers talk to patients about alcohol: a qualitative study. Presented at the Society of Medicine Annual Meeting in Chicago, IL. May 12–15, 2004.

[29] Anderson P, Laurant M, Kaner E, et al. Engaging general practitioners in the management of hazardous and harmful alcohol consumption: results of a meta-analysis. 2004;65(2):191–9.

[30] Kazis L, Kalman D, Lee A, et al. Large health survey. Washington (DC): Veterans Health Administration; 2002.

[31] Burman M, Buchbinder M, Kivlahan D, et al. Alcohol-related advice for VA primary care patients: who gets it, who gives it? J Stud Alcohol 2004;65(5):621–30.

[32] Williams E, Kivlahan D, Saitz R, et al. Are primary care patients with at-risk drinking ready to change? Presented at the Society of Medicine Annual Meeting in Chicago, IL. May 12–15, 2004.

[33] Bien T, Miller W, Tonigan J. Brief interventions for alcohol problems: a review [comment appears in: Addiction 1995;90(8):1118–21]. Addiction 1993;88(3):315–35.

[34] Kahan M, Wilson L, Becker L. Effectiveness of physician-based interventions with problem drinkers. Can Med Assoc J 1995;152(6):851–9.

[35] Wilk AJNM, Havighurst T. Meta-analysis of randomized control trials addressing brief interventions in heavy alcohol drinkers. J Gen Intern Med 1997;12:274–83.

[36] Poikolainen K. Effectiveness of brief interventions to reduce alcohol intake in primary health care populations: a meta-analysis. Prev Med 1999;28:503–9.

[37] Moyer A, Finney J, Swearingen C, et al. Brief interventions for alcohol problems: a meta-analytic review of controlled investigations in treatment-seeking and non-treatment-seeking populations. Addiction 2002;97:279–92.

[38] Chick J, Lloyd G, Crombie E. Counseling problem drinkers in medical wards: a controlled study. BMJ 1985;290(6473):965–7.

[39] Persson J, Magnusson PH. Early intervention in patients with excessive consumption of alcohol: a controlled study. Alcohol 1989;6(5):403–8.

[40] Fleming M, Barry K, Manwell L, et al. Brief physician advice for problem alcohol drinkers: a randomized controlled trial in community-based primary care practices. JAMA 1997;277: 1039–45.

[41] Miller W, Hester R. Treating addictive behaviors: processes of change. New York: Plenum Press; 1986.

[42] Miller W, Rollnick S. Motivational interviewing: preparing people to change addictive behavior. New York: The Guilford Press; 1991.

[43] Saitz R, Ellison R, Conigliario J, et al. Alcohol screening and brief intervention curriculum. 2004: Alcohol Clinical Training (ACT) project. Available at: http://www.bu.edu/act/mdalcoholtraining/curriculum_top.html. Accessed January 24, 2005.

[44] Whitlock E, Polen M, Green C, et al. Behavioral counseling interventions in primary care to reduce risky/harmful alcohol use by adults: a summary of the evidence for the US Preventive Services Task Force. Ann Intern Med 2004;140:557–68.

[45] Fleming MF, Manwell LB, Barry KL, et al. Brief physician advice for alcohol problems in older adults: a randomized community-based trial. J Fam Pract 1999;48(5):378–84.

[46] Fleming MF, Mundt MP, French MT, et al. Brief physician advice for problem drinkers: long-term efficacy and benefit-cost analysis. Alcohol Clin Exp Res 2002;26(1):36–43.

[47] Blow F. Brief interventions in the treatment of at-risk drinking in older adults. Personal communication, October 24, 2005.

[48] Lemke S, Moos RH. Treatment and outcomes of older patients with alcohol use disorders in community residential programs. J Stud Alcohol 2003;64(2):219–26.

[49] Lemke S, Moos RH. Outcomes at 1 and 5 years for older patients with alcohol use disorders. J Subst Abuse Treat 2003;24(1):43–50.

[50] Oslin DW, Pettinati H, Volpicelli JR. Alcoholism treatment adherence: older age predicts better adherence and drinking outcomes. Am J Geriatr Psychiatry 2002;10(6):740–7.

[51] Satre DD, Mertens JPA, Arean PA, et al. Contrasting outcomes of older versus middle-aged and younger adult chemical dependency patients in a managed care program. J Stud Alcohol 2003;64(4):520–30.

[52] Kofoed LL, Tolson RL, Atkinson RM, et al. Treatment compliance of older alcoholics: an elder-specific approach is superior to "mainstreaming.". J Stud Alcohol 1987;48:47–51.

[53] Pettinati HM, Volpicelli JR, Pierce JD Jr, et al. Improving naltrexone response: an intervention for medical practitioners to enhance medication compliance in alcohol dependent patients. J Addict Dis 2000;19(1):71–83.

[54] Oslin DW, Slaymaker VJ, Blow FC, et al. Treatment outcomes for alcohol dependence among middle aged and older adults. Addict Behav 2005;30(7):1431–6.

[55] Kashner TM, Rodell DI, Ogden SR, et al. Outcomes and costs of two VA inpatient treatment programs for older alcoholic patients. Hosp Community Psychiatry 1992;43(10):985–9.

[56] Volpicelli JR, Alterman AI, Hayashida M, et al. Naltrexone in the treatment of alcohol dependence. Arch Gen Psychiatry 1992;49:876–80.

[57] O'Malley SS, Jaffe AJ, Chang G, et al. Naltrexone and coping skills therapy for alcohol dependence: a controlled study. Arch Gen Psychiatry 1992;49:881–7.

[58] Oslin D, Liberto JG, O'Brien J, et al. Naltrexone as an adjunctive treatment for older patients with alcohol dependence. Am J Geriatr Psychiatry 1997;5(4):324–32.

[59] Pelc I, Verbanck P, Le Bon O, et al. Efficacy and safety of acamprosate in the treatment of detoxified alcohol-dependent patients: a 90-day placebo-controlled dose-finding study. Br J Psychiatry 1997;171:73–7.

[60] Sass H, Soyka M, Mann K, et al. Relapse prevention by acamprosate: results from a placebo-controlled study in alcohol dependence. Arch Gen Psychiatry 1996;53:673–80.

[61] Brower KJ, Mudd S, Blow FC, et al. Severity and treatment of alcohol withdrawal in elderly versus younger patients. Alcohol Clin Exp Res 1994;18:196–201.

[62] Orleans CT, Resch N, Noll E, et al. Use of transdermal nicotine in a state-level prescription plan for the elderly: a first look at "real-world" patch users. JAMA 1994;271:601–7.

[63] Hurt RD, Sachs DP, Glover ED, et al. A comparison of sustained-release bupropion and placebo for smoking cessation. N Engl J Med 1997;337:1195–202.

[64] Hall SM, Reus VI, Munoz RF, et al. Nortriptyline and cognitive-behavioral therapy in the treatment of cigarette smoking. Arch Gen Psychiatry 1998;55:683–90.

[65] Maxwell CJ, Hirdes JP. The prevalence of smoking and implications for quality-of-life among the community-based elderly. Am J Prev Med 1993;9:338–45.

[66] Paganinihill A, Hsu G. Smoking and mortality among residents of a California retirement community. Am J Public Health 1994;84:992–5.
[67] Rickels K, Case W, Schweizer E, et al. Long-term benzodiazepine users 3 years after participation in a discontinuation program. Am J Psychiatry 1991;148:757–61.
[68] Schweizer E, Case WG, Rickels K. Benzodiazepine dependence and withdrawal in elderly patients. Am J Psychiatry 1989;146(4):529–31.
[69] Oslin DW. The treatment of late life depression complicated by alcohol dependence. Am J Geriatr Psychiatry 2005;13(6):491–500.
[70] Osterling A, Berglund M. Elderly first time admitted alcoholics: a descriptive study on gender differences in a clinical population. Alcohol Clin Exp Res 1994;18:1317–21.
[71] Liberto JG, Oslin DW, Ruskin PE. Alcoholism in older persons: a review of the literature. Hosp Community Psychiatry 1992;43(10):975–84.
[72] Barry KL, Blow FC, Walton MA, et al. Elder-specific brief alcohol intervention: 3-month outcomes. Alcohol Clin Exp Res 1998;22:32A.
[73] Oslin DW. Late-life alcoholism: issues relevant to the geriatric psychiatrist. Am J Geriatr Psychiatry 2004;12(6):571–83.

ELSEVIER
SAUNDERS

Psychiatr Clin N Am
28 (2005) 913–939

PSYCHIATRIC
CLINICS
OF NORTH AMERICA

Evidence-Based Review of Pharmacologic and Nonpharmacologic Treatments for Older Adults with Schizophrenia

Aricca D. Van Citters, MS[a], Sarah I. Pratt, PhD[a],
Stephen J. Bartels, MD, MS[a],*, Dilip V. Jeste, MD[b]

[a]New Hampshire-Dartmouth Psychiatric Research Center, 2 Whipple Place,
Suite 202, Lebanon, NH 03755, USA
[b]Department of Psychiatry, Veterans Affairs San Diego Healthcare System,
3350 La Jolla Village Drive, 116A-1, San Diego, CA 92161, USA

Longitudinal studies of the course of schizophrenia show that a majority of individuals affected by this disorder experience clinically significant reduction and even remission of symptoms with aging [1], yet many individuals with schizophrenia continue to experience debilitating symptoms in older age. Furthermore, approximately 20% of middle-aged and older persons who have schizophrenia experience the first onset of their symptoms after the age of 45 [2]. Schizophrenia has a negative impact on the functioning and well-being of many older affected adults [1,3] and is associated with heightened morbidity, health care use, and costs and even increased mortality [4–6]. Demographic projections indicate that the aging of the "baby boom" generation will increase the proportion of Americans over age 65 from 13% currently to 20% by the year 2030 [7]. This percentage represents an expected increase in the number of people over age 65, from 35 million to 71 million people [7]. Moreover, the number of older people who have psychiatric disorders including schizophrenia will likely increase disproportionately compared with older people in the general population, in part because improved treatments may lower mortality rates in younger adults who have

This work was supported in part by funding from National Institutes of Mental Health Grant K24 MH66282 (to S.J. Bartels) and P30 MH66248 (to D.V. Jeste) and by the US Department of Veterans Affairs.
* Corresponding author.
E-mail address: sbartels@dartmouth.edu (S.J. Bartels).

serious mental illnesses, allowing more of them to live to old age [8]. Approximately 140,000 persons or 0.4% of older Americans have a diagnosis of schizophrenia [9]. If population projections are accurate, within 25 years this figure will more than double to nearly 300,000.

Several evidence-based reviews have been published evaluating the effectiveness of treatments for schizophrenia, that focus on younger adults [10–14], and over 56 topic reviews exist in the Cochrane Database of Systematic Reviews. Only one Cochrane Database review evaluates the treatment of older adults who had schizophrenia [15]. This 1990 review is limited to the evaluation of a randomized clinical trial (RCT) of remoxipride [16], an agent that was pulled from the market because of safety concerns. Evidence-based reviews of treatment for younger adults who had schizophrenia, combined with general reviews of treatment for older adults who had schizophrenia [17–19], indicate that antipsychotic drugs coupled with psychosocial interventions should be the mainstay of treatment for persons who have schizophrenia.

Despite an extensive literature on effective interventions for younger adults who have schizophrenia, the results of these studies do not necessarily translate to older adults because of age-associated changes in physiologic, social, and cognitive functioning. Changes in cognition, metabolism, receptor sensitivity, and psychologic development can alter the effects of both psychotherapeutic interventions and pharmacologic responses. The additional burden of medical comorbidity and potential drug–drug interactions associated with polypharmacy further complicate treatment. Older people experience increased sensitivity and a greater likelihood of medication side effects [20]. For example, compared with their younger counterparts, older adults who have schizophrenia experience more severe extrapyramidal symptoms (EPS) and higher rates of tardive dyskinesia [21]. Antipsychotic medications may also differentially cause problems such as cognitive impairment and cardiovascular effects in older people. Generally, physicians may attempt to adjust for these risk factors by prescribing lower daily doses of antipsychotic and anticholinergic medications [1]. The selection of appropriate and optimal treatments for older patients who have schizophrenia should accommodate age-associated pharmacokinetic and pharmacodynamic changes and reflect a critical ascertainment of the evidence supporting alternative treatment options.

This review evaluates the evidence for the provision of pharmacologic and nonpharmacologic treatments for older persons who have schizophrenia. Specifically, this review addresses whether treatments for older adults who have schizophrenia are effective in improving symptoms and are well tolerated.

Data sources and search strategy

To identify relevant articles for this review, two strategies were followed. A review of pharmacologic studies was conducted using the following strategy. PubMed, PsychINFO, CINAHL, and BIOSIS were searched within three topic areas for English language articles indexed through May 2005: pharmacologic treatment (keywords: antipsychotic, aripiprazole, clozapine, olanzapine, quetiapine, risperidone, and ziprasidone), schizophrenia, and older adults (keywords "geri," late-life, senile, elder, "gero," and older in the title). Additional articles were identified through a bibliographic review and through PubMed and Web-of-Science "related records" searches. The review of nonpharmacologic intervention studies was conducted through the following strategy. PubMed and PsychINFO were searched within three topic areas for English language articles indexed through May 2005: psychosocial treatment (keywords psychosocial, skills training, and cognitive behavioral), schizophrenia, and older adults (keywords elder, geri, older, and older adults). Additional articles were identified through a bibliographic review.

Criteria for selected studies

Studies were included if they evaluated the efficacy and safety of pharmacologic and nonpharmacologic interventions in older adults who had schizophrenia or schizoaffective disorder. Pharmacologic trials included those that focused entirely on older adults (age ≥ 50) who had schizophrenia or schizoaffective disorder. This review excluded literature examining heterogeneous samples and the limited literature on treatment for paraphrenia. Nonpharmacologic interventions included studies with samples in which 50% or more of participants were diagnosed with schizophrenia or schizoaffective disorder or studies in which outcomes were separately reported for these disorders in middle-aged or older persons (age ≥ 40). The distinction in diagnostic inclusion criteria was developed because of the nature of interventions that focus on functional impairment, as opposed to biological mechanisms. The distinction in age criteria reflects the availability of interventions targeting older persons who had schizophrenia.

Eligible pharmacologic studies consisted of RCTs, quasi-experimental studies, or longitudinal outcome studies consisting of 100 or more patients. Fourteen pharmacologic studies fulfilled all inclusion criteria. Eligible nonpharmacologic studies consisted of two RCTs, two quasi-experimental studies, and one uncontrolled prospective cohort study. To our knowledge, this represents all of the studies of psychosocial interventions for older adults that have been published to date, in which samples included at least some percentage of individuals who had schizophrenia.

Data extraction and analysis

Descriptive characteristics, outcome, and tolerability data were abstracted from all of the studies selected for this review. The data included study type, agent and dose or model descriptions, sample characteristics, duration and completeness of follow-up, study measures and outcomes, and strengths and weaknesses. Primary outcomes of interest included improvement in psychiatric symptoms, functioning, and tolerability. The statistical aggregation of data was not feasible because of the lack of similarity among studies with respect to study design, intervention characteristics, inclusion criteria, and outcome measures.

Pharmacologic studies

Identification of studies

Among the fourteen pharmacologic studies that met inclusion criteria, five studies were double-blind RCTs [22–27], two studies reported the results of open-label RCTs [28,29], two studies were quasi-experimental studies [30,31], and two studies reported on noncontrolled prospective cohort studies [32,33]. In addition, two randomized controlled augmentation studies were identified, including one double [34] and one single blind [35] trial. Finally, one additional RCT was identified [16]; however, it was not included in this review because it examined the effectiveness of an agent (remoxipride) that has been removed from the market [36].

Antipsychotic agents

As shown in Table 1, five unique double-blind RCTs evaluated the effectiveness of antipsychotic agents for older adults who had schizophrenia. Two studies examined the effectiveness and safety of conventional antipsychotic agents [22,23]; two studies compared the results of atypical antipsychotic agents with conventional antipsychotic agents [24,25]; and one recent trial compared the effectiveness of olanzapine with risperidone [26,27]. Results from all of these studies generally showed improvement in psychiatric symptoms. Studies comparing atypical and conventional antipsychotics have suggested that olanzapine has superior efficacy and less severe EPS compared with haloperidol [25] and that clozapine and chlorpromazine are equally efficacious [24]. However, the available studies evaluating clozapine and conventional antipsychotics had small sample sizes [22–25] and were restricted to inpatients [22,24] and largely male Veterans Affairs populations [23,24]. These limitations warranted caution in the interpretation and generalizability of these studies. A head-to-head comparison of two atypical antipsychotic agents (olanzapine and risperidone) suggests that these agents have similar effects on cognitive [27] and psychiatric symptoms [26]. There were no significant differences in side effects between these two drugs, except for greater weight gain with olanzapine [26]. Of note, only one study included a placebo group; however, this study evaluated relapse and hospitalization after the discontinuation of antipsychotic treatment and did not evaluate the side effects or effectiveness of pharmacologic treatment for reducing psychopathology or improving functioning [23].

Table 1
Double-blind randomized controlled trials of antipsychotic medications in older adults with schizophrenia

Study	Study design	Agent	Sample	Follow-up	Outcome measures and results	Limitations and comments
Branchey et al 1978 [22]	Double-blind crossover design FLU/THIO: n = 30	FLU mean dose at endpoint 285 mg/wk THIO mean dose at endpoint 5 mg/wk	Hospitalized pts; age, 67; Female, 53.3%; Dx, chronic schizophrenia	4-wk washout period; first 8-wk active phase (half received THIO, half received FLU); 4-week washout period; second 8-wk active phase (half received FLU, half received THIO)	CGI improved in both groups; no difference between groups; BPRS anergia and total improved in both groups; BPRS emotional withdrawal improved in THIO; THIO better than FLU in reducing tension but had more severe motor retardation; rigidity and tremor increased with both drugs; FLU had more rigidity than THIO; THIO had decreased blood pressure and weight gain	Small sample size; no mention of dropout rate

(continued on next page)

Table 1 (*continued*)

Study	Study design	Agent	Sample	Follow-up	Outcome measures and results	Limitations and comments
Ruskin and Nyman, 1991 [23]	Double-blind RCT; HAL: n = 11 PBO: n = 12	All stabilized on HAL, then randomized to HAL or PBO HAL: mean dose not stated PBO stabilized dose of HAL cut in half for 2 wk and then terminated	VA outpatients; age, 60.1; female, 0%; Dx, schizophrenia, receiving neuroleptics	6 mo; Discontinued: HAL, 27.3%; PBO, 16.6% (35 people entered trial; prior to randomization, 2 decided to drop out, 10 could not tolerate HAL)	Relapse: HAL, 12.5%; PBO, 50% Hospitalized: HAL, 0%; PBO, 10% Relapse was predicted by age, dose of neuroleptic prior to study entry, placebo, BPRS psychosis score, and years since last hospitalization	Small sample size; symptom outcomes not reported; side effects not reported
Howanitz et al 1999 [24]	Double-blind RCT; CLOZ: 24 CHLOR: 18	Flexible dose schedule: CLOZ began at 12.5 mg/d, increased to 300 mg/d: mean dose 300 mg/d CHLOR began at 25 mg/d, increased to 600 mg/d: mean dose 600 mg/d	VA inpatients CLOZ: age, 65; female, 8.3% CHLOR: age, 68.5; female, 5.6%; Dx, chronic schizophrenia/ schizoaffective and PANSS ≥ 60	Efficacy assessed after 12 wk Discontinued: CLOZ, 12.5%; CHLOR, 38.9%	PANSS total, positive, negative, and global scores and CGI improved in both groups; no between-group differences	Small sample size; 16/42 patients had hematologic abnormalities; percentage of adverse events equal in both groups; benztropine and chloral hydrate administered when needed for side effects and agitation

| Kennedy et al 2003 [25] | Double-blind RCT OLZ: n = 83 HAL: n = 34 | OLZ mean modal dose 11.9 mg/d HAL mean modal dose 9.4 mg/d | Age, 66.0 ($\pm$4.6); female, 61.5%; Dx, schizophrenia | 6-week; Discontinuation: because of adverse event: OLZ: 1%; HAL, 3%; lack of efficacy, OLZ, 22%; HAL, 44%; those with $\geq$40% BPRS reduction continued for 52 weeks | OLZ greater improvement than HAL on BPRS total and negative factor, and PPCT, psychosis core total, delusions item, ANX/DEP, and NEG factor; clinical response ($\geq$40% decrease in BPRS score) achieved by 51% of OLZ and 29% of HAL (p = .08); no change in CGI, MADRS, SF-36, QLS, PANSS hallucinations, agitation, positive, or cognitive factor; less EPS for OLZ vs HAL with treatment by age effect | Post-hoc analysis; small sample size; safety; OLZ superior to HAL for SAS and BAS |
| Jeste et al 2003 [26] | Double-blind RCT; OLZ: n = 88 RIS: n = 87 | OLZ mean modal dose 11.1 mg/d RIS mean modal dose 1.9 mg/d | OLZ: age, 71.4 ($\pm$ 5.6); female, 68.2% RIS: age, 70.9 ($\pm$ 5.6); female, 60.9%; Dx, schizophrenia/ schizoaffective and PANSS 50–120 | 8 wk; Discontinued: OLZ, 19.3%; RIS, 27.6% | Ham-D, CGI, and PANSS total and POS, NEG, DIS, and ANX/DEP subscales improved in both groups; clinical improvement $\geq$ 20% reduction in PANSS total, OLZ, 59%; RIS, 58%; also, 32.5% of RIS and 36.0% of OLZ rated as much or very much improved at endpoint; no difference between OLZ and RIS | Adverse events: RIS, 9.2%; OLZ, 15.9%; weight gain in both groups but less frequent in RIS; no change in PANSS hostility/ excitement scale |

(continued on next page)

Table 1 (*continued*)

Study	Study design	Agent	Sample	Follow-up	Outcome measures and results	Limitations and comments
Harvey et al 2003 [27] (same study and sample as Jeste et al 2003 [26])	Double-blind RCT; OLZ: n = 89 RIS: n = 87	OLZ mean dose 11.5 mg/d RIS mean dose 2 mg/d	OLZ: age, 71.4 (± 5.9); female, 66% RIS: age, 71.2 (± 6.0); female, 62%; Dx, schizophrenia/ schizoaffective and PANSS 50–120	8 wk; 87.4% completed ≥ 1 post-baseline cognitive tests (OLZ = 79; RIS = 74); Discontinued: OLZ, 30.4%; RIS, 27.0%	Attention and memory improved in both groups (TMT-A and SVLT); substantial improvement on TMT-A seen for 25% of OLZ and 18% of RIS; executive function and verbal fluency improved in RIS but not OLZ (TMT-B, WCST total error score, VFE sum of categories and letters); no differences between OLZ and RIS	Side effects of treatment and symptom outcomes reported in Jeste et al 2003 [26]; no change in CPT total scores or WCST categories score

Abbreviations: ANX/DEP, anxiety and depression; BAS, Barnes Akathisia Scale; BPRS, Brief Psychiatric Rating Scale; CGI, Clinical Global Impression Scale; CHLOR, chlorpromazine; CLOZ, clozapine; CMAI, Cohen-Mansfield Agitation Inventory; CPT, Continuous Performance Test (measure of attention); DIS, disorganized thoughts; Dx, diagnosis; EPS, extrapyramidal symptoms; FLU, fluphenazine; HAL, haloperidol; Ham-D, Hamilton Depression Scale; MADRS, Montgomery-Asberg Depression Rating Scale; NEG, negative; OLZ, olanzapine; PANSS, Positive and Negative Syndrome Scale; PBO, placebo; POS, positive; PPCT, PANSS Psychosis Core Total; QLS, Heinrichs-Carpenter Quality of Life Scale; QOL, World Health Organization Quality of Life questionnaire; RIS, risperidone; SAS, Simpson-Angus Scale; SF-36, medical outcomes study 36-item short form; SVLT, Serial Verbal Learning Test (measure of memory); THIO, thioridazine; TMT-A, Trail Making Test, part A, visuomotor speed (measure of attention); TMT-B, Trail Making Test, part B, visuomotor speed and the ability to alternate between sets (measure of executive function); TYP, typical or conventional antipsychotics; VA, Veterans Affairs; VFE, verbal fluency examination; WCST, Wisconsin Card Sorting Test (measure of executive function).

Open-label RCTs [28,29], quasi-experimental studies [30,31], and large prospective single-agent trials [32,33] of antipsychotic treatment for older adults who had schizophrenia are shown in Table 2. These studies help to further establish the evidence base for antipsychotic treatment in this population. The open-label RCTs have indicated that olanzapine and risperidone were associated with less parkinsonism and a greater improvement in negative and depressive symptoms after crossover from conventional antipsychotics [29], and olanzapine was associated with a greater improvement than haloperidol in reducing Positive and Negative Syndrome Scale (PANSS [37]) total scores, negative symptoms, and the clinical global severity of disease [28]. A prospective quasi-experimental study found no difference in symptom improvement between a large sample receiving olanzapine and a smaller sample receiving either risperidone or a conventional antipsychotic [31]. A retrospective quasi-experimental study has indicated that risperidone had fewer side effects and was more effective in improving PANSS total scores, positive symptoms, and clinical global severity, compared with conventional antipsychotics [30]. In addition, two large prospective single-agent studies of risperidone have indicated that it was associated with improved positive and negative symptoms as well as improved clinical global impression [32,33]. This set of studies should be interpreted with caution because of a variety of study characteristics, including the lack of blinded evaluation [28–33], small sample sizes [28–30], a lack of randomization [30,31], the retrospective nature of the evaluation [30], and the absence of a comparison group [32,33].

In addition to the literature reviewed above, several small single-agent open-label studies have evaluated the use of aripiprazole [38], clozapine [39,40], fenfluramine [41], haloperidol [42], olanzapine [43,44], quetiapine [45,46], risperidone [47–49], and thiothixene [50] in older adults who have schizophrenia. Moreover, several studies have examined clozapine [51–56], haloperidol [57], olanzapine [58–60], quetiapine [61–63], risperidone [59,60,64–66], and thioridazine [57] in heterogeneous samples that included older adults who had schizophrenia.

Dosing of antipsychotic agents

Generally, the dosing of antipsychotic agents in the studies that met inclusion criteria for this review began at low levels and then increased to a targeted level. Mean olanzapine dosages were similar across studies (9.9–13.1 mg/d) [25–29,31]. Mean risperidone dosages were similar in the three RCTs (1.7–2.0 mg/d) [26,27,29] but were higher in nonrandomized studies (2.3–4.2 mg/d) [31–33,67]. Among the studies evaluating the effectiveness of haloperidol, mean dosages ranged from 7.2 to 9.4 mg/d [25,28]. Finally, mean antipsychotic dosages for those agents that were evaluated in only one of the reviewed studies included clozapine at 300 mg/d [24], chlorpromazine at 600 mg/d [24], fluphenazine at 285 mg/d [22], and thioridazine at 5 mg/d [22].

Table 2
Open-label RCTs, quasi-experimental studies, and large prospective Studies (n ≥ 100) of antipsychotic medications in older adults with schizophrenia

Study	Study design	Agent	Sample	Follow-up	Outcome measures and results	Limitations and comments
Open-label RCT						
Barak et al 2002 [28]	Open-label RCT; OLZ: n = 10 HAL: n = 10	OLZ, mean dose 13.1 mg/d (range 5.0–25.0 mg/d); HAL mean dose 7.2 mg/d	Age 69.2 (±6.1); female 50%; Dx, schizophrenia and PANSS ≥ 50	≥3 mo; mean duration 15 ± 8 mo; Discontinued: OLZ, 40% (3 no response, 1 administrative); HAL, 40% (1 no response, 3 EPS)	OLZ, decrease in PANSS total and negative scores; HAL, no change in PANSS subscales or CGI; OLZ superior to HAL in reducing PANSS total and negative scores and CGI; No between-group differences on PANSS positive and general subscales	Small sample sizes; evaluators not blind to treatment; OLZ had fewer EPS than HAL; mean weight increase in both groups

| Ritchie et al 2003 [29] | Open-label RCT; crossover from TYP; OLZ: n = 34 RIS: n = 32 | Started switch at 5 mg/d OLZ or 0.5 mg/d RIS; after switch, OLZ mean dose 9.9 mg/d; RIS mean dose 1.7 mg/d | Age 69.6 (± 6.2); female 71.2%; Dx, schizophrenia | Switch completed after 4 weeks, plus 2 consecutive visits on same dose and no TYP; mean length to crossover: OLZ, 40.6 d; RIS, 40.4 d; Early treatment failures (death, side effects, non-compliance, marked deterioration, protocol violation) OLZ, 11.8%, RIS, 31.2% | BPRS, SANS, and MADRS scores improved during crossover in both groups; no between-group differences; OLZ, improved QOL on psychologic, physical well-being, and perceived health status; RIS, no effect on QOL; OLZ better than RIS on psychologic domain on QOL; switching from TYP to RIS or OLZ both associated with improved parkinsonism, and OLZ alone associated with reduced dyskinetic symptoms | Small sample sizes; evaluators not blind to treatment; both had improved parkinsonism; OLZ had reduction in dyskinetic symptoms |

(continued on next page)

Table 2 (*continued*)

Study	Study design	Agent	Sample	Follow-up	Outcome measures and results	Limitations and comments
Quasi-experimental studies						
Barak, et al 2002 [30]	Retrospective quasi-experimental; RIS: n = 26; TYP: n = 25	RIS mean dose 2.3 mg/d; TYP mean dose 280.7 mg/d chlorpromazine equivalents (36% of TYP sample received HAL)	Inpatients: age 72.7 (5.9); female 59%; Dx, schizophrenia/ schizoaffective and PANSS ≥ 55	6 and 18 months; Discontinuation: RIS, 19% (n = 1 EPS, n = 2 lack of efficacy, n = 2 treatment no longer needed); TYP, 12% (n = 3, severe EPS)	CGI and PANSS total improved in both groups at 6 and 18 mo; RIS, PANSS POS, NEG, GEN subscales improved at 6 and 18 mo; TYP, PANSS POS subscale improved at 6 and 18 mo; RIS improved more than TYP in PANSS positive and total score and CGI; clinical improvement (CGI ≤ 3) for 58% RIS and 29% TYP; no differences in weight gain	No randomization; no washout period; retrospective evaluation; evaluators not blind to treatment; more frequent side effects in TYP (64%) vs RIS (15%); Benzodiaz-epines more frequent with RIS; anti-parkinsonian meds more frequent in TYP
Ciudad et al 2004 [31]	Prospective quasi-experimental; OLZ: n = 105; RIS/TYP: n = 30	OLZ mean dose 11.7 mg/d OTHER: RIS (n = 15, mean dose 4.2 mg/d) and TYP (n = 15, mean dose not stated)	OLZ: age 65.8 (± 5.9); female 63.8% RIS/TYP: age 65.6 (± 5.3); female 46.7%; Dx, schizophrenia	6 mo; Discontinuation: OLZ, 16%, RIS/TYP, 13%	No differences between OLZ and RIS/TYP in CGI, GAF, EQ-5D, and Awad scores	No randomization; evaluators not blind to treatment; Safety, RIS/TYP more likely to have adverse event than OLZ (72% vs 58%)

Open-label prospective

Study	Design	Dose	Population	Duration/Discontinuation	Results	Comments
Madhusoodanan et al 1999 [32]	Prospective open-label, multicenter; RIS: n = 103	RIS: Mean dose 2.4 mg/d; most patients (73%) received a mean dose ≤ 3 mg/d	Inpatients; age 71 (±5.4); female: 49.5%; Dx, schizophrenia/schizoaffective	12-wk study; Discontinuation (25%): adverse events (11), patient choice to discontinue (7), administrative reasons or inadequate response (8)	BPRS and PANSS total and POS, NEG, GEN subscales were improved; clinical improvement, 45% were improved according to criteria of ≥20% reduction in PANSS total and a CGI score ≥3	No control group; short washout period; high use of concurrent meds; Safety, ESRS scores reduced; no changes in labs, vitals, or EKG
Davidson et al 2000 [33]	Prospective open-label, multicenter; RIS: n = 180	RIS: mean dose 3.7 mg/d	Mean age 73; female 62%; Dx, schizophrenia/schizoaffective and PANSS 60–120	12-mo; Discontinuation (46%): adverse event (n = 30); insufficient response (n = 26)	Improvement on PANSS total and POS, NEG, and GEN subscales and cognition cluster scores; PANSS clinical improvement achieved by 54% at endpoint; CGI clinical improvement achieved by 59% at endpoint	No control group; Safety, 22% of patients had EPS-like adverse events; no significant weight gain [67]

Abbreviations: Awad, 10-item scale used to evaluate patients attitude toward medication; BPRS, Brief Psychiatric Rating Scale; CGI, Clinical Global Impression Scale; Dx, diagnosis; EPS, Extrapyramidal symptoms; EQ-5D, European Quality of Life questionnaire; GAF, Global Assessment of Functioning scale; GEN, general; HAL, haloperidol; MADRS, Montgomery-Asberg Depression Rating Scale; NEG, negative; OLZ, olanzapine; PANSS, Positive and Negative Syndrome Scale; POS, positive; QOL, World Health Organization Quality of Life questionnaire; RIS, risperidone; TYP, Typical or conventional antipsychotics.

Augmentation studies

Table 3 describes two RCTs of antidepressant augmentation of antipsychotic agents. The first double-blind, placebo-controlled study has indicated that mianserin and trazodone were associated with improved affective flattening and alogia [34]. In addition, a single-blind RCT of citalopram augmentation has suggested improvements in depression and clinical global impression [35]. Both studies had small sample sizes [34,35], and one study was conducted only among male Veterans Affairs patients [35]. Two recent small pilot studies have evaluated augmentation therapy with donepezil (N = 6) [68] and rivastigmine (N = 13) [69] among persons who had chronic schizophrenia and comorbid dementia and found improvements in cognitive functioning.

Pharmaceutical company support

Of note, all but three of the fourteen pharmacologic studies meeting inclusion criteria were supported by funding from pharmaceutical companies. The studies without pharmaceutical support included the RCT of clozapine and chlorpromazine [24] and the two augmentation studies of antidepressant agents [34,35]. Pharmaceutical support should be considered in evaluating studies because of the potential for conflicts of interest associated with the study design, data analysis, and publication bias [70].

Nonpharmacologic interventions: identification of studies

Among the five evaluations of nonpharmacologic interventions, two studies described results of RCTs [71,72], two studies reported on quasi-experimental studies [73,74], and one study reported on a noncontrolled prospective cohort study [75]. Three promising psychosocial interventions for older adults who had schizophrenia and other psychotic disorders have been developed and described within these reports. These interventions included a combined skills training and cognitive behavioral treatment for middle-aged and older adults who had schizophrenia [71,72,75]; a social skills training program for middle-aged and older adults who had chronic psychotic disorders [73]; and a combined skills training and health management intervention for community-dwelling older adults who had serious mental illness [74]. Each represents a manualized intervention with prospective outcome data. These models are summarized in Table 4.

The modular Cognitive Behavioral Social Skills Training (CBSST) program, consisting of group training in cognitive restructuring and illness self-management skills, was used throughout the program to challenge patients' convictions regarding delusional beliefs and to explore the resistance to treatment recommendations, including medication nonadherence and homework noncompliance. McQuaid and colleagues [75] have described

Table 3
Randomized trials of other psychoactive medications in older adults with schizophrenia

Study	Study design	Agent	Sample	Follow-up	Outcome measures and results	Limitations and comments
Hayashi et al 1997 [34]	Double-blind, RCT; augmentation with MIA, n = 13; TRZ, n = 13; PBO, n = 13	MIA mean dose 58.5 mg/d; TRZ mean dose 192.3 mg/d	Age 62.7; female 39.5%; Dx, schizophrenia with moderate to severe negative symptoms, based on PANSS	5 wk; Discontinued: MIA, 0%; TRZ, 8% (n = 1) for agitation; PBO, 0%	MIA and TRZ improved in affective flattening and blunting and alogia; MIA, SANS total decreased; No differences between MIA and TRZ on SANS scores; TRZ, improved AIMS score; no change in BPRS total, POS factor, or ANX/DEP factor	No severe side effects caused by MIA or TRZ; small sample size; augmentation in addition to a range of conventional antipsychotics
Kasckow et al 2001 [35]	Single-blind RCT; CIT, n = 9; No CIT, n = 10	CIT augmentation starting dose, 20 mg/d; maximal dose did not exceed 40 mg/d	Male veterans; CIT: age, 65.4 (±12.7) No CIT: age, 59.2 (±8.2) Dx, chronic schizophrenia and PANSS ≥ 45, Ham-D ≥ 12	10 wk; Discontinued: CIT, 0%; No CIT, 20%	PANSS total, Ham-D, and CGI improved in both groups; CIT improved more than No CIT in Ham-D and CGI; no change in MMSE	Small sample size; mean dose not reported; no major adverse events; No CIT group did not receive a placebo pill; augmentation to conventional and atypical antipsychotics

Abbreviations: AIMS, abnormal Involuntary Movement Scale; ANX/DEP, anxiety and depression; BPRS, Brief Psychiatric Rating Scale; CGI, Clinical Global Impression Scale; CIT, citalopram augmentation; Dx, diagnosis; Ham-D, Hamilton Depression Scale; MIA, mianserin; MMSE, mini-mental state examination; PANSS, Positive and Negative Syndrome Scale; PBO, placebo; SANS, scale for the Assessment of Negative Symptoms; TRZ, trazodone.

Table 4
Psychosocial interventions in older adults with schizophrenia

Study	Study design	Model and conditions	Sample	Follow-up	Outcome measures and results	Limitations and comments
McQuaid et al 2000 [75]	Non-controlled, prospective cohort, n = 9	CBSST (12 wk)	Age 62.6 (±8.7); female 22%; Dx, 100% schizophrenia	3 mo; 1 dropped out before groups began	Good attendance and compliance with homework	Small sample size; only 1 assessment tool administered; no data presented on the assessment tool (3-item self-report measure); mostly male participants
Granholm et al 2002 [71]	Single-blind RCT, CBSST, n = 8; TAU, n = 7	CBSST (12 wk) vs TAU	CBSST: age 55.0 (±5.9); female 12.5%; Dx, 100% schizophrenia TAU: age 56.3 (±7.7); female 14.3%; Dx, 100% schizophrenia	3 mo; retention rate not specifically mentioned	Greater reduction in positive and depressive symptoms for CBSST; greater reduction in negative symptoms for TAU	Small sample size; no between-group differences are significant; no age ranges provided; no functional impairment inclusion criterion; mostly male subjects
Patterson et al 2003 [73]	Quasi-experimental, 2 FAST sites, n = 16; 2 TAU sites, n = 16	Skills training (24 wk) in social skills and illness self-management (FAST) vs TAU	FAST: age 47.9 (±5.3); female 31%; Dx, 81% schizophrenia TAU: age 51.7 (±8.5); female 31%; Dx, 69% schizophrenia	9 mo; 20% dropped out after baseline assessment	Greater improvement for FAST in independent living skills and negative symptoms (PANSS); no changes in positive symptoms or quality of well being	Small sample size; no measurement of social functioning; includes patients in their 40s; no functional impairment inclusion criterion

| Bartels et al 2004 [74] | Quasi-experimental, ST+HM, n = 12; HM only, n = 12 | Skills training in illness self-management and ST + assistance from a nurse (HM) vs HM only for 12 mo | ST+HM: age: 65 (±4.6); female 75%; Dx, 66% schizophrenia; TAU: age 67.9 (±6.4); female 67%; Dx, 66% schizophrenia | ST+HM vs HM (n = 12 vs n = 12) 12 mo; HM (n = 24) 24 mo | Greater improvement for ST+HM in independent living skills and social functioning; HM resulted in identification of previously undetected medical conditions and greater receipt of preventive health care | Small sample size; no TAU comparison; HM only were dropouts from ST+HM; mostly female subjects |
| Granholm et al 2005 [72] | Single-blind RCT, CBSST, n = 37; TAU, n = 39 | Cognitive behavioral therapy + skills training (24 wk) in illness self-management (CBSST) vs TAU | CBSST: age 54.5 (±7.0); female 30%; Dx, 100% schizophrenia TAU: age 53.1 (±7.5); female 23%; Dx, 100% schizophrenia | 6 mo; 86% retention | Greater improvement for CBSST in cognitive insight (Beck Cognitive Insight Scale), mastery of skills (Comprehensive Module Test), and leisure skills (Independent Living Skills Survey) | Includes patients in their 40s; No measurement of social functioning; no follow-up beyond post-treatment; no functional impairment inclusion criterion; measure of skill acquisition represents teaching to the task; mostly male subjects |

Abbreviations: CBSST, cognitive behavioral therapy plus social skills training; Dx, diagnosis; FAST, Functional Adaptation Skills Training; HM, health management; PANSS, Positive and Negative Syndrome Scale; ST, skills training; TAU, treatment as usual.

an early evaluation of the CBSST intervention. This noncontrolled, prospective cohort study included only nine participants but established the feasibility of recruiting older adults who have schizophrenia to consistently attend the group sessions and actively participate in activities both in and out of the group setting [75]. An early pilot RCT of the CBSST intervention included 15 participants [71]. Although functional outcomes were not reported in this trial, the authors have noted greater reductions in positive and depressive symptoms for the CBSST group compared with the usual care group. More recently, Granholm and colleagues [72] conducted a randomized, controlled trial of the CBSST program that included 76 outpatients who had schizophrenia or schizoaffective disorder ranging in age from 42 to 74 years old. One half of the patients were randomly assigned to receive CBSST and the other half to care as usual. The authors have reported significant improvements in the CBSST group compared with the care as usual group in "social functioning," cognitive insight (insight about beliefs), and performance on a comprehensive module test but no improvements for either group in symptoms, number of hospitalizations, or living skills.

Two quasi-experimental studies of skills training interventions have been conducted by Patterson and colleagues [73], who have described an evaluation of the Functional Adaptation Skills Training (FAST) program, a 24-week modular skills training intervention to improve community functioning in middle-aged and older adults who have chronic psychotic disorders. The FAST intervention includes modules related to medication self-management, social skills, communication skills, organization and planning, transportation, and financial management. Four board-and-care homes were randomly assigned to serve as either intervention or usual care research sites. A total of 32 board-and-care residents aged 42 to 69 years participated in the trial. Positive findings from this study included significantly greater improvement in community functioning skills for the FAST group compared with the care as usual group, both at post-treatment and at 3-month follow-up [73]. There were no significant differences between the groups in the improvement of psychiatric symptoms.

Bartels and colleagues [74] have reported on an evaluation of the Skills Training and Health Management (ST+HM) intervention, which was developed for older adults who have serious mental illness, with the aim of enhancing independent functioning and health care outcomes [74]. A pilot study of the ST+HM intervention included 24 outpatients over the age of 60, of whom two thirds had schizophrenia or schizoaffective disorder and one third had bipolar disorder. Half of the sample received weekly ST focusing on medication self-management and social skills plus assistance from a nurse with accessing preventive and chronic medical care (HM) for 1 year, whereas the other half received HM alone for 1 year. A greater improvement in independent living skills was obtained for individuals who received ST+HM compared with individuals who received only HM. Medium to large effect sizes were found for individuals who received ST+HM compared with

HM alone in several specific skill areas, including self care and health management skills. Compared with those who received HM alone, older adults who received ST+HM also demonstrated a significant improvement in social functioning. Positive findings from the HM component, which all participants received, included the identification of several previously undetected medical conditions in approximately one third of the sample and improvement in the receipt of preventive health care services. An adaptation of the ST+HM model is currently being evaluated in a multisite RCT [76].

Discussion

This review identified 14 studies of pharmacologic trials and five studies of three nonpharmacologic interventions that were evaluated among older adults who had schizophrenia. Published data from RCTs support the effectiveness of antipsychotic medications in the treatment of schizophrenia in older adults, although only modest differences exist between individual antipsychotic agents in effectiveness. Overall, the studies comparing atypical and conventional antipsychotics found modest advantages favoring the effectiveness and lower incidence of parkinsonism for atypical antipsychotics, although similar rates of discontinuation have been reported. The three RCTs comparing the effectiveness of atypical and conventional antipsychotics included two studies that found modest advantages of atypical antipsychotics over conventional antipsychotics [25,28] and one study that found no differences [24]. In addition, less parkinsonism was associated with risperidone and olanzapine compared with conventional antipsychotics [29]. In contrast, no consistent differences were found in the effectiveness and incidence of side effects in an RCT comparing two different atypical antipsychotics. A comparison of risperidone and olanzapine did not detect significant differences in effectiveness in improving psychotic symptoms [26] or cognitive outcomes [27]. In addition to the findings supporting the effectiveness of pharmacologic interventions, a limited literature suggests that nonpharmacologic interventions, particularly skills training, hold promise for enhancing skills required for community functioning.

The largest RCT comparing the effectiveness of two different atypical antipsychotic agents in the treatment of older adults who had schizophrenia includes separate reports on symptom outcomes by Jeste and colleagues [26] and cognitive outcomes by Harvey and colleagues [27]. The 8-week double-blind study randomly assigned 175 persons who had schizophrenia or schizoaffective disorder (ages 60 and older) to receive olanzapine or risperidone. Similar improvements in positive symptoms, negative symptoms, disorganized thoughts, and affective symptoms were found for both groups. Clinical global impression scores also improved in both groups [26]. Evidence for the improvement of attention and memory was obtained for both groups; however, executive function and verbal fluency improved only in the group receiving risperidone [27]. No change was found in uncontrolled hostility or excitement on the PANSS.

Among the small group of studies that have specifically examined the effectiveness of antipsychotic medications in older adults who had schizophrenia, findings on effective dosages provide some guidance to practicing clinicians. Generally, dosages for older adults who have schizophrenia are approximately twice those recommended in the treatment of older persons who have behavioral symptoms of dementia [77,78]. For example, dosages of approximately 2 mg/d for risperidone and 10 mg/d for olanzapine in older adults who have schizophrenia are twice those reported to be useful in dementia patients (1 mg/d for risperidone and 5 mg/d for olanzapine).

There is no compelling evidence supporting an advantage of any one antipsychotic agent or class of antipsychotic agents over another with respect to discontinuation rates. These rates varied widely across different studies and interventions. Among the pharmacologic studies, 19% to 46% of persons receiving risperidone discontinued treatment before the end of the study [26,27,29,30,32,33]; 12% to 40% of persons receiving olanzapine discontinued treatment before the end of the study [25–29,31]; and 27% to 47% of persons receiving haloperidol discontinued treatment before study completion [23,28]. Among nonpharmacologic studies, dropout rates were only 10% to 20%. However, retention rates for all of these studies should be considered with caution because of small sample sizes and large variations in study duration (6 weeks to 1 year).

There are a small number of differences with respect to the overall incidence of significant side effects between different agents. For example, olanzapine, risperidone, and haloperidol have been associated with weight gain in older adults who have schizophrenia [26,28], although weight gain is most pronounced among patients receiving olanzapine. The study by Jeste and colleagues [26] has noted that clinically relevant weight gain ($\geq 7\%$) was three times more common among persons receiving olanzapine compared with risperidone, and an open-label study has found no weight gain associated with use of risperidone over 1 year for 127 older persons who had schizophrenia [67]. The US Food and Drug Administration (FDA) has recently issued a warning regarding the association between atypical antipsychotics and the risk for weight gain and diabetes [79,80]. American Diabetes Association and American Psychiatric Association (ADA/APA) guidelines identify different levels of risk of these two adverse effects associated with different atypical antipsychotic agents, with clozapine and olanzapine having the highest risk, followed by quetiapine and risperidone. Aripiprazole and ziprasidone reportedly have the lowest risk, although the data on these two drugs are limited [81].

The only study comparing clozapine (n = 24) to a conventional antipsychotic (n = 18; chlorpromazine augmented with benzotropine) has found no difference in terms of safety or efficacy over a 3-month period, although both agents were associated with significant hematologic events [24]. Although there were no differences with respect to positive and negative symptoms and global clinical severity, the discontinuation rate was higher in persons receiving chlorpromazine (39% versus 13%). Of note, 33% (8/24) of the patients who received clozapine and 44% (8/18) of those who received chlorpromazine developed hematologic abnormalities [24]. This finding reinforces the need to monitor white blood cell counts for persons receiving these agents. The risk for clozapine-associated agranulocytosis is heightened among older adults (compared with younger adults) and should be closely monitored [55,82]. No other studies have compared clozapine to other agents in this population. One small case study of clozapine use in five older persons who had schizophrenia found improvements in symptoms but also identified substantial side effects, including agranulocytosis, sedation, orthostasis, and worsening of congestive heart failure [40].

To date, there have been no aggregate analyses of serious adverse events, including mortality across multiple studies of atypical antipsychotics in older persons who had schizophrenia. Of note, the FDA has recently issued a warning regarding the use of all atypical antipsychotic agents in older adults who have dementia. Fifteen of seventeen placebo-controlled studies of olanzapine, risperidone, quetiapine, and aripiprazole have shown numerical increases in mortality, compared with placebo, for older adults who had behavioral disorders of dementia. These studies involved 5106 patients and identified mortality rates of 4.5% among patients who received atypical antipsychotics, compared with 2.6% among those who received placebo ($P < .05$). These data demonstrate a 1.6 to 1.7 fold increase in mortality, most commonly caused by cardiovascular events or infections such as pneumonia [83,84]. Because these studies were almost entirely populated by elderly persons (including many with psychotic symptoms), a systematic evaluation of serious adverse events in older adults who have schizophrenia receiving atypical antipsychotics is indicated.

The current findings on augmentation therapy are suggestive but not definitive with respect to the potential benefits of adding antidepressants or cholinesterase inhibitors to antipsychotic medications. For example, Hayashi and colleagues [34] have found that trazodone and mianserin were associated with a reduction in negative symptoms (affective flattening or blunting and alogia). Trazodone was also associated with decreased EPS. However, neither treatment was associated with an improvement in psychotic symptoms or affective symptoms [34]. In contrast, Kasckow and colleagues [35] have reported that older adults receiving citalopram augmentation had significantly greater improvement in depressive symptoms and clinical global severity, compared with a control group. Augmentation with cholinesterase inhibitors was evaluated in two small case series of patients who had schizophrenia and comorbid dementia [68,69]. Stryer and colleagues [68] conducted a 4-week single-blind administration of donepezil (5 mg/d) augmentation for six patients. Significant improvements were seen in cognitive impairment and Clinical Global Impression Scale scores. Similarly, Mendelsohn and colleagues [69] conducted a 12-week open-label examination of 13 patients who received rivastigmine augmentation (9 mg/d). Improvements were seen in cognitive impairment, activities of daily living, and negative symptoms. These open-label studies give preliminary evidence supporting cholinesterase inhibitors in improving cognitive symptoms among persons who have comorbid dementia and schizophrenia. In addition, as shown by the RCT conducted by Harvey and colleagues [27], olanzapine and risperidone may also positively affect cognitive functioning in some older persons who have schizophrenia. At this stage, however, the value of these drugs in improving cognition in schizophrenia is unclear.

There are several limitations to the evidence base for the pharmacologic treatment of older adults who have schizophrenia. First, there are few well-designed head-to-head comparisons of antipsychotic agents or psychosocial interventions. Second, to our knowledge, no studies have evaluated the cost effectiveness of any treatment modality for older adults who have schizophrenia. Third, only five of 14 studies have evaluated long-term effects (≥ 3 months), tolerability, or safety of pharmacologic interventions [23,28,30,31,33]. In contrast, psychosocial interventions have been evaluated over a period of 3 months to 1 year [71–75]. This difference is, in part, associated with the progressive learning approach used in the skills training interventions. Fourth, clinical trials of antipsychotic medications among older adults who had schizophrenia have often been limited by small sample sizes and inadequate control over doses, duration of treatment, and concomitant medications. Finally, little is known about the effectiveness or safety of newer antipsychotics such as quetiapine, ziprasidone, or aripiprazole among older adults who have schizophrenia or schizoaffective disorder. Quetiapine was approved for use among persons who have schizophrenia by the FDA in 1997, but limited research has evaluated its effectiveness and safety among older adults. One small pilot study has evaluated quetiapine among six older persons (ages 61–72) who had schizophrenia or schizoaffective disorder [45]. Three patients experienced reductions in positive and negative symptoms. Pre-existing EPS decreased in three of five persons; transient hypotension, dizziness, and somnolence developed in two patients; and patient weight increased by an average of 2 pounds [45]. A larger mixed-sample study (N = 151) has evaluated the effectiveness of quetiapine in older adults who had psychotic disorders. This study focused on older individuals with Alzheimer's and Parkinson's disease but did not specifically report outcomes on the smaller sample with schizophrenia (N = 33) [46]. Aripiprazole (approved by the FDA in 2002) has been evaluated in a recent case study of 10 hospitalized older adults who had schizophrenia or schizoaffective disorder (ages 62–85). Seven of 10 patients responded to aripiprazole and showed improvements in positive and negative symptoms as well as global clinical impression. Pre-existing EPS decreased in three of four patients, and four of 10 patients developed postural hypotension that resolved over time. Six of the 10 patients lost an average of 5.25 pounds, although one patient gained 18 pounds [38]. This preliminary evidence suggests that quetiapine and aripiprazole may be similar to other atypical antipsychotics in effectiveness and safety among older adults who have schizophrenia and schizoaffective disorder. To our knowledge, there are no published reports on the effectiveness or safety of ziprasidone (approved by the FDA in 2001) in the treatment of older adults who have schizophrenia. Further evaluation of these agents is warranted.

Compared with pharmacologic trials, the evaluation of psychosocial interventions for older persons who have schizophrenia has been even more limited. Several interventions have been developed that have been specifically tailored to improve functioning in aging individuals with schizophrenia. These interventions have been manualized and delivered in community settings with mental health consumers. The interventions were well tolerated, had low dropout rates, and were associated with positive outcomes. Nevertheless, several caveats are in order. First, sample sizes in the evaluations of these interventions were very small, in which four of the five studies included fewer than 35 participants [71,73–75]. Second, four of the five studies described interventions for "middle-aged and older adults" and included individuals as young as age 42 [71–73,75]. Finally, two of the five studies included diagnoses other than schizophrenia [73,74]. Although a majority of these samples consisted of persons who had schizophrenia, subanalyses of individuals with schizophrenia alone were not conducted. Overall, it is likely that older adults can tolerate psychosocial interventions and benefit from them, although larger randomized trials are needed to establish effectiveness.

This review examines the evidence base for pharmacologic and nonpharmacologic interventions that have been evaluated among older adults who have schizophrenia. Because of age-related differences in medical comorbidity, stressors, cognitive function, and other factors, pharmacologic and psychosocial interventions for older adults who have schizophrenia are different from those used for treating younger adults. Although several database studies support the use of medications and psychosocial interventions to improve the psychiatric symptoms and functioning of older persons who have schizophrenia, to date there has been a lack of rigorous evaluation for many of the newer antipsychotic agents, and few nonpharmacologic interventions have been developed or evaluated. Furthermore, many of the published reports have methodological limitations and potential difficulties with generalizability. Despite these limitations, this review identifies the evidence base for both classes of interventions and shows that older adults can improve with pharmacologic and psychosocial interventions. Further research conducted through well-designed studies is needed to identify optimal treatments for different subgroups of older persons who have schizophrenia.

References

[1] Jeste DV, Twamley EW, Eyler Zorrilla LT, et al. Aging and outcome in schizophrenia. Acta Psychiatr Scand 2003;107(5):336–43.

[2] Harris MJ, Jeste DV. Late-onset schizophrenia: an overview. Schizophr Bull 1988;14(1): 39–55.

[3] Bartels SJ, Mueser KT, Miles KM. Functional impairments in elderly patients with schizophrenia and major affective illness in the community: social skills, living skills, and behavior problems. Behav Ther 1997;28(1):43–63.

[4] Bartels SJ. Caring for the whole person: integrated health care for older adults with severe mental illness and medical comorbidity. J Am Geriatr Soc 2004;52(12):S249–57.

[5] Jeste DV, Gladsjo JA, Lindamer LA, et al. Medical comorbidity in schizophrenia. Schizophr Bull 1996;22(3):413–30.

[6] Bartels SJ, Clark RE, Peacock WJ, et al. Medicare and Medicaid costs for schizophrenia patients by age cohort compared with depression, dementia, and medically ill patients. Am J Geriatr Psychiatry 2003;11(6):648–57.

[7] United States Census Bureau. US interim projections by age, sex, race, and Hispanic origin: table 2a. projected population of the united states, by age and sex: 2000 to 2050. Aug 26, 2004. Available at: http://www.census.gov/ipc/www/usinterimproj/. Accessed May 16, 2005.

[8] Jeste DV, Alexopoulos GS, Bartels SJ, et al. Consensus statement on the upcoming crisis in geriatric mental health: research agenda for the next 2 decades. Arch Gen Psychiatry 1999; 56(9):848–53.

[9] Narrow WE, Rae DS, Robins LN, et al. Revised prevalence estimates of mental disorders in the United States: using a clinical significance criterion to reconcile 2 survey's estimates. Arch Gen Psychiatry 2002;59(2):115–23.

[10] Lehman AF, Buchanan RW, Dickerson FB, et al. Evidence-based treatment for schizophrenia. Psychiatr Clin North Am 2003;26(4):939–54.

[11] Camprubi M, Dratcu L. Evidence-based management of schizophrenia. Hosp Med 2004; 65(4):201–5.

[12] Emsley R, Oosthuizen P. Evidence-based pharmacotherapy of schizophrenia. Int J Neuropsychopharmacol 2004;7(2):219–38.

[13] Margison F. Evidence-based medicine in the psychological treatment of schizophrenia. J Am Acad Psychoanal Dyn Psychiatry 2003;31(1):177–90.

[14] Drake RE, Mueser KT, Torrey WC, et al. Evidence-based treatment of schizophrenia. Curr Psychiatry Rep 2000;2(5):393–7.

[15] Arunpongpaisal S, Ahmed I, Aqeel N, et al. Antipsychotic drug treatment for elderly people with late-onset schizophrenia. Cochrane Database Syst Rev 2003;2:CD004162.

[16] Phanjoo AL, Link C. Remoxipride versus thioridazine in elderly psychotic patients. Acta Psychiatr Scand 1990;82(Suppl 358):S181–5.

[17] Tune LE, Salzman C. Schizophrenia in late life. Psychiatr Clin North Am 2003;26(1):103–13.

[18] Sable JA, Jeste DV. Antipsychotic treatment for late-life schizophrenia. Curr Psychiatry Rep 2002;4(4):299–306.

[19] Salzman C, Tune L. Neuroleptic treatment of late-life schizophrenia. Harv Rev Psychiatry 2001;9(2):77–83.

[20] Banerjee S, Dickinson E. Evidence based health care in old age psychiatry. Int J Psychiatry Med 1997;27(3):283–92.

[21] Jeste DV, Rockwell E, Harris MJ, et al. Conventional vs. newer antipsychotics in elderly patients. Am J Geriatr Psychiatry 1999;7(1):70–6.

[22] Branchey MH, Lee JH, Amin R, et al. High- and low-potency neuroleptics in elderly psychiatric patients. JAMA 1978;239(18):1860–2.

[23] Ruskin PE, Nyman G. Discontinuation of neuroleptic medication in older, outpatient schizophrenics: a placebo-controlled, double-blind trial. J Nerv Ment Dis 1991;179(4):212–4.

[24] Howanitz E, Pardo M, Smelson DA, et al. The efficacy and safety of clozapine versus chlorpromazine in geriatric schizophrenia. J Clin Psychiatry 1999;60(1):41–4.

[25] Kennedy JS, Jeste D, Kaiser CJ, et al. Olanzapine vs haloperidol in geriatric schizophrenia: analysis of data from a double-blind controlled trial. Int J Geriatr Psychiatry 2003;18(11): 1013–20.

[26] Jeste DV, Barak Y, Madhusoodanan S, Grossman F, et al. International multisite double-blind trial of the atypical antipsychotics risperidone and olanzapine in 175 elderly patients with chronic schizophrenia. Am J Geriatr Psychiatry 2003;11(6):638–47 [erratum appears in: Am J Geriatr Psychiatry. 2004;12(1):49].

[27] Harvey PD, Napolitano JA, Mao L, et al. Comparative effects of risperidone and olanzapine on cognition in elderly patients with schizophrenia or schizoaffective disorder. Int J Geriatr Psychiatry 2003;18(9):820–9.

[28] Barak Y, Shamir E, Zemishlani H, et al. Olanzapine vs. haloperidol in the treatment of elderly chronic schizophrenia patients. Prog Neuropsychopharmacol Biol Psychiatry 2002; 26(6):1199–202.

[29] Ritchie CW, Chiu E, Harrigan S, et al. The impact upon extra-pyramidal side effects, clinical symptoms and quality of life of a switch from conventional to atypical antipsychotics (risperidone or olanzapine) in elderly patients with schizophrenia. Int J Geriatr Psychiatry 2003; 18(5):432–40.

[30] Barak Y, Shamir E, Weizman R. Would a switch from typical antipsychotics to risperidone be beneficial for elderly schizophrenic patients? a naturalistic, long-term, retrospective, comparative study. J Clin Psychopharmacol 2002;22(2):115–20.

[31] Ciudad A, Montes JM, Olivares JM, et al. Safety and tolerability of olanzapine compared with other antipsychotics in the treatment of elderly patients with schizophrenia: a naturalistic study. Eur Psychiatry 2004;19(6):358–65.

[32] Madhusoodanan S, Brecher M, Brenner R, et al. Risperidone in the treatment of elderly patients with psychotic disorders. Am J Geriatr Psychiatry 1999;7(2):132–8.

[33] Davidson M, Harvey PD, Vervarcke J, et al on behalf of the Risperidone Working Group. A long-term, multicenter, open-label study of risperidone in elderly patients with psychosis. Int J Geriatr Psychiatry 2000;15(6):506–14.

[34] Hayashi T, Yokota N, Takahashi T, et al. Benefits of trazodone and mianserin for patients with late-life chronic schizophrenia and tardive dyskinesia: an add-on, double-blind, placebo-controlled study. Int Clin Psychopharmacol 1997;12(4):199–205.

[35] Kasckow JW, Mohamed S, Thallasinos A, et al. Citalopram augmentation of antipsychotic treatment in older schizophrenia patients. Int J Geriatr Psychiatry 2001;16(12):1163–7.

[36] Friedman MA, Woodcock J, Lumpkin MM, et al. The safety of newly approved medicines: do recent market removals mean there is a problem? JAMA 1999;281(18):1728–34.

[37] Kay SR, Opler LA, Fiszbein A. The positive and negative syndrome scale (PANSS) for schizophrenia. Schizophr Bull 1987;13(2):261–76.

[38] Madhusoodanan S, Brenner R, Gupta S, et al. Clinical experience with aripiprazole treatment in ten elderly patients with schizophrenia or schizoaffective disorder: retrospective case studies. CNS Spectr 2004;9(11):862–7.

[39] Saitz R, Helmuth ED, Aromaa SE, et al. Web-based screening and brief intervention for the spectrum of alcohol problems. Prev Med 2004;39(5):969–75.

[40] Herst L, Powell G. Is clozapine safe in the elderly? Aust N Z J Psychiatry 1997;31(3):411–7.

[41] Alphs LD, Lafferman JA, Ross L, et al. Fenfluramine treatment of negative symptoms in older schizophrenic inpatients. Psychopharmacol Bull 1989;25(1):149–53.

[42] Weisbard JJ, Pardo M, Pollack S. Symptom change and extrapyramidal side effects during acute haloperidol treatment in chronic geriatric schizophrenics. Psychopharmacol Bull 1997; 33(1):119–22.

[43] Sajatovic M, Perez D, Brescan D, et al. Olanzapine therapy in elderly patients with schizophrenia. Psychopharmacol Bull 1998;34(4):819–23.

[44] Madhusoodanan S, Brenner R, Suresh P, et al. Efficacy and tolerability of olanzapine in elderly patients with psychotic disorders: a prospective study. Ann Clin Psychiatry 2000;12(1): 11–8.

[45] Madhusoodanan S, Brenner R, Alcantra A. Clinical experience with quetiapine in elderly patients with psychotic disorders. J Geriatr Psychiatry Neurol 2000;13(1):28–32.

[46] Yeung PP, Tariot PN, Schneider LS, et al. Quetiapine for elderly patients with psychotic disorders. Psychiatr Ann 2000;30(3):197–201.

[47] Berman I, Merson A, Sison C, et al. Regional cerebral blood flow changes associated with risperidone treatment in elderly schizophrenia patients: a pilot study. Psychopharmaco Bull 1996;32(1):95–100.

[48] Lasser RA, Bossie CA, Zhu Y, et al. Efficacy and safety of long-acting risperidone in elderly patients with schizophrenia and schizoaffective disorder. Int J Geriatr Psychiatry 2004;19(9) 898–905.

[49] Bullock R, Libretto S. Risperidone in the treatment of psychoses in the elderly: a case repor series. Eur Psychiatry 2002;17(2):96–103.

[50] Mohler G. Clinical trial of thiothixene (Navane) in elderly chronic schizophrenics. Curr The Res Clin Exp 1970;12(6):377–86.

[51] Chengappa KN, Baker RW, Kreinbrook SB, et al. Clozapine use in female geriatric patient with psychoses. J Geriatr Psychiatry Neurol 1995;8(1):12–5.

[52] Pitner JK, Mintzer JE, Pennypacker LC, et al. Efficacy and adverse effects of clozapine in four elderly psychotic patients. J Clin Psychiatry 1995;56(5):180–5.

[53] Salzman C, Vaccaro B, Lieff J, et al. Clozapine in older patients with psychosis and behav ioral disruption. Am J Geriatr Psychiatry 1995;3(1):26–33.

[54] Sajatovic M, Ramirez LF, Garver D, et al. Clozapine therapy for older veterans. Psychiat Serv 1998;49(3):340–4.

[55] Barak Y, Wittenberg N, Naor S, et al. Clozapine in elderly psychiatric patients: tolerability safety, and efficacy. Compr Psychiatry 1999;40(4):320–5.

[56] Oberholzer AF, Hendriksen C, Monsch AU, et al. Safety and effectiveness of low-dose clo zapine in psychogeriatric patients: a preliminary study. Int Psychogeriatr 1992;4(2):187–95

[57] Tsuang MM, Lu LM, Stotsky BA, et al. Haloperidol versus thioridazine for hospitalized psychogeriatric patients: double-blind study. J Am Geriatr Soc 1971;19(7):593–600.

[58] Solomons K, Geiger O. Olanzapine use in the elderly: a retrospective analysis. Can J Psychi atry 2000;45(2):151–5.

[59] Madhusoodanan S, Suresh P, Brenner R, et al. Experience with the atypical antipsychotics risperidone and olanzapine in the elderly. Ann Clin Psychiatry 1999;11(3):113–8.

[60] Verma S, Orengo CA, Kunik ME, et al. Tolerability and effectiveness of atypical antipsy chotics in male geriatric inpatients. Int J Geriatr Psychiatry 2001;16(2):223–7.

[61] McManus D, Arvanitis L, Kowalcyk B for the Seroquel Trial 48 Study Group. Quetiapine a novel antipsychotic: experience in elderly patients with psychotic disorders. J Clin Psychi atry 1999;60(5):292–8.

[62] Tariot PN, Salzman C, Yeung PP, et al. Long-term use of quetiapine in elderly patients with psychotic disorders. Clin Ther 2000;22(9):1068–84.

[63] Jaskiw GE, Thyrum PT, Fuller MA, et al. Pharmacokinetics of quetiapine in elderly patient with selected psychotic disorders. Clin Pharmacokinet 2004;43(14):1025–35 [erratum ap pears in: Clin Pharmacokinet 2004;43(15):1178].

[64] Sajatovic M, Ramirez LF, Vernon L, Brescan D, et al. Outcome of risperidone therapy in elderly patients with chronic psychosis. Int J Psychiatry Med 1996;26(3):309–17.

[65] Jeste DV, Lacro JP, Bailey A, et al. Lower incidence of tardive dyskinesia with risperidone compared with haloperidol in older patients. J Am Geriatr Soc 1999;47(6):716–9.

[66] Kiraly SJ, Gibson RE, Ancill RJ, et al. Risperidone: treatment response in adult and geriatric patients. Int J Psychiatry Med 1998;28(2):255–63.

[67] Barak Y. No weight gain among elderly schizophrenia patients after 1 year of risperidone treatment. J Clin Psychiatry 2002;63(2):117–9.

[68] Stryjer R, Strous RD, Bar F, et al. Beneficial effect of donepezil augmentation for the man agement of comorbid schizophrenia and dementia. Clin Neuropharmacol 2003;26(1):12–7.

[69] Mendelsohn E, Rosenthal M, Bohiri Y, et al. Rivastigmine augmentation in the management of chronic schizophrenia with comorbid dementia: an open-label study investigating effects

on cognition, behaviour and activities of daily living. Int Clin Psychopharmacol 2004;19(6): 319–24.

[70] Bodenheimer T. Uneasy alliance: clinical investigators and the pharmaceutical industry. N Engl J Med 2000;342(20):1539–44.

[71] Granholm E, McQuaid JR, McClure FS, et al. A randomized controlled pilot study of cognitive behavioral social skills training for older patients with schizophrenia. Schizophr Res 2002;53(1–2):167–9.

[72] Granholm E, McQuaid JR, McClure FS, et al. A randomized, controlled trial of cognitive behavioral social skills training for middle-aged and older outpatients with chronic schizophrenia. Am J Psychiatry 2005;162(3):520–9.

[73] Patterson TL, McKibbin C, Taylor M, et al. Functional adaptation skills training (FAST): a pilot psychosocial intervention study in middle-aged and older patients with chronic psychotic disorders. Am J Geriatr Psychiatry 2003;11(1):17–23.

[74] Bartels SJ, Forester B, Mueser KT, et al. Enhanced skills training and health care management for older persons with severe mental illness. Community Ment Health J 2004;40(1): 75–90.

[75] McQuaid JR, Granholm E, McClure FS, et al. Development of an integrated cognitive-behavioral and social skills training intervention for older patients with schizophrenia. J Psychother Pract Res 2000;9(3):149–56.

[76] Pratt SI, Forester B, Bartels S. Integrating psychosocial rehabilitation and health care for older adults with SMI: from pilot study to randomized controlled trial. Paper presented at the 16th Annual Meeting of the American Association for Geriatric Psychiatry. Honolulu (HI), March 1–4, 2003.

[77] Weintraub D, Katz I. Pharmacologic interventions for psychosis and agitation in neurodegenerative diseases: evidence about efficacy and safety. Psychiatr Clin North Am 2005;28(4): 941–83.

[78] Alexopoulos GS, Streim J, Carpenter D, et al. Using antipsychotic agents in older patients. J Clin Psychiatry 2004;65(Suppl):S25–99 [discussion: 100–2; quiz: 103–4].

[79] Rosack J. FDA to require diabetes warning on antipsychotics. Psychiatr News 2003;38(20): 1–a-27.

[80] FDA's proposed diabetes warning. Psychiatr News 2003;38(20):26.

[81] Consensus development conference on antipsychotic drugs and obesity and diabetes. Diabetes Care 2004;27(2):596–601.

[82] Alvir JM, Lieberman JA, Safferman AZ, et al. Clozapine-induced agranulocytosis: incidence and risk factors in the United States. N Engl J Med 1993;329(3):162–7.

[83] US Food and Drug Administration. FDA public health advisory: deaths with antipsychotics in elderly patients with behavioral disturbances. April 11, 2005. Available at: http:// www.fda.gov/cder/drug/advisory/antipsychotics.htm. Accessed May 28, 2005.

[84] Kuehn BM. FDA warns antipsychotic drugs may be risky for elderly. JAMA 2005;293(20): 2462.

ELSEVIER
SAUNDERS

Psychiatr Clin N Am
28 (2005) 941–983

PSYCHIATRIC
CLINICS
OF NORTH AMERICA

Pharmacologic Interventions for Psychosis and Agitation in Neurodegenerative Diseases: Evidence About Efficacy and Safety

Daniel Weintraub, MD, Ira R. Katz, MD, PhD*

Department of Psychiatry, University of Pennsylvania, 3535 Market Street, Philadelphia, PA 19104, USA

Approximately 5% of community-dwelling elderly individuals have dementia, and the prevalence of dementia will quadruple by the year 2050 [1]. Alzheimer's disease (AD), vascular dementia (VaD), mixed dementia (AD plus VaD), and dementia with Lewy bodies (DLB) account for a majority of dementia cases [2,3]. In addition, dementia may occur as a late complication in over 50% of patients with Parkinson's disease (PD) [4].

Neuropsychiatric symptoms are common in both dementia and PD and tend to persist or recur [5–9]. These noncognitive symptoms include psychosis (delusions and hallucinations), mood disturbances (depression or euphoria), irritability and lability, disinhibition, agitation, aggression, and apathy. Approximately 50% of dementia patients living in the community [10] and as many as 80% of those living in a residential care environment [11] exhibit clinically significant neuropsychiatric complications. Approximately 23% to 37% of AD patients [12], 15% of VaD patients [13], 15% to 40% of PD patients [14], and 90% of DLB patients [15] experience delusions or hallucinations. In addition, approximately 30% of patients with AD [10] and VaD [8] and 20% of those with PD [7] exhibit agitation. In patients with AD, psychosis and agitation are associated with increased caregiver burden, more rapid rates of decline, and an increased risk of nursing home placement [16,17], with the latter also being true for PD [17].

This study was supported by Grants MH067894 and MH066270 from the National Institute of Mental Health and by the Veterans Affairs Mental Illness Research, Education and Clinical Center.

* Corresponding author.
 E-mail address: katzi@mail.med.upenn.edu (I.R. Katz).

Medications from numerous classes have been investigated as potential treatments for the neuropsychiatric symptoms of dementia and PD, but currently there are no clear standards of care. This article reviews the evidence base of the pharmacologic treatment of psychosis and agitation in dementia and PD, focusing on the potential benefits versus risks for each major class that has been studied. There is a body of research evaluating the effectiveness of behavioral, psychosocial, and environmental treatments, but a review of that information is beyond the scope of this article. Also, dementia and its behavioral complications are chronic conditions, and the need to guide treatment should include information that goes beyond the efficacy of individual agents in relatively short-term studies to include findings that validate algorithms for combining or sequencing treatments over time, depending on the individual patient's responses. However, until now, little research has been conducted to address questions about long-term management.

Treatment studies in this area can be divided into two groups based on the type of symptoms and neurodegenerative disease. The first group consists of subjects with AD, either exclusively or primarily. Because AD patients frequently also have vascular disease, many of the subjects included in these studies have comorbid VaD, or mixed dementia [18]. Because the samples in most of these studies are mixed (ie, including patients with AD, VaD, or mixed dementia), this review considers these studies together. Within these conditions, psychosis and agitation are addressed in parallel because they frequently co-occur in patients and are often considered together in the design of treatment studies and the evaluation of outcomes. Moreover, for a substantial number of patients with psychosis or agitation, observations of hallucinations or delusions can vary substantially from week to week, even during placebo treatment [19].

The other group of treatment studies includes patients with either PD or DLB. Many experts have suggested that PD with dementia (PDD) and DLB may not be distinct diseases may lie on a continuum (PD presenting initially with predominantly motor symptoms and DLB presenting additionally with prominent cognitive and psychiatric symptoms) [6]. Compared with AD and DLB, dementia is not a diagnostic feature of PD, but the cumulative prevalence of dementia in PD may be as high as 75% [4]. For these disorders, psychoses, rather than psychoses or agitation, have been the primary targets for treatment studies.

Method

A review of literature was conducted of English language studies published between January 1, 1965 through June 30, 2005 that reported results (either primary or secondary analyses) for the pharmacologic treatment of psychosis or agitation in dementia or PD using online databases (MEDLINE and the Cochrane Database of Systematic Reviews) and reference lists from retrieved articles. In MEDLINE, results of searches in three separate domains were combined: dementia (MeSH terms dementia, Alzheimer disease, dementia, vascular, Lewy body disease, or Parkinson's disease) [1]; psychosis or agitation (MeSH terms psychotic disorders, hallucinations, delusions, paranoid disorders, neurobehavioral manifestations, psychomotor agitation, or the keyword agitation or aggression) [2]; and pharmacologic treatment (MeSH terms drug therapy, psychotropic drugs, antipsychotic agents, cholinesterase inhibitors, antidepressive agents, or anticonvulsants) [3].

A study was included in Tables 1 through 6 if it was a randomized, double-blind, placebo-controlled trial or a meta-analysis of randomized, controlled trials (RCTs) [1]; tested a pharmacologic intervention [2]; enrolled subjects with dementia or PD [3]; and reported outcomes for psychosis or agitation specifically or neuropsychiatric symptoms in general [4]. Trials included those that tested a single agent versus placebo and those that had an active comparator group in addition to placebo. Although they are not included in the tables, active comparator studies without a placebo group are discussed below if they were believed to impart important findings. All articles were reviewed by both of the present authors, and a consensus was reached on which articles to include.

Meta-analyses are included at the top of each table; otherwise, the tables are organized chronologically, citing the earliest studies first. If a study tested two active treatments from different medication classes, it is included in tables for both classes. Dosages for active treatment are presented as the mean milligrams per day. When reporting results, priority was given to primary outcome measures that reported specifically on psychosis or agitation and then neuropsychiatric symptoms in general; relevant secondary outcome measures are also included, when informative. When reporting adverse events, priority was given to clinically relevant and significant results, and in PD and DLB, particular attention was paid to the impact of treatment on motor symptoms. When they were provided in a study, P values are included in the tables for both results and adverse events. Box 1 lists the rating instruments that were used in the tabulated studies.

Results

Alzheimer's disease, vascular dementia, and mixed dementia

Antipsychotic agents, both typical and atypical, are the medications that have been studied most intensively as treatments for psychosis and agitation. Other agents that have been evaluated include cholinesterase inhibitors, antidepressants, and mood stabilizers. Antipsychotic drug studies typically have enrolled patients with either psychosis or agitation. In contrast, studies of mood stabilizers have specifically targeted agitation or

Table 1
Placebo-controlled studies of antipsychotics in Alzheimer's disease, vascular dementia, and mixed dementia

Study	Study design	Number of subjects/completers	Length of study	Active treatment	Setting	Diagnosis	Relevant outcome measures and results	Adverse events and comments for study medication
Schneider et al 1990 [20]	Meta-analysis of 7 placebo-controlled studies of neuroleptics for agitation in dementia	252	3–8 wk	7 different typical antipsychotics used (66–267 mg/d [chlorpromazine equivalents])	Nursing facilities and inpatient	Senile dementia or VaD ± psychosis	Effect size (correlation coefficient r) = .18 (P = .004) BESD = .41–.59 No individual study in meta-analysis showed superiority of treatment	Authors' assessment that improvement reliably seen in agitation and hallucinations with treatment Adverse events not accounted for in metaanalysis
Lanctot et al 1998 [35]	Meta-analysis of 16 double-blind, placebo-controlled or active comparator studies of neuroleptics for behavioral disorders	499	3–12 wk	7 different typical antipsychotics used (0.05–0.9 defined daily dose)	Nursing facilities and outpatient	Dementia in ≥70% of patients	Mean % of patients improved was 61% for neuroleptics and 34% for placebo Therapeutic effect = 26% (P < .001) No differences in improvement between neuroleptic classes	Treatment emergent side effects more common with neuroleptics than placebo (difference, 25%) No detectable differences in adverse events between neuroleptic classes No differences between neuroleptics and placebo in pooled mean dropout rates

Lonergan et al 2002 [25]	Review of 5 double-blind, placebo-controlled studies	573	3–16 wk	Haloperidol (0.25–6 mg/d)	Nursing facilities and outpatient	AD and VaD	Haloperidol useful in reducing aggression but no treatment effect for other manifestations of agitation	No increase in study discontinuation rate with haloperidol. Adverse events, particularly EPS, more common with haloperidol in most studies
Finkel et al 1995 [21]	Double-blind, placebo-controlled crossover	33/30 (phase I)	17 wk (11-wk phase, then 6-wk phase)	Thiothixene (mean 4.6 mg/d during phase I)	Nursing facility	Dementia	Positive treatment effect for change in CMAI score at end of phase I ($P < .001$)	Sedation and lack of energy more common with thiothixene at 2 time points during phase I
Auchus and Bissey-Black 1997 [26]	Double-blind, placebo-controlled and active comparator	15/12	6 wk	Haloperidol (3 mg/d) and fluoxetine (20 mg/d)	Outpatient	AD	No treatment effect for haloperidol on change in CMAI score ($P = .82$)	Adverse symptoms more common with haloperidol than placebo ($P = .05$)

(continued on next page)

Table 1 (continued)

Study	Study design	Number of subjects/ completers	Length of study	Active treatment	Setting	Diagnosis	Relevant outcome measures and results	Adverse events and comments for study medication
Devanand et al 1998 [24]	Double-blind, placebo-controlled crossover	71/60 (phase I)	12 wk (two 6-wk phases)	Haloperidol (0.5–0.75 or 2–3 mg/d)	Outpatient	AD	Positive treatment effect for higher dose haloperidol change in 5 efficacy measures in phase I ($P \leq .04$) Response rates 55%–60% for higher dose haloperidol, 25%–35% for lower dose haloperidol, and 25%–30% for placebo on 3 outcome measures in phase I ($P \geq .05$)	Moderate-severe EPS occurred in 20% of subjects on higher dose haloperidol and no subjects on lower dose haloperidol or placebo in phase I

Study	Design	N	Duration	Drug	Setting	Dementia	Response	Adverse effects
Allain et al 1999 [23]	Double-blind, placebo-controlled and active comparator	306/259	3 wk	Tiapride (mean 175 mg/d) and haloperidol (mean 3.5 mg/d)	Nursing facilities and inpatient	Dementia	Response rates (≥25% decrease in MOSES agitation subscore) greater with tiapride (63%, $P = .04$) and haloperidol (69%, $P = .004$) than with placebo (49%)	Increase in EPS with haloperidol ($P = .008$) but not tiapride ($P = .73$) compared with placebo. Study discontinuation due to adverse events higher in haloperidol (n = 17) than in tiapride (n = 5) and placebo (n = 6) groups
Katz et al 1999 [28]	Double-blind, placebo-controlled	625/435	12 wk	Risperidone (0.5, 1, or 2 mg/d)	Nursing facilities	AD, VaD, or mixed dementia	Positive treatment effect for change in BEHAVE-AD score at 1 mg ($P = .02$) and 2 mg/d ($P < .001$). Positive treatment effect for change in BEHAVE-AD psychosis and aggressiveness subscales at 1 and 2 mg/d	42% study discontinuation rate for risperidone 2 mg/d. Significantly more extrapyramidal symptoms for risperidone 2 mg/d
De Deyn et al 1999 [29]	Double-blind, placebo controlled and active comparator	334/223	12 wk	Risperidone (mean 1.1 mg/d) and haloperidol (mean 1.2 mg/d)	Nursing facilities	AD, VaD, or mixed dementia	No treatment effect for risperidone ($P = .25$) or haloperidol ($P = .13$) for ≥ 30% decrease in BEHAVE-AD score	Somnolence more common with haloperidol. Increase in EPS adverse events with haloperidol ($P = .023$), but not risperidone

(continued on next page)

Table 1 (continued)

Study	Study design	Number of subjects/completers	Length of study	Active treatment	Setting	Diagnosis	Relevant outcome measures and results	Adverse events and comments for study medication
Teri et al 2000 [27]	Double-blind, placebo-controlled and active comparator versus open BMT	149/91	16 wk	Haloperidol (mean 1.8 mg/d), trazodone, and BMT	Outpatient	AD	No treatment effect for haloperidol in ADCS-CGIC score ($P = .81$) No treatment effect for haloperidol for change in CMAI, BRSD, or ABID scores ($P > .25$ for all scores)	Worsening in physical and instrumental ADLs with haloperidol compared with placebo ($P \le .05$) No increase in adverse events in haloperidol compared with placebo
Street et al 2000 [31]	Double-blind, placebo-controlled	206/152	6 wk	Olanzapine (5, 10, or 15 mg/d)	Nursing facilities	AD	Positive treatment effect for change in NPI-NH core total (agitation and psychosis) at 5 mg ($P \le .001$) and 10 mg/d ($P = .006$)	Increase in study discontinuations due to adverse events with olanzapine Somnolence and gait disturbance more common with olanzapine No increase in extrapyramidal symptoms with olanzapine
Meehan et al 2002 [33]	Double-blind, placebo-controlled and active comparator	272/245	24 h	Olanzapine (intramuscular 2.5 or 5 mg) and lorazepam	Nursing facilities and inpatient	AD, VaD, or mixed dementia	Positive treatment effect for olanzapine 2.5 mg ($P < .05$) and 5.0 mg ($P < .05$) on change in	No increase in adverse events or extrapyramidal symptoms with olanzapine

Pollock et al 2002 [22]	Double-blind, placebo-controlled and active comparator	85/39	Up to 17 d	Perphenazine (mean 7 mg/d) and citalopram	Inpatient	AD, VaD, or mixed dementia	No treatment effect for perphenazine on change in NRS score ($P = .14$)	No increase in adverse events or extrapyramidal symptoms with perphenazine
Brodaty et al 2003 [30]	Double-blind, placebo-controlled	345/236	12 wk	Risperidone (mean 1 mg/d)	Nursing facilities	AD, VaD, or mixed dementia	Positive treatment effect for change in CMAI aggression subscale score ($P < .001$) Positive treatment effect for change in BEHAVE-AD total ($P < .001$) and psychotic subscale ($P = .004$) scores	Increase in serious cerebrovascular adverse events in risperidone group (16.8% vs 8.8%), including 5 strokes and 1 TIA Somnolence and urinary tract infection more common with risperidone
De Deyn et al 2004 [32]	Double-blind, placebo-controlled	652/465	10 wk	Olanzapine (1, 2.5, 5, or 7.5 mg/d)	Nursing facilities	AD	No treatment effect for change in NPI/NH psychosis score on primary analysis ($P = .142$)	No increase in study discontinuation rate or worsening of motor function with olanzapine Weight gain, anorexia, and urinary incontinence more common with olanzapine
Ballard et al 2005 [34]	Double-blind, placebo-controlled and active comparator	93/80 completed at least 6 wk of treatment	26 wk	Quetiapine (most on 100 mg/d) and rivastigmine	Nursing facilities	AD	No treatment effect for quetiapine on change in CMAI score ($P = .50$)	Worsening cognition on severe impairment battery with quetiapine compared with placebo ($P = .01$)

Abbreviations: BESD, binomial effect-size display; BMT, behavioral management techniques; TIA, transient ischemic attack.

Table 2
Placebo-controlled studies of cognitive enhancing agents with behavioral outcomes in Alzheimer's disease, vascular dementia, and mixed dementia

Study	Study design	Number of subjects/ completers	Length of study	Active treatment	Setting	Diagnosis	Relevant outcome measures and results	Adverse events and comments for study medication
Trinh et al 2003 [42]	Meta-analysis of 16 double-blind, placebo-controlled studies of cholinesterase inhibitors	5529	6 weeks–1 year	Metrifonate, tacrine, galantamine, donepezil, velnacrine, and physostigmine	Outpatient	AD	Positive treatment effect for change in NPI score, but no treatment effect for change in ADAS-noncog score. Outcomes for NPI psychosis and agitation subscales not presented	NPI improvement driven by metrifonate, which is not available in US. Donepezil and galantamine not superior or neurobehavioral outcomes
Feldman et al 2001 [43]	Double-blind, placebo-controlled	290/247	24 weeks	Donepezil (5 or 10 mg/d)	Assisted living and outpatient	AD	Positive treatment effect for change in NPI score (P < .001). Positive treatment effect for change in NPI depression, anxiety, and apathy subscales, but not psychosis or agitation	No increase in study discontinuation rate with donepezil. Diarrhea, headaches, vomiting and arthralgias more common with donepezil

Study	Design	N	Duration	Drug (dose)	Setting	Diagnosis	Efficacy	Comments
Tariot et al 2001 [41]	Double-blind, placebo-controlled	208/162	24 weeks	Donepezil (mean 10 mg/d)	Nursing facilities	AD	No treatment effect for change in NPI-NH score On secondary analysis, positive treatment effect for categorical change in agitation ($P = .044$)	No increase in study discontinuation rate with donepezil Weight loss, nausea, abdominal pain and tremor more common with donepezil
Erkinjuntti et al 2002 [46]	Double-blind, placebo-controlled	592/457	24 weeks	Galantamine (24 mg/d)	Outpatient	Mixed dementia or VaD	Positive treatment effect for change in NPI score ($P = .016$)	Nausea and vomiting associated led to higher study discontinuation rate with galantamine Outcomes for NPI psychosis and agitation subscales not presented
Reisberg et al 2003 [47]	Double-blind, placebo-controlled	252/181	28 weeks	Memantine (20 mg/d)	Outpatient	AD	No treatment effect for change in NPI score ($P = .33$)	No increase in study discontinuation rate or adverse events with memantine

(continued on next page)

Table 2 (*continued*)

Study	Study design	Number of subjects/ completers	Length of study	Active treatment	Setting	Diagnosis	Relevant outcome measures and results	Adverse events and comments for study medication
AD2000 Collaborative Group 2004 [44]	Double-blind, placebo-controlled	565/152	2 years	Donepezil (5 or 10 mg/d)	Outpatient	AD or mixed dementia	No treatment effect for change in NPI score at any point in time ($P = .60$) No treatment effect for subjects with highest baseline NPI scores ($P = .40$)	Increase in study discontinuation rate due to adverse events during 12-wk run-in with donepezil ($P = .001$)
Holmes et al 2004 [45]	Double-blind, placebo-controlled withdrawal study	96/80	12 weeks	Donepezil (10 mg/d)	Outpatient	AD	Positive treatment effect for change in NPI score ($P = .02$) Outcomes for NPI psychosis and agitation subscales not presented	No increase in study discontinuation rate during randomized withdrawal with donepezil
Tariot et al 2004 [48]	Double-blind, placebo-controlled add-on study	404/322	24 weeks	Memantine (20 mg/d) or placebo added to donepezil	Outpatient	AD	Positive treatment effect for change in NPI score ($P = .002$) Outcomes for NPI psychosis and agitation subscales not presented	Decrease in study discontinuation rate with memantine ($P = .01$) Confusion more common with memantine ($P = .01$)
Ballard et al 2005 [34]	Double-blind, placebo-controlled and active	93/80 completed at least 6 wk of treatment	26 weeks	Rivastigmine (most on ≥ 9 mg/d) and quetiapine	Nursing facilities	AD	No treatment effect for rivastigmine on change in CMAI score ($P = .30$)	No information on adverse events with rivastigmine

Table 3
Placebo-controlled studies of mood stabilizers with behavioral outcomes in Alzheimer's disease, vascular dementia, and mixed dementia

Study	Study design	Number of subjects/ completers	Length of study	Active treatment	Setting	Diagnosis	Relevant outcome measures and results	Adverse events and comments for study medication
Tariot et al 1998 [50]	Double-blind, placebo-controlled	51/47	6 wk	Carbamazepine (mean 304 mg/d)	Nursing facilities	AD, VaD, or mixed dementia	Positive treatment effect for change in total BPRS score ($P \leq .001$) and BPRS agitation factor ($P \leq .001$)	Increase in adverse events with carbamazepine ($P = .03$) Ataxia and disorientation more common with carbamazepine
Porsteinsson et al 2001 [52]	Double-blind, placebo-controlled	56/49	6 wk	Divalproex sodium (mean 826 mg/d)	Nursing facilities	AD, VaD, or mixed dementia	No treatment effect for change in BPRS score ($P = .61$)	Increase in adverse events with divalproex sodium ($P = .03$) Sedation, gastrointestinal side effects, and respiratory problems more common with divalproex sodium

(continued on next page)

Table 3 (continued)

Study	Study design	Number of subjects/ completers	Length of study	Active treatment	Setting	Diagnosis	Relevant outcome measures and results	Adverse events and comments for study medication
Tariot et al 2001 [54]	Double-blind, placebo-controlled	172/100	6 wk	Divalproex sodium (median 1000 mg/d)	Nursing facilities	AD, VaD, or mixed dementia	No treatment effect for change in BRMS ($P = .941$) or BPRS ($P = .690$) scores Positive treatment effect for change in CMAI score ($P = .035$)	Higher study discontinuation rate with divalproex sodium due to adverse events (primarily sedation) ($P \leq .001$) Study terminated early due to higher discontinuation rate with divalproex
Olin et al 2001 [51]	Double-blind, placebo-controlled	21/16	6 wk	Carbamazepine (mean 388 mg/d)	Outpatient	AD	No treatment effect for change in BPRS score ($P = .519$)	Mild adverse events in 4 of 9 subjects taking carbamazepine
Sival et al 2002 [53]	Double-blind, placebo-controlled	42/39	3 wk	Sodium valproate (mean 480 mg/d)	Inpatient	AD, VaD, PD, or mixed dementia	No treatment effect for change in SDAS-9 score	Data for specific adverse events not presented

Table 4
Placebo-controlled studies of antidepressants with behavioral outcomes in Alzheimer's disease, vascular dementia, and mixed dementia

Study	Study design	Number of subjects/completers	Length of study	Active treatment	Setting	Diagnosis	Relevant outcome measures and results	Adverse events and comments for study medication
Nyth and Gottfries 1990 [56]	Double-blind, placebo-controlled phase with complex follow-up	98/61	4 wk double-blind treatment	Citalopram (up to 30 mg/d)	Nursing facilities, inpatient, and outpatient	AD or VaD	Positive treatment effect for citalopram on GBS irritability ($P = .02$) and depressed mood ($P = .03$) subscores at end of phase I	No drug-placebo differences in side effects. No drug-placebo differences were observed in symptoms of withdrawal during citalopram discontinuation
Auchus and Bissey-Black 1997 [26]	Double-blind, placebo-controlled and active comparator	15/12	6 wk	Fluoxetine (20 mg/d) and haloperidol	Outpatient	AD	No treatment effect for fluoxetine on change in CMAI score ($P = .82$)	Increase in adverse events with fluoxetine ($P = .05$)
Levkovitz et al 2001 [57]	Double-blind, placebo-controlled, crossover add-on study	20/20	7 wk	Fluvoxamine (50 mg/d) or placebo added to perphenazine	Outpatient	AD	Positive treatment effect for change in BPRS score ($P = .03$). Outcomes for BPRS psychosis and agitation subscales not presented	No examination of possible carry-over effect from cross-over design. Minimal adverse events with fluvoxamine

(continued on next page)

Table 4 (*continued*)

Study	Study design	Number of subjects/completers	Length of study	Active treatment	Setting	Diagnosis	Relevant outcome measures and results	Adverse events and comments for study medication
Teri et al 2000 [27]	Double-blind, placebo-controlled and active comparator versus open behavioral management techniques (BMT)	149/91	16 wk	Trazodone (mean 200 mg/d), haloperidol, and BMT	Outpatient	AD	No treatment effect for trazodone in ADCS-CGIC score ($P = .99$) No treatment effect for trazodone on change in CMAI, BRSD, or ABID scores ($P \geq .25$ for all scores)	Worsening in physical and instrumental ADLs with trazodone compared with placebo ($P < .05$) Worsening in MMSE score with trazodone compared with BMT ($P < .05$) No increase in adverse events with trazodone compared with placebo
Pollock et al 2002 [22]	Double-blind, placebo-controlled and active comparator	85/39	Up to 17 d	Citalopram (20 mg/d) and perphenazine	Inpatient	AD, VaD, or mixed dementia	Positive treatment effect for citalopram on change in total NRS score ($P = .002$) Positive treatment effect for citalopram on NRS agitation subscale ($P < .03$), but not psychosis subscale	No increase in adverse events or extrapyramidal symptoms with citalopram

| Lyketsos et al 2003 [55] | Double-blind, placebo-controlled | 44/36 | 12 wk | Sertraline (mean 95 mg/d) | Outpatient | AD | No treatment effect for change in NPI score ($P = .32$) | Study designed to treat depression in AD. No increase in adverse events with sertraline |
| Finkel et al 2004 [58] | Double-blind, placebo-controlled add-on study | 245/200 | 12 wk | Sertraline (mean 126 mg/d) or placebo added to donepezil | Outpatient | AD | No treatment effect for change in NPI ($P = .54$) | No increase in study discontinuation rate with sertraline. Diarrhea more common with sertraline ($P < .05$) |

Abbreviation: **BMT**, behavioral management techniques.

Table 5
Placebo-controlled studies of antipsychotics in Parkinson's disease and dementia with Lewy bodies

Study	Study design	Number of subjects/ completers	Length of study	Active treatment	Setting	Diagnosis	Relevant outcome measures and results	Adverse events and comments for study medication
Wolters et al 1990 [60]	Double-blind, placebo-substitution	6/3	40 d	Clozapine (mean 171 mg/d)	Inpatient	PD with psychosis	3/6 patients responded by clinical evaluation	Worsening parkinsonism in 3/6 patients and delirium in 4/6 patients treated with clozapine
French Clozapine Study Group 1999 [61]	Double-blind, placebo-controlled	60/46	4 wk	Clozapine (mean 36 mg/d)	Outpatient	PD with psychosis	Positive treatment effect change in PANSS positive score ($P < .001$)	Somnolence and worsening parkinsonism more commonly reported as adverse events with clozapine. No change in UPDRS motor or MMSE scores with clozapine
Parkinson Study Group 1999 [62]	Double-blind, placebo-controlled	60/54	4 wk	Clozapine (mean 25 mg/d)	Outpatient	PD with psychosis	Positive treatment effect for change in BPRS ($P = .002$) and SAPS ($P = .01$) scores	Improved tremor with clozapine. Leukopenia in one clozapine patient
Breier et al 2002 [64]	Double-blind, placebo-controlled	87/60	4 wk	Olanzapine (mean modal 4 mg/d)	Outpatient	PD with psychosis	No treatment effect for change in BPRS ($P = .96$) or NPI ($P = .78$) scores	Higher study discontinuation rate with olanzapine. Increased parkinsonism with olanzapine

Study	Design	N	Duration	Drug	Setting	Diagnosis	Results	Comments
Breier et al 2002 [64]	Double-blind, placebo-controlled	78/59	4 wk	Olanzapine (mean modal 4 mg/d)	Outpatient	PD with psychosis	No treatment effect for change in BPRS ($P = .61$) or NPI ($P = .50$) scores	Increased parkinsonism with olanzapine
Ondo et al 2002 [65]	Double-blind, placebo-controlled	30/27	9 wk	Olanzapine (mean dosage 5 mg/d)	Outpatient	PD with psychosis	No treatment effect for change in UPDRS item 2 ($P = .16$) or structured interview for hallucinations in PD (no P value provided)	Increased parkinsonism with olanzapine
Cummings et al 2002 [67]	Double-blind, placebo-controlled (post hoc analysis of AD study)	29/25	6 wk	Olanzapine (5, 10, or 15 mg/d)	Nursing facilities	DLB (post hoc diagnosis)	Positive treatment effect for change in BPRS score at 5 mg/d ($P = .03$) Positive treatment effect for change in NPI/NH hallucinations at 5 mg/d ($P = .009$) and delusions at 5 ($P = .009$) and 10 mg/d ($P = .02$)	No change in parkinsonism or MMSE score with olanzapine

(continued on next page)

Table 5 (*continued*)

Study	Study design	Number of subjects/completers	Length of study	Active treatment	Setting	Diagnosis	Relevant outcome measures and results	Adverse events and comments for study medication
Pollak et al 2004 [63]	Double-blind, placebo-controlled	60/46	4 wk	Clozapine (mean 36 mg/d)	Outpatient	PD with psychosis	Positive treatment effect for change in PANSS positive score ($P \leq .001$)	Somnolence, worsening of parkinsonism, and sialorrhea more commonly reported as adverse events with clozapine Neutropenia (n = 2) and seizures (n = 1) with clozapine No change in UPDRS motor or MMSE scores with clozapine
Ondo et al 2005 [66]	Double-blind, placebo-controlled	31/26	12 wk	Quetiapine (mean 170 mg/d)	Outpatient	PD with psychosis	No treatment effect for change in BPRS (no *P* value provided) or Baylor PD Hallucination Questionnaire ($P = .19$) scores	No change in UPDRS motor score with quetiapine

Table 6
Placebo-controlled studies of cognitive enhancing agents with behavioral outcomes in Parkinson's disease and dementia with Lewy bodies

Study	Study design	Number of subjects/ completers	Length of study	Active treatment	Setting	Diagnosis	Relevant outcome measures and results	Adverse events and comments for study medication
McKeith et al 2000 [70]	Double-blind, placebo-controlled	120/92	20 wk	Rivastigmine (mean 9 mg/d)	Outpatient	DLB	Positive treatment effect for change in NPI-4 on 2 of 3 analyses (ITT $P = .09$, LOCF $P = .05$, OC $P = .01$) Outcomes for NPI psychosis and agitation subscales only not presented	Greatest improvement seen in NPI apathy subscale Higher study discontinuation rate with rivastigmine More nausea, vomiting, anorexia, and somnolence with rivastigmine No change in UPDRS motor score with rivastigmine
Aarsland et al 2002 [71]	Double-blind, placebo-controlled crossover	14/12	20 wk	Donepezil (5 and 10 mg/d)	Outpatient	PD with cognitive impairment	Outcome data not presented for NPI	Low NPI scores at baseline No change in mean UPDRS motor score with donepezil
Leroi et al 2004 [72]	Double-blind, placebo-controlled	16/10	18 wk	Donepezil (6 mg/d)	Outpatient	PD with cognitive impairment	No treatment effect for change in NPI score ($P = .99$)	Study discontinuation in 5/7 donepezil patients No change in mean UPDRS motor score with donepezil

(continued on next page)

Table 6 (continued)

Study	Study design	Number of subjects/ completers	Length of study	Active treatment	Setting	Diagnosis	Relevant outcome measures and results	Adverse events and comments for study medication
Emre et al 2004 [73]	Double-blind, placebo-controlled	541/410	24 wk	Rivastigmine (8.6 mg/d)	Outpatient	PD with dementia	Positive treatment effect for change in NPI score ($P = .02$) Positive treatment effect for fewer hallucinations as adverse event ($P = .04$)	Higher study discontinuation rate with rivastigmine More nausea, vomiting, tremor, anorexia, and dizziness with rivastigmine No between-group differences in UPDRS motor scores

---

Box 1. Rating instruments used in the tabulated studies

ADAS-noncog, Alzheimer Disease Assessment Scale (noncognitive)

ADCS-CGIC, Alzheimer's Disease Cooperative Study Clinical Global Impression of Change

ABID, Agitated Behavior Inventory for Dementia

ADLs, Activities of Daily Living

BEHAVE-AD, Behavior Pathology in Alzheimer's Disease Rating Scale

BPRS, Brief Psychiatric Rating Scale

BRMS, Bech-Rafaelsen Mania Scale

BRSD, Behavioral Rating Scale for Dementia

CMAI, Cohen-Mansfield Agitation Inventory

EPS, Extrapyramidal symptoms (used synonymously with parkinsonism, ie, increase in tremor, rigidity, or bradykinesia)

GBS, Gottfries-Brane-Steen geriatric rating scale

MMSE, Mini-Mental State Examination

MOSES, Multidimensional Observation Scale for the Elderly Subjects

NBS, Neurobehavioral Rating Scale

NPI, Neuropsychiatric Inventory

NPI/NH, Neuropsychiatric Inventory-Nursing Home version

NPI-4, Neuropsychiatric Inventory cluster of delusions, hallucinations, apathy, and depression

PANSS, Positive and Negative Syndrome Scale

PANSS-EC, Positive and Negative Syndrome Scale-Excited Component

SAPS, Scale for the Assessment of Positive Symptoms

SDAS-9, Social Dysfunction and Aggression scale 9

---

agitation as a component of a putative manic syndrome. Many of the cholinesterase inhibitor studies have examined changes in neuropsychiatric symptoms, not in patient samples selected as having psychotic or behavioral symptoms that require treatment but in those selected for inclusion in studies that focused primarily on cognitive or functional outcomes. Studies of antidepressants are included in the present review because these agents have been evaluated for their effects on psychosis and agitation as well as depression.

Antipsychotic drugs

A classic 1990 review and meta-analysis on the use of typical antipsychotic agents identified seven placebo-controlled studies (published between

1960 and 1982) for the treatment of psychosis and agitation in dementia and found a small to moderate but statistically and clinically significant benefit for neuroleptic treatment (Table 1) [20–35]. Since then, two additional meta-analyses and 13 placebo-controlled clinical trials have been published, and a number of additional trials have been completed. When the literature as a whole is reviewed, the conclusions about efficacy with small to moderate treatment effects remain valid.

Since the 1990 review, there have been several studies of typical antipsychotic agents, comparing them with placebo and, in a number of cases, with newer atypical agents or other treatments. Findings from the initial treatment arm of a small-scale crossover study found thiothixene to be superior to placebo in decreasing agitation [21]. Another study found no drug–placebo difference for perphenazine for psychotic symptoms or agitation [22]. The typical agent that has been studied most intensively is haloperidol, but findings on its efficacy have been mixed. Findings from several studies [23,24] and a 2002 meta-analysis [25] demonstrated efficacy, but other studies did not [26,27]. One well-designed study randomized patients to dosages of haloperidol that were higher (2–3 mg/d) or lower (0.5–0.75 mg/d) or placebo and found efficacy for the treatment of behavioral symptoms only with the higher doses [24].

The first randomized studies of atypical antipsychotic agents were published in 1999. One study [28] randomized subjects to risperidone, 0.5, 1.0, and 2.0 mg/d, or placebo and found that the 1.0 and 2.0 mg/d dosages were superior to placebo in reducing psychosis and agitation. In this study there were dose-related increases in extrapyramidal symptoms (EPS) and somnolence, and a dosage of 1 mg/d offered the best balance between efficacy and adverse events. Another placebo-controlled comparison trial [29] of risperidone and haloperidol reported that neither drug was superior to placebo in the primary outcome measure (improvement of 30% or more in the BEHAVE-AD total score). However, drug–placebo differences for both agents were apparent in a number of secondary analyses, with no consistent differences between agents. With respect to adverse events, risperidone caused less sedation and EPS than haloperidol did. Finally, a study [30] of risperidone versus placebo for nursing home residents with aggressive symptoms found active medication to be superior for aggression, agitation, and psychosis. However, there was an increase in the number of serious adverse events in the risperidone group, including cerebrovascular adverse events (CVAEs) (discussed in greater detail below). In addition to these placebo-controlled studies, there was a report [36] of a double-blind active comparator study of risperidone versus haloperidol that found no significant differences between these agents in outcomes on the CMAI and BEHAVE-AD scales; however, patients given haloperidol exhibited greater EPS at the endpoint.

An early study [37] of variable doses of olanzapine versus placebo, described only in abstract form, found no placebo differences; however, the doses achieved may have been subtherapeutic. The first published placebo-controlled study [31] of olanzapine randomized patients with psychosis or agitation to fixed dosages of 5, 10, and 15 mg/d or placebo and demonstrated significant improvement in psychosis and agitation for olanzapine compared with placebo at dosages of 5 and 10 mg/d but not at 15 mg/d. However, olanzapine treatment also was associated with more somnolence and gait disturbance. The most recent placebo-controlled study [32] of olanzapine for treating psychosis with or without agitation randomized patients to four fixed doses ranging from 1.25 to 7.5 mg/d or placebo and found no drug–placebo differences in primary outcomes, although secondary analyses demonstrated scattered suggestions of drug–placebo differences. There were higher rates of weight gain, anorexia, and urinary incontinence with olanzapine treatment.

Olanzapine has also been studied as a potential treatment for the short-term management of acute agitation. In a placebo-controlled active comparator study of intramuscular olanzapine versus lorazepam and placebo for the treatment of acute agitation, olanzapine, 2.5 and 5 mg, demonstrated greater short-term benefit (ie, at 2 and 24 hours) than placebo did, and it appeared to be well tolerated [33]. This study also demonstrated the efficacy of lorazepam over the short term.

In the only published randomized study [34] of quetiapine for the treatment of psychosis or agitation in AD, treatment with quetiapine did not lead to a significant improvement in agitation. This study also found worsened cognition with quetiapine compared with placebo.

Complementing these treatment studies, three studies have reported on double-blind studies of neuroleptic discontinuation [38–40]. All of them found that a substantial proportion of the patients who are stabilized on these conditions can be withdrawn from the drugs without worsening of symptoms. These findings support current clinical practice and United States policy for nursing home care, which recommend periodic trials of dose reduction or discontinuation in patients who are stabilized on antipsychotic medications. However, one of these studies [40] found that higher levels of residual symptoms may predict worsening when active medications are discontinued. This finding clearly demonstrates the need for additional research on the effectiveness of treatment algorithms and longer-term strategies for managing psychotic and behavioral symptoms in dementia.

Cognitive enhancing agents

The literature includes findings on the outcomes of cognitive enhancing agents (ie, cholinesterase inhibitors and memantine) in two separable types of studies (Table 2) [34,41–48]. Two published studies recruited subjects with significant behavioral symptoms. However, the majority of reports are observations of the effects of treatment on behavioral symptoms in subjects who were recruited for studies designed to evaluate cognitive and functional measures as primary outcomes. In general, inclusion in these studies did not require behavioral symptoms that were severe enough to require treatment; in fact, clinically significant behavioral symptoms may have been exclusions.

One study randomized residential care subjects with dementia and agitation to treatment with rivastigmine, quetiapine, or placebo and reported that neither active treatment was superior to placebo [34]. Another study evaluated the outcomes of treatment with donepezil versus placebo in nursing home residents with AD for whom at least one behavioral symptom on the NPI occurred at least several times per week [41]. Although there was no drug–placebo difference in the NPI total score (the primary study endpoint), secondary analyses demonstrated effects of active treatment on agitation and aggression but not other neurobehavioral symptoms.

A larger number of studies considered behavioral symptoms as outcomes. Findings from 16 placebo-controlled studies (published between 1992 and 2001) of cholinesterase inhibitors in mild to moderate dementia were summarized in a meta-analysis that found significant benefit for active treatment in those studies that used the NPI as the neurobehavioral outcome measure but not in those that used another instrument, such as the ADAS (noncognitive) [42]. Overall NPI scores decreased by approximately 15% to 20%, suggesting that there may be either a modest treatment effect or an effect of these agents in preventing the onset or worsening of behavioral symptoms. However, between-group differences on NPI psychosis and agitation subscales were not presented. In addition, it is important to note that the biggest improvements in NPI scores came in studies that used metrifonate, an agent that is not available in the United States. There have been three additional placebo-controlled studies of donepezil that reported neuropsychiatric outcomes [43–45]. None of these studies reported drug–placebo differences in psychosis or agitation. One additional placebo-controlled study [46] of galantamine reported a significant decrease in total NPI score with active treatment, but it did not report on between-group differences for psychosis and agitation and aggression subscales. Finally, an analysis [49] of pooled data from 3 studies that included 1347 subjects randomized to galantamine and 686 randomized to placebo reported that there were small, but statistically significant drug–placebo differences in agitation and aggression and anxiety.

Two studies of memantine for the treatment of moderate to severe AD have reported on neuropsychiatric outcome measures [47,48]. In the first study, memantine did not lead to a significant improvement in neuropsychiatric symptoms compared with placebo [47]. In the second study, the combination of memantine plus donepezil was reported to be superior to placebo plus donepezil in reducing overall neuropsychiatric symptoms; however, specific outcomes for psychosis and agitation were not presented [48]. Although there was a decrease in the discontinuation rate with memantine treatment, it was associated with increased confusion.

Mood stabilizers

There have been five randomized studies of mood stabilizers for the treatment of agitation in dementia, involving either carbamazepine or sodium valproate/divalproex sodium. The first study, published in 1998, found carbamazepine to be superior to placebo for the treatment of agitation and aggression, although there were significantly more side effects, including ataxia and disorientation, in the carbamazepine group (Table 3) [50–54]. A subsequent study of agitated patients who were resistant to antipsychotic treatment reported that carbamazepine, although well tolerated, was not significantly better than placebo on the primary outcome measure for agitation [51].

Three studies used either sodium valproate or divalproex sodium to treat agitation in dementia. Two of the three studies were negative on the primary outcome measure [52,53], and the third study was negative on two of the three agitation inventories that were used to assess outcomes [54]. In addition, somnolence and gastrointestinal side effects were more common with divalproex sodium in the two studies that reported adverse event data [52,54], leading to early termination of one of the studies [54].

Antidepressants

Antidepressants have been evaluated as treatments for the depression of AD and for other neuropsychiatric symptoms. One recent study confirmed the efficacy of sertraline in patients with AD and depression (Table 4) [22,26,27,55–58]; secondary analyses did not demonstrate statistically significant effects on a wider array of neuropsychiatric symptoms as assessed with the NPI.

There have been six other placebo-controlled studies of antidepressants that evaluated treatment responses on neuropsychiatric symptoms, all of them using serotonergic agents. The first was a study [56] of citalopram versus placebo in patients with AD or vascular dementia, unselected for behavioral symptoms; the study found drug–placebo differences in depression and irritability on the GBS scale. A more recent small-scale pilot study [26] that evaluated fluoxetine versus haloperidol and placebo found no difference between active treatment and placebo in the treatment of agitation. In addition, there were significantly more adverse events, most frequently nervousness, worsening of confusion, and tremor, in the fluoxetine group. Another small study [57] of fluvoxamine or placebo as adjuncts to perphenazine treatment reported that the fluvoxamine–perphenazine combination was superior with respect to placebo–perphenazine for outcomes as evaluated with the BPRS; however, outcome data for psychosis and agitation specifically were not presented. One recent study [58] evaluated sertraline versus placebo as an adjunct to donepezil treatment for subjects with AD and at least mild behavioral symptoms. There were no significant drug–placebo differences on the primary outcome measures; however, post hoc analyses in subjects with more severe behavioral symptoms suggested a possible benefit in that subgroup. A citalopram study [22] in dementia found it to be well tolerated and better than placebo in improving neurobehavioral symptoms overall and for agitation specifically but not for psychotic symptoms.

In the only placebo-controlled study [27] of trazodone for the treatment of agitation and behavioral disturbances in patients with AD, it was evaluated (at a dosage of approximately 200 mg/d) versus haloperidol, placebo, and behavioral management therapy. Neither trazodone nor the other active treatments were found to be superior to placebo in behavioral outcomes; however, dizziness was more common with trazodone treatment. A recent smaller scale double-blind, placebo-controlled study [59] of trazodone for patients with frontotemporal dementia suggested that it could improve behavioral symptoms associated with this disorder.

Parkinson's disease and dementia with Lewy bodies

There have been 13 randomized pharmacologic trials in patients who have PD or DLB that reported outcomes for symptoms of psychosis or agitation, including one post hoc analysis of a subset of patients with possible DLB who participated in an AD study. All of these studies tested antipsychotic drugs or cholinesterase inhibitors. In PD patients, the earliest antipsychotic drug studies used clozapine, and more recent ones tested newer atypical antipsychotic agents. Recently, cholinesterase inhibitors have been studied for the effects on psychosis and agitation in both DLB and PD patients. There have been no randomized studies of either mood stabilizers or antidepressants for psychosis or agitation in PD or DLB.

Antipsychotic drugs

The first study of clozapine for the treatment of PD psychosis was published in 1990 (Table 5) [60–67]. It was not possible to assess efficacy in this placebo-substitution study because of the very small sample size, but the authors noted that the dosage of clozapine used (mean, 171 mg/d) led to a worsening of parkinsonism in all patients and that it induced delirium in most patients.

In 1999, the first two placebo-controlled studies of low-dose clozapine for the treatment of PD psychosis were published. In a study by the French Clozapine Parkinson Study Group [61], clozapine was found to be significantly better than placebo in reducing positive symptoms of psychosis. It did not, on average, worsen parkinsonism or global cognition. In the other study, conducted by the Parkinson Study Group [62], clozapine was superior to placebo on all three outcome measures, again with no deleterious effect on the severity of parkinsonism or global cognition. However, one clozapine patient had to discontinue treatment secondary to the development of leukopenia. One more recent placebo-controlled study [63] of clozapine for PD psychosis found active treatment to be superior to placebo on all efficacy measures, with no significant worsening in motor or cognitive scores.

In 2000, the first study [68] of a newer atypical antipsychotic agent for PD psychosis was published. In a very small, randomized active comparator study of risperidone versus clozapine, risperidone but not clozapine led to an improvement in psychosis, although the between-group difference was not significant. Parkinsonism worsened in the risperidone group and improved with clozapine treatment, but again, the between-group difference was not significant. Soon thereafter, two publications reported results from three olanzapine studies that found no significant differences between active and placebo treatment for any efficacy measures [64,65]. However, olanzapine was associated with significant worsening of parkinsonism in all three studies and with a higher dropout rate in one. In a randomized, single-blind, active comparator study [69] of quetiapine versus clozapine, there was no difference between the two treatments in therapeutic response. Over the course of the study, parkinsonism did not worsen and dyskinesia decreased significantly in both groups, with no significant differences between them. Finally, in a recently published placebo-controlled trial [66] of quetiapine in dosages up to 200 mg/d for PD psychosis, no significant differences between active and placebo treatment were reported for any efficacy measures. In this study, no worsening of parkinsonism was found with quetiapine treatment.

One study [67] reported a post hoc analysis of a subgroup of patients from a placebo-controlled trial of olanzapine for the treatment of psychosis in AD who were retrospectively diagnosed with DLB. In these patients, olanzapine, 5 and 10 mg/d, led to a decrease in positive symptoms of psychosis without worsening either parkinsonism or cognition.

Cholinesterase inhibitors

The first placebo-controlled study of cholinesterase inhibitors in DLB was published in 2000 (Table 6) [70–73]. Subjects treated with rivastigmine had a significantly greater improvement in a cluster of neuropsychiatric symptoms that included delusions and hallucinations, although the greatest improvement was in apathy. Additionally, rivastigmine-treated subjects showed significant improvement on tests of attention, working memory, and episodic secondary memory compared with controls [74]. The first two placebo-controlled studies of cholinesterase inhibitors for the treatment of PDD did not demonstrate superiority for donepezil relative to placebo for psychiatric symptoms; however, both studies were small, designed to evaluate cognitive outcomes, and entered only subjects with limited psychiatric comorbidity [71,72]. Finally, a recent large placebo-controlled study [73] of rivastigmine versus placebo for PDD found that rivastigmine-treated patients had a significantly greater decrease in neuropsychiatric symptoms than controls with treatment and were less likely to report hallucinations as an adverse event. However, there were significantly more adverse events (including nausea, vomiting, tremor, and dizziness) and a higher study discontinuation rate with rivastigmine.

Efficacy

Alzheimer's disease, vascular dementia, and mixed dementia

Four classes of medications have been studied for the treatment of psychosis and agitation in AD, VaD, or mixed dementia. Regarding antipsychotic drugs, the findings for older typical agents suggest modest efficacy. A meta-analysis that considered studies published before 1990 concluded that treatment effects translate into an increment of approximately 18% of patients who benefit from typical antipsychotic treatment compared with placebo [20]. Subsequent findings on typical agents serve, in general, to confirm this estimate of the magnitude of the benefits [75]. For atypical antipsychotics, the published evidence for efficacy is most compelling for risperidone, for which there are two published reports of positive results for the treatment of psychosis and agitation and aggression [28,30]. There have been two published studies of olanzapine for the treatment of persistent psychosis and agitation, with one positive [31]. The only published study of quetiapine was negative [34]. As of the time of the present review, no reports of placebo-controlled, randomized trials have been published for aripiprazole or ziprasidone. However, there have been presentations at meetings or other reports of additional placebo-controlled studies on risperidone, olanzapine, quetiapine, and aripiprazole. The current pipeline of investigations also includes the Clinical Antipsychotic Trials of Intervention Effectiveness study [76] sponsored by the National Institute of Mental Health that evaluated olanzapine, quetiapine, and risperidone versus placebo as first-line and alternative treatment sequences for psychosis or agitation in AD. The literature is likely to evolve at a rapid rate. Presently, the most appropriate way to summarize may be to observe that positive findings have been reported for the treatment of psychosis, agitation, or aggression with both risperidone and olanzapine compared with placebo and that the effect sizes for treatment are within the ranges previously reported for typical antipsychotic medications.

There are no published studies demonstrating the effects of cholinesterase inhibitors or other cognitive-acting medications in which patients were recruited specifically for the evaluation of behavioral outcomes. However, a meta-analysis that reviewed secondary behavioral outcomes found that cholinesterase inhibitor treatment was better than placebo in reducing neuropsychiatric symptoms on one of two primary outcome measures (ie, the NPI but not the ADAS-cognitive), but results for psychosis and agitation specifically were not presented [42]. Findings on secondary analyses from other studies of cholinesterase inhibitors [34,41,43–46] or memantine [47,48] do not provide further evidence for significant treatment benefits. Thus, the available published literature does not support the efficacy of cholinesterase inhibitors or memantine as effective treatments for clinically significant symptoms of psychosis or agitation. However, it does suggest that treatment with these cognitive-acting agents may improve less severe behavioral symptoms and highlight the importance of further research on the extent to which treatment can prevent or delay the onset of clinically significant symptoms. There is little evidence to support the use of mood stabilizers as a treatment for agitation in dementia. Positive findings from early research on carbamazepine support the concept that mood-stabilizing anticonvulsants may be effective, but more recent studies using sodium valproate or divalproex sodium have not demonstrated efficacy [52–54]. Serotonin reuptake inhibitors may be effective for the treatment of depression of AD. In addition, findings from other research on the use of serotonin uptake inhibitors in the treatment of psychosis and agitation in AD suggest the value of further research in this area [22,57].

Parkinson's disease and dementia with Lewy bodies

Studies of antipsychotic medications in PD have used psychosis as the primary inclusion criterion. The only positive placebo-controlled studies of antipsychotics in PD have involved clozapine, which has demonstrated efficacy at low dosages in three studies [61–63]. There have been three negative placebo-controlled studies of olanzapine [64,65] and an equivocal active comparator study of risperidone versus clozapine [68]. Clinically, quetiapine is the antipsychotic agent used most commonly in PD because it is perceived to be effective and better tolerated from a motor standpoint than other atypical antipsychotics (eg, risperidone and olanzapine). Results from several open-label studies and a recent randomized, single-blind, active comparator study of quetiapine versus clozapine [69] lends support to clinicians' favorable impression of quetiapine for PD psychosis, but the only published placebo-controlled study of quetiapine was negative [66].

Regarding cholinesterase inhibitors, secondary analyses from a recent large-scale cholinesterase inhibitor study for PDD found that rivastigmine-treated patients had a significant improvement in neuropsychiatric symptoms (NPI) compared with placebo and that they were less likely to report psychosis as an adverse event [73].

Even though DLB is a relatively common condition in which psychotic symptoms are almost universal, there has only been one prospective randomized study for the treatment of neuropsychiatric complications in this population [70]. In the one study to date, rivastigmine led to significant improvement in most analyses on a composite neuropsychiatric score that included delusions, hallucinations, depression, and apathy, although it was not clear that significant between-group differences were seen for either delusions or hallucinations alone. Cholinesterase inhibitors are the recommended first-line treatment for DLB because of their benefit for cognitive symptoms [74] and lack of toxicity compared with antipsychotic medications.

In summary, clozapine is efficacious in the treatment of PD psychosis. Further research is needed to evaluate the possible role of cholinesterase inhibitors in the treatment or prevention of psychotic symptoms. For patients with DLB, there is evidence that rivastigmine may decrease neuropsychiatric symptoms, suggesting that it may be an appropriate first-line treatment for psychotic and behavioral symptoms as well as cognitive deficits.

Safety and tolerability

Alzheimer's disease, vascular dementia, and mixed media

The atypical antipsychotics were developed in research programs designed to find agents that were effective in treating schizophrenia and other psychoses with a decreased propensity to induce EPS and tardive dyskinesia [29,36,77]. Subsequent research has confirmed the relative safety of these agents with respect to drug-induced parkinsonism and tardive dyskinesia in older as well as younger patients. However, these findings must be tempered by research showing that adverse events, sometimes serious, are more varied and common than previously believed with this medication class.

Individual clinical trials of atypical antipsychotic agents in patients with dementia have demonstrated several relatively common side effects, including somnolence or sedation and gait disturbance, particularly at higher doses. Somnolence and sedation can be disabling, and treatment can be limiting. Together with even subtle gait disturbances, they can be risk factors for falls and resultant fractures or other injuries. However, a finely structured evaluation of falls in one clinical trial of risperidone demonstrated that behavioral symptoms, specifically wandering or pacing, as well as drug side effects can be associated with falls and that there are conditions (high wandering, moderate dose) under which treatment is associated with a decreased risk of falls and others (low wandering, high dose) under which falls are increased [78].

The atypical antipsychotic agents differ significantly in their pharmacologic profiles. Ziprasidone has not been studied systematically in older patients, probably because of concerns about its propensity to increase QTc intervals. Among the atypical agents, olanzapine has the strongest interactions with muscarinic cholinergic receptors. However, clinical trials have not consistently demonstrated the cognitive deficits that would be expected for an agent with significant muscarinic blocking activity. On the other hand, the only published placebo-controlled trial of quetiapine reported a worsening of cognition in patients with severe dementia [34]. Finally, as emphasized in the manufacturers' product labels, all of the atypical antipsychotic agents can lead to hyperglycemia and diabetes. However, there has been relatively little research on these metabolic effects, specifically in older patients.

More significant concerns about the use of atypical antipsychotic agents have arisen recently, brought to public attention through regulatory mechanisms. Concerns about cerebrovascular adverse events (CVAEs or strokes) began when an Australian nursing home study found an increased risk of CVAEs, transient ischemic attacks, and related adverse events in patients randomized to risperidone versus placebo [30]. The difference was of a magnitude that was likely to be clinically significant; however, evaluations of statistical significance were complicated by methodological questions about statistical inference regarding unexpected side effects. Specifically, there are no clear guidelines about how issues of multiple comparisons should be addressed when increased rates of one out of many possible adverse effects are observed. Pooling data from all available risperidone studies, including the additional subjects from other studies, did not alter the finding of an increased risk of CVAE. Based on all available data, the risks of CVAEs (including those judged to be serious adverse events and others) is 3.3% for subjects randomized to risperidone and 1.1% for those randomized to placebo, with a relative risk (95% CI) of 3.2 (1.4, 7.2) [75,79]. However, it is possible to approach the problem in a different way, considering the reports from the Australian study as hypothesis-generating, and asking if data from other studies confirm the "CVAE hypothesis." From this perspective, when findings from the other studies were considered separately, they did not provide independent confirmation of an increased risk of CVAEs with risperidone treatment.

As isolated findings, the data from risperidone trials may have been difficult to interpret. However, subsequent analyses of the rates of CVAEs in placebo-controlled clinical analyses led the US Food and Drug Administration (FDA) and the manufacturers of olanzapine and aripiprazole to agree on warnings about increased risks of strokes and related events with these agents. Taken together, these independent findings provide confirmation of the increased risks and suggest they represent a class effect.

Only a component of the findings that led to these warnings has been published, and in the absence of data, it is difficult to draw conclusions about what factors may increase or decrease the risks of CVAEs. Reports on the clinical features of the patients who experienced CVAEs during the risperidone trials found that almost all of the patients had significant risk factors for stroke, including hypertension, atrial fibrillation, previous stroke, and diabetes [72,73]. Observations that subjects who experienced CVAEs had significant risk factors for stroke cannot be used to argue against the association of the drug with CVAEs; the findings were derived from randomized clinical trials, so it is reasonable to assume that these and other risk factors were evenly distributed across those assigned to drug versus placebo. Nevertheless, these observations do suggest that the medications can lead to stroke by mechanisms that are additive or interactive with known risk factors. Accordingly, the number of patients in any setting who are likely to experience CVAEs as a result of drug exposure will depend on the baseline risk in the population. There have been suggestions that pooling results from patients who may have relatively low baseline risks (eg, subjects with AD) and high baseline risks (eg, subjects with VaD) may lead to inappropriate treatment recommendations (eg, avoiding antipsychotic use in all patients with dementia) [73]. However, in the absence of additional data, it is not possible to evaluate these or alternative suggestions about patients who may be at greater or lesser risk of CVAEs during treatment with atypical antipsychotics.

Even less background scientific and clinical information is available to support recent FDA warnings about an increased risk of mortality in older patients with dementia treated with atypical antipsychotics (www.fda.gov/cder/drug/advisory/antipsychotics.htm). As stated: "The Food and Drug Administration has determined that the treatment of behavioral disorders in elderly patients with dementia with atypical (second generation) antipsychotic medications is associated with increased mortality. Of a total of seventeen placebo-controlled trials performed with olanzapine (Zyprexa), aripiprazole (Abilify), risperidone (Risperdal), or quetiapine (Seroquel) in elderly demented patients with behavioral disorders, fifteen showed numerical increases in mortality in the drug-treated group compared with the placebo-treated patients. These studies enrolled a total of 5106 patients, and several analyses have demonstrated an approximately 1.6-1.7 fold increase in mortality in these studies. Examination of the specific causes of these deaths revealed that most were the result of either heart-related events (eg, heart failure, sudden death) or infections (mostly pneumonia).

The atypical antipsychotics fall into three drug classes based on their chemical structure. Because the increase in mortality was seen with atypical antipsychotic medications in all three chemical classes, the Agency has concluded that the effect is probably related to the common pharmacologic effects of all atypical antipsychotic medications, including those that have not been systematically studied in the dementia population.... Because of these findings, the Agency will ask the manufacturers of these drugs to include a Boxed Warning in their labeling describing this risk and noting that these drugs are not approved for this indication.... The Agency is also considering adding a similar warning to the labeling for older antipsychotic medications because the limited data available suggest a similar increase in mortality for these drugs."

Other information released by the FDA provides an alternative way to express the magnitude of the increased risks: "Over the course of these trials averaging about 10 weeks in duration, the rate of death in drug-treated patients was about 4.5%, compared with a rate of about 2.6% in the placebo group."

As with the concerns over CVAEs, the FDA findings alert providers and consumers to the need for caution. However, without publication of the evidence that led to the conclusions, it is difficult to know whether the risks are uniform or there are definable subgroups of patients who may be at greater or lesser risk for drug-related mortality. Critical questions that remain unanswered include how the risks of atypical antipsychotic agents interact with those associated with aging and related medical conditions. It is important to recognize that the FDA estimates were derived primarily from studies with large numbers of "old-old" nursing home residents with high degrees of medical comorbidity and at high mortality risk, even in the absence of specific treatment. There is no evidence about whether patients with specific medical comorbidities are at greater risk and no evidence about how to apply the warning in patients who are relatively healthy.

Research on other medication classes have confirmed expected patterns of side effects. For example, studies of sodium valproate or divalproex sodium in patients with dementia have identified somnolence and ataxia as significant side effects; and studies of cholinesterase inhibitors identified significant gastrointestinal side effects. However, because there is less evidence for the efficacy of these other medications in the treatment of psychosis and agitation in dementia, there has been less attention to conducting the research and analyses that would be necessary to balance the potential benefits versus risks.

Parkinson's disease and dementia with Lewy bodies

In PD, concerns about worsening parkinsonism and dyskinesia are paramount. Clozapine and possibly quetiapine at low dosages do not appear to worsen motor symptoms, although higher dosages of either agent may not be as well tolerated [60,69]. Results from randomized studies of olanzapine suggest that it is not well tolerated from a motor standpoint in PD [64,65]. The only randomized study of risperidone in PD found worsening parkinsonism with risperidone and an improvement with clozapine treatment [68]; although the differences were not statistically significant, this may have been related to a small sample size. The results from open-label studies with risperidone in PD have been mixed [80], but it is rarely used in clinical practice, probably because of clinical impressions that it frequently worsens parkinsonism.

One of the defining features of DLB is the extreme sensitivity to antipsychotic medications, both typical [81] and even newer atypical agents [82]. There have been no prospective, randomized studies of antipsychotic use in this population.

Despite theoretical concerns that cholinesterase inhibitors may worsen parkinsonism, adverse events on motor symptoms have not been observed in randomized clinical trials in either PD or DLB. However, study discontinuation rates have been higher with cholinesterase inhibitor treatment compared with placebo treatment, and gastrointestinal adverse events are common.

Treatment recommendations

Alzheimer's disease, vascular dementia, and mixed dementia

The evidence for the efficacy of drug treatment in reducing psychosis and behavioral symptoms in dementia is greatest for antipsychotic agents.

Although the efficacy of the newer atypical agents appears to be comparable to that of the older typical agents, they are associated with lower risks of extrapyramidal symptoms and tardive dyskinesia. Recent estimates of the overall benefit observed in randomized clinical trials for antipsychotic treatment above that of placebo are approximately 20% [83], similar to the 18% benefit reported in a meta-analysis of typical antipsychotics [20]. The risks, as estimated by the FDA, include an increment of approximately 2% in mortality. Using these figures, for every 100 demented patients treated for psychosis or agitation with an atypical antipsychotic, approximately 20 would benefit from treatment, but approximately 2 would die. The number of patients who must be treated for one patient to benefit (ie, the number needed to treat) is approximately five, whereas the number who must be treated for one to die (ie, the number needed to harm) is approximately 50. The observed ratio of benefit to risk, approximately 10:1, must be a matter of grave concern.

In the absence of any more specific data, one principle that follows from the warning must be that the use of atypical antipsychotic agents in dementia should be reserved for those patients who have severe psychotic symptoms or agitation, in which severity is evaluated with respect to the extent to which symptoms represent sources of suffering, excess disability, or danger. There have been recommendations that even among patients with severe symptoms, the use of atypical antipsychotic medications may be most appropriate for those in whom symptoms are sources of potential danger. In other cases, the use of these agents may be most appropriate only after behavioral, psychosocial, environmental, and possibly other pharmacologic approaches to treatment (eg, cognitive enhancing agents or serotonin reuptake inhibitors) have been tried and found to be ineffective.

A number of questions arise in applying this principle. One question is whether it is possible to manage patients with psychotic or behavioral symptoms without antipsychotic medication. The answer is yes, at least for most of the patients in nursing homes with symptoms of the type and severity that were addressed in the randomized clinical trials. The best evidence for this comes from the reports of the randomized clinical trials themselves. In the published randomized trials of risperidone, the number of subjects with early withdrawals from treatment for any reason in those who were assigned to placebo was 27% [28], 35% [29], and 33% [30]. For the olanzapine studies, they were 24% [37] and 29.5% [31]. For the risperidone studies for which information was available, the proportions of placebo patients who withdrew because of a lack of efficacy were 5.5% [28] and 19.4% [30]; for the olanzapine studies the proportion were 6.5% [37] and 5.7% [31]. Admittedly, it is possible that a lack of efficacy could have contributed to dropouts that were attributed to other causes. Furthermore, there are no reports on how early termination from placebo treatment varied with symptom severity. Nevertheless, it is clear that a large majority of the subjects included in the available studies could be managed while receiving placebo without any specific treatment, and the number of patients who were terminated because of lack of efficacy was small. However, it is important to recognize that patients with the most severe symptoms would not have been entered into a study in which there was a chance of randomization to placebo treatment.

Another question is whether the estimates of treatment benefits and risks derived from the available clinical trials apply equally to patients with varying degrees of symptom severity. It may be reasonable, for example, to hypothesize that drug–placebo differences and the benefits of treatment may be greater in patients with or without psychosis who have severe symptoms of agitation and aggression. However, the published literature does not address this question. It is also possible that severe behavioral symptoms may be associated with increased risks of medical morbidity and mortality and that these may be attenuated with treatment. In fact, some studies [84,85], but not others [86,87], have reported that psychotic or behavioral symptoms are associated with increased morality, but there have been no studies of the impact of symptom severity on this risk. Answers to these questions are within the data that are available to the FDA and the pharmaceutical companies. Hopefully the relevant analyses will be reported in the near future. At present, however, it is important to observe that the published data and the FDA warnings are adequate to recommend limiting the use of atypical antipsychotic medication to patients with severe psychotic and behavioral symptoms but not to allow estimates of the potential benefits versus the risks in these patients.

The evidence for the efficacy of cognitive enhancing agents and serotonin reuptake inhibitors for psychosis and agitation in dementia is equivocal. Nevertheless, cautious administration of these agents may be a useful strategy for the management of mild to moderate psychosis and agitation that are not responsive to nonpharmacologic interventions. For patients whose symptoms include depression, anxiety, or irritability, the use of antidepressants may be particularly useful.

Clinicians working with patients who have psychosis and agitation associated with dementia have a difficult task: applying scientific evidence and general principles to estimate the benefits versus the risks of alternative treatments for an individual patient even in the face of critical gaps in the information that is available to them. Nevertheless, the conduct of such individualized benefit-risk analyses must be the cornerstone of treatment planning. Presently, there is no alternative but to fill in the gaps in scientific knowledge with clinical judgement.

Specifically, before initiating treatment with atypical antipsychotic agents, clinicians should document their clinical judgement regarding the potential risks and benefits of treatment. This should include (1) an evaluation of the quality and severity of the symptoms, including estimates of the risk and costs of not treating patients (eg, danger to the patient or others, excess disability, impairments in quality of life, and the magnitude of the patient's suffering). For patients living in the community, other considerations include the burden to family caregivers and the value of maintaining the patient in the community; (2) an assessment of the potential benefits of alternative treatments, including outcomes of previous trials and clinical estimation of the likely benefit of a specific treatment; (3) documentation of the clinician's awareness of the potential risks associated with treatment, including the overall risks and the provider's judgement of the clinical characteristics of the individual patient that may modify risks; (4) a statement documenting the provider's overall judgement about whether or not the potential benefits outweigh potential risks in this case; (5) discussion of the risk:benefit ratio with the patient's family or health care proxy; and (6) establishment of a clear treatment plan, with close monitoring of both neurobehavioral and medical outcomes.

There is no empirical evidence about the duration of treatment that is required for patients with dementia and psychotic or behavioral symptoms. The current practice is to initiate trials of dose reduction or withdrawal after patients have responded to treatment and have been stable for several months. When symptoms recur in such patients, a further risk-benefit analysis is necessary. However, in conducting such an evaluation, it is reasonable to assume that the probability of treatment benefits may be greater than for those without previous treatment.

Parkinson's disease and dementia with Lewy bodies

In PD, clozapine is the best established medication for the treatment of psychosis. However, the potential risk for agranulocytosis is of concern, and the requirement for frequent blood monitoring is burdensome. Clozapine is best reserved for severe psychosis in PD that persists after attempts to control symptoms by modifying dopaminergic treatments for motor symptoms. Based on limited evidence, mainly anecdotal and from open-label studies, quetiapine may be considered as a possible antipsychotic medication in PD at this time. Because psychosis in PD frequently occurs in association with dementia, cholinesterase inhibitors should be considered as possible alternative or adjunctive treatments.

For DLB, cholinesterase inhibitors are the only class of psychiatric medication that has been evaluated in randomized clinical trials. Even on the basis of the limited evidence that is available, these agents appear to have positive effects on both neuropsychiatric symptoms and cognition. The evidence supports the recommendation that patients with DLB should have a trial of a cholinesterase inhibitor. Given the possibility of severe antipsychotic sensitivity in DLB, this class of medications cannot be recommended for use in this population.

Summary

Despite a significant body of research in this area, there are critical gaps in the evidence base on the treatment of the psychotic and behavioral symptoms associated with Alzheimer's disease and vascular dementia. This problem has been exacerbated by recent FDA warnings on the risks of increased CVAEs and mortality with atypical antipsychotic treatment, without the release of the scientific evidence on which these warnings are based. At present, the evidence for treatment benefits are greatest for risperidone and olanzapine, but these are the agents for which there have been warnings about the increased risks of CVAEs as well as mortality. Use of these agents should be reserved for those cases in which psychotic or behavioral symptoms are severe and associated with secondary complications. Their use should require an evaluation of the balance between the potential benefits and risks of treatment for the individual patient, and the provider's judgement that the balance is in favor of treatment.

The published clinical trials provide evidence in support of the use of clozapine for clinically significant psychotic symptoms in PD for patients who have not responded or cannot tolerate modifications to their PD medication regimen. In DLB, there is evidence in support of the use of cholinesterase inhibitors as treatments for both cognitive impairment and neuropsychiatric symptoms.

References

[1] Fitzpatrick AL, Kuller AH, Ives DG, et al. Incidence and prevalence of dementia in the Cardiovascular Health Study. J Am Geriatr Soc 2004;52:195–204.

[2] Stevens T, Livingston G, Kitchen G, et al. Islington study of dementia subtypes in the community. Br J Psychiatry 2002;180:270–6.

[3] Rahkonen T, Eloniemi-Sulkava U, Rissanen S, et al. Dementia with Lewy bodies according to the consensus criteria in a general population aged 75 years or older. J Neurol Neurosurg Psychiatry 2003;74:720–4.

[4] Aarsland D, Andersen K, Larsen JP, et al. Prevalence and characteristics of dementia in Parkinson disease: an 8-year prospective study. Arch Neurol 2003;60:387–92.

[5] Mega MS, Cummings JL, Fiorello T, et al. The spectrum of behavioral changes in Alzheimer's disease. Neurology 1996;46:130–5.

[6] McKeith I, Mintzer JE, Aarsland D. Dementia with Lewy bodies. Lancet Neurol 2004;3: 19–28.

[7] Aarsland D, Larsen JP, Lim NG, et al. Range of neuropsychiatric disturbances in patients with Parkinson's disease. J Neurol Neurosurg Psychiatry 1999;67:492–6.

[8] Lyketsos CG, Steinberg M, Tschanz JT, et al. Mental and behavioral disturbances in dementia: findings from the Cache County Study on Memory in Aging. Am J Psychiatry 2000;157: 708–14.

[9] Steinberg M, Tschanz JT, Corcoran C, et al. The persistence of neuropsychiatric symptoms in dementia: the Cache County Study. Int J Geriatr Psychiatry 2004;19:19–26.

[10] Lyketsos CG, Lopez O, Jones B, et al. Prevalence of neuropsychiatric symptoms in dementia and mild cognitive impairment: results from the Cardiovascular Health Study. JAMA 2002; 288:1475–83.

[11] Margallo-Lana M, Swann A, O'Brien J, et al. Prevalence and pharmacological management of behavioural and psychological symptoms amongst dementia sufferers living in care environments. Int J Geriatr Psychiatry 2001;16:39–44.

[12] Bassiony MM, Lyketsos CG. Delusions and hallucinations in Alzheimer's disease: review of the brain decade. Psychosomatics 2003;44:388–401.

[13] Leroi I, Voulgari A, Breitner JC, et al. The epidemiology of psychosis in dementia. Am J Geriatr Psychiatry 2003;11:83–91.

[14] Marsh L, Williams JR, Rocco M, et al. Psychiatric comorbidities in patients with Parkinson disease and psychosis. Neurology 2004;63:293–300.

[15] Baskys A. Lewy body dementia: the litmus test for neuroleptic sensitivity and extrapyramidal symptoms. J Clin Psychiatry 2004;65(Suppl 11):S16–22.

[16] Steele C, Rovner B, Chase GA, et al. Psychiatric symptoms and nursing home placement of patients with Alzheimer's disease. Am J Psychiatry 1990;147:1049–51.

[17] Goetz CG, Stebbins GT. Risk factors for nursing home placement in advanced Parkinson's disease. Neurology 1993;43:2227–9.

[18] Snowdon DA, Greiner LH, Mortimer JA, et al. Brain infarction and the clinical expression of Alzheimer disease: the Nun Study. JAMA 1997;277:813–7.

[19] Schneider LS, Katz IR, Park S, et al. Psychosis of Alzheimer disease: validity of the construct and response to risperidone. Am J Geriatr Psychiatry 2003;11:414–25.

[20] Schneider LS, Pollock VE, Lyness SA. A meta-analysis of controlled trials of neuroleptic treatment in dementia. J Am Geriatr Soc 1990;38:553–63.

[21] Finkel SI, Lyons JS, Anderson RL, et al. A randomized, placebo-controlled trial of thiothixene in agitated, demented nursing home patients. Int J Geriatr Psychiatry 1995;10:129–36.

[22] Pollock BG, Mulsant BH, Rosen J, et al. Comparison of citalopram, perphenazine, and placebo for the acute treatment of psychosis and behavioral disturbances in hospitalized, demented patients. Am J Psychiatry 2002;159:460–5.

[23] Allain H, Dautzenberg PHJ, Maurer K, et al. Double blind study of tiapride versus haloperidol and placebo in agitation and aggressiveness in elderly patients with cognitive impairment. Psychopharmacology (Berl) 2000;148:361–6.

[24] Devanand DP, Marder K, Michaels KS, et al. A randomized, placebo-controlled dose-comparison trial of haloperidol for psychosis and disruptive behaviors in Alzheimer's disease. Am J Psychiatry 1998;155:1512–20.

[25] Lonergan E, Luxenberg J, Colford J. Haloperidol for agitation in dementia. Cochrane Database Syst Rev 2002;2:CD002852.

[26] Auchus AP, Bissey-Black C. Pilot study of haloperidol, fluoxetine, and placebo for agitation in Alzheimer's disease. J Neuropsychiatry Clin Neurosci 1997;9:591–3.

[27] Teri L, Logsdon RG, Peskind E, et al. Treatment of agitation in AD: a randomized, placebo-controlled clinical trial. Neurology 2000;55:1271–8.

[28] Katz IR, Jeste DV, Mintzer JE, et al. Comparison of risperidone and placebo for psychosis and behavioral disturbances associated with dementia: a randomized, double-blind trial. J Clin Psychiatry 1999;60:107–15.

[29] De Deyn PP, Rabheru K, Rasmussen A, et al. A randomized trial of risperidone, placebo, and haloperidol for behavioral symptoms of dementia. Neurology 1999;53:946–55.

[30] Brodaty H, Ames D, Snowden JS, et al. A randomized placebo-controlled trial of risperidone for the treatment of aggression, agitation, and psychosis of dementia. J Clin Psychiatry 2003; 64:134–43.

[31] Street JS, Clark WS, Gannon KS, et al. Olanzapine treatment of psychotic and behavioral symptoms in patients with Alzheimer disease in nursing care facilities: a double-blind, randomized, placebo-controlled trial. Arch Gen Psychiatry 2000;57:968–76.

[32] De Deyn PP, Carrasco MM, Deberdt W, et al. Olanzapine versus placebo in the treatment of psychosis with or without associated behavioral disturbances in patients with Alzheimer's disease. Int J Geriatr Psychiatry 2004;19:115–26.

[33] Meehan KM, Wang H, David SR, et al. Comparison of rapidly acting intramuscular olanzapine, lorazepam, and placebo: a double-blind, randomized study in acutely agitated patients with dementia. Neuropsychopharmacology 2002;26:494–504.

[34] Ballard C, Margallo-Lana M, Juszcak E, et al. Quetiapine and rivastigmine and cognitive decline in Alzheimer's disease: randomised double blind placebo controlled trial. BMJ 2005;330:874–8.

[35] Lanctôt KL, Best TS, Mittmann N, et al. Efficacy and safety of neuroleptics in behavioral disorders associated with dementia. J Clin Psychiatry 1998;59:550–61.

[36] Chan W, Lam LC, Choy CN, et al. A double-blind randomised comparison of risperidone and haloperidol in the treatment of behavioural and psychological symptoms in Chinese dementia patients. Int J Geriatr Psychiatry 2001;16:1156–62.

[37] Satterlee WG, Reams SG, Burns PR, et al. A clinical update on olanzapine treatment in schizophrenia and in elderly Alzheimer's disease patients. Psychopharmacol Bull 1995; 31:534.

[38] van Reekum R, Clarke D, Conn D, et al. A randomized, placebo-controlled trial of the discontinuation of long-term antipsychotics in dementia. Int Psychogeriatr 2002;14: 197–210.

[39] Bridges-Parlet S, Knopman D, Steffes S. Withdrawal of neuroleptic medications from institutionalized dementia patients: results of a double-blind, baseline-treatment-controlled pilot study. J Geriatr Psychiatry Neurol 1997;10:119–26.

[40] Ballard CG, Thomas A, Fossey J, et al. A 3-month, randomized, placebo-controlled, neuroleptic discontinuation study in 100 people with dementia: the neuropsychiatric inventory median cutoff is a predictor of clinical outcome. J Clin Psychiatry 2004;65:114–9.

[41] Tariot PN, Cummings JL, Katz IR, et al. A randomized, double-blind, placebo-controlled study of the efficacy and safety of donepezil in patients with Alzheimer's disease in the nursing home setting. J Am Geriatr Soc 2001;49:1590–9.

[42] Trinh NH, Hoblyn J, Mohanty S, et al. Efficacy of cholinesterase inhibitors in the treatment of neuropsychiatric symptoms and functional impairment in Alzheimer disease: a meta-analysis. JAMA 2003;289:210–6.

[43] Feldman H, Gauthier S, Hecker J, et al. A 24-week, randomized, double-blind study of donepezil in moderate to severe Alzheimer's disease. Neurology 2001;57:613–20.

[44] AD2000 Collaborative Group. Long-term donepezil treatment in 565 patients with Alzheimer's disease (AD2000): randomised double-blind trial. Lancet 2004;363:2105–15.

[45] Holmes C, Wilkinson D, Dean C, et al. The efficacy of donepezil in the treatment of neuropsychiatric symptoms in Alzheimer disease. Neurology 2004;63:214–9.

[46] Erkinjuntti T, Kurz A, Gauthier S, et al. Efficacy of galantamine in probable vascular dementia and Alzheimer's disease combined with cerebrovascular disease: a randomised trial. Lancet 2002;359:1283–90.

[47] Reisberg B, Doody R, Stöffler A, et al. Memantine in moderate-to-severe Alzheimer's disease. N Engl J Med 2003;348:1333–41.

[48] Tariot PN, Farlow MR, Grossberg GT, et al. Memantine treatment in patients with moderate to severe Alzheimer disease already receiving donepezil. JAMA 2004;291:317–24.

[49] Herrmann N, Rabheru K, Wang J, et al. Galantamine treatment of problematic behavior in Alzheimer disease: post-hoc analysis of pooled data from three large trials. Am J Geriatr Psychiatry 2005;13:527–34.

[50] Tariot PN, Erb R, Podgorski CA, et al. Efficacy and tolerability of carbamazepine for agitation and aggression in dementia. Am J Psychiatry 1998;155:54–61.

[51] Olin JT, Fox LS, Pawluczyk S, et al. A pilot randomized trial of carbamazepine for behavioral symptoms in treatment-resistant outpatients with Alzheimer disease. Am J Geriatr Psychiatry 2001;9:400–5.

[52] Porsteinsson AP, Tariot PN, Erb R, et al. Placebo-controlled study of divalproex sodium for agitation in dementia. Am J Geriatr Psychiatry 2001;9:58–66.

[53] Sival RC, Haffmans PMJ, Jansen PAF, et al. Sodium valproate in the treatment of aggressive behavior in patients with dementia-a randomized placebo controlled clinical trial. Int J Geriatr Psychiatry 2002;17:579–85.

[54] Tariot PN, Schneider LS, Mintzer JE, et al. Safety and tolerability of divalproex sodium in the treatment of signs and symptoms of mania in elderly patients with dementia: results of a double-blind, placebo-controlled trial. Current Therapeutic Research 2001; 62:51–67.

[55] Lyketsos CG, DelCampo L, Steinberg M, et al. Treating depression in Alzheimer disease: efficacy and safety of sertraline therapy, and the benefits of depression reduction: the DIADS. Arch Gen Psychiatry 2003;60:737–46.

[56] Nyth AL, Gottfries CG. The clinical efficacy of citalopram in treatment of emotional disturbances in dementia disorders: a Nordic multicentre study. Br J Psychiatry 1990;157:894–901.

[57] Levkovitz Y, Bloch Y, Kaplan D, et al. Fluvoxamine for psychosis in Alzheimer's disease. J Nerv Ment Dis 2001;189:126–9.

[58] Finkel SI, Mintzer JE, Dysken M, et al. A randomized, placebo-controlled study of the efficacy and safety or sertraline in the treatment of the behavioral manifestations of Alzheimer's disease in outpatients treated with donepezil. Int J Geriatr Psychiatry 2004; 19:9–18.

[59] Lebert F, Stekke W, Hasenbroekx C, et al. Frontotemporal dementia: a randomised, controlled trial with trazodone. Dement Geriatr Cogn Disord 2004;17:355–9.

[60] Wolters EC, Hurwitz TA, Mak E, et al. Clozapine in the treatment of parkinsonian patients with dopaminomimetic psychosis. Neurology 1990;40:832–4.

[61] The French Clozapine Parkinson Study Group. Clozapine in drug-induced psychosis in Parkinson's disease. Lancet 1999;353:2041–2.

[62] The Parkinson Study Group. Low-dose clozapine for the treatment of drug-induced psychosis in Parkinson's disease. N Engl J Med 1999;340:757–63.

[63] Pollak P, Tison F, Rascol O, et al. Clozapine in drug induced psychosis in Parkinson's disease: a randomised, placebo controlled study with open follow up. J Neurol Neurosurg Psychiatry 2004;75:689–95.

[64] Breier A, Sutton VK, Feldman PD, et al. Olanzapine in the treatment of dopamimetic-induced psychosis in patients with Parkinson's disease. Biol Psychiatry 2002;52:438–45.

[65] Ondo WG, Levy JK, Vuong KD, et al. Olanzapine treatment for dopaminergic-induced hallucinations. Mov Disord 2002;17:1031–5.

[66] Ondo WG, Tintner R, Voung KD, et al. Double-blind, placebo-controlled, unforced titration parallel trial of quetiapine for dopaminergic-induced hallucinations in Parkinson's disease. Mov Disord 2005;20:958–63.

[67] Cummings JL, Street JS, Masterman DL, et al. Efficacy of olanzapine in the treatment of psychosis in dementia with Lewy bodies. Dement Geriatr Cogn Disord 2002;13:67–73.

[68] Ellis T, Cudkowicz ME, Sexton PM, et al. Clozapine and risperidone treatment of psychosis in Parkinson's disease. J Neuropsychiatry Clin Neurosci 2000;12:364–9.

[69] Morgante L, Epifanio A, Spina E, et al. Quetiapine and clozapine in parkinsonian patients with dopaminergic psychosis. Clin Neuropharmacol 2004;27:153–6.

[70] McKeith I, Del Ser T, Spano PF, et al. Efficacy of rivastigmine in dementia with Lewy bodies: a randomised, double-blind, placebo-controlled international study. Lancet 2000;356: 2031–6.

[71] Aarsland D, Laake K, Larsen JP, et al. Donepezil for cognitive impairment in Parkinson's disease: a randomised controlled study. J Neurol Neurosurg Psychiatry 2002;72:708–12.

[72] Leroi I, Brandt J, Reich SG, et al. Randomized placebo-controlled trial of donepezil in cognitive impairment in Parkinson's disease. Int J Geriatr Psychiatry 2004;19:1–8.

[73] Emre M, Aarsland D, Albanese A, et al. Rivastigmine for dementia associated with Parkinson's disease. N Engl J Med 2004;351:2509–18.

[74] Wesnes KA, McKeith IG, Ferrara R, et al. Effects of rivastigmine on cognitive function in dementia with Lewy bodies: a randomised placebo-controlled international study using the Cognitive Drug Research computerized assessment system. Dement Geriatr Cogn Disord 2002;13:183–92.

[75] Bullock R. Treatment of behavioural and psychiatric symptoms in dementia: implications of recent safety warnings. Curr Med Res Opin 2005;21:1–10.

[76] Schneider LS, Tariot PN, Lyketsos CG, et al. National Institutes of Mental Health Clinical Antipsychotic Trials of Intervention Effectiveness (CATIE): Alzheimer disease trial methodology. Am J Geriatr Psychiatry 2001;9:346–60.

[77] Jeste DV, Okamoto A, Napolitano J, et al. Low incidence of persistent tardive dyskinesia in elderly patients with dementia treated with risperidone. Am J Psychiatry 2000;157:1150–5.

[78] Katz IR, Rupnow M, Kozma C, et al. Risperidone and falls in ambulatory nursing home residents with dementia and psychosis or agitation: secondary analysis of a double-blind, placebo-controlled trial. Am J Geriatr Psychiatry 2004;12:499–508.

[79] Herrmann N, Lanctôt KL. Do atypical antipsychotics cause stroke? CNS Drugs 2005;19: 91–103.

[80] Tarsy D, Baldessarini RJ, Tarazi FI. Effects of newer antipsychotics on extrapyramidal function. CNS Drugs 2002;16:23–45.

[81] McKeith I, Fairbairn A, Perry R, et al. Neuroleptic sensitivity in patients with senile dementia of Lewy body type. BMJ 1992;305:673–8.

[82] McKeith IG, Ballard CG, Harrison RW. Neuroleptic sensitivity to risperidone in Lewy body dementia. Lancet 1995;346:699.

[83] Lawlor BA. Behavioral and psychological symptoms in dementia: the role of atypical antipsychotics. J Clin Psychiatry 2004;65(Suppl 11):S5–10.

[84] Walsh JS, Welch HG, Larson EB. Survival of outpatients with Alzheimer-type dementia. Ann Intern Med 1990;113:429–34.

[85] Moritz DJ, Fox PJ, Luscombe FA, et al. Neurological and psychiatric predictors of mortality in patients with Alzheimer disease in California. Arch Neurol 1997;54:878–85.

[86] Carlson MC, Brandt J, Steele C, et al. Predictor index of mortality in dementia patients upon entry in long-term care. J Gerontol A Biol Sci Med Sci 2001;56:M567–70.

[87] Lopez OL, Wisniewski SR, Becker JT, et al. Psychiatric medication and abnormal behavior as predictors of progression in probable Alzheimer disease. Arch Neurol 1999;56:1266–72.

ELSEVIER
SAUNDERS

Psychiatr Clin N Am
28 (2005) 985–1005

PSYCHIATRIC
CLINICS
OF NORTH AMERICA

Evidence-Based Interventions for Nursing Home Residents with Dementia-Related Behavioral Symptoms

Nipali Bharani, MD*, Mark Snowden, MD, MPH

Department of Psychiatry and Behavioral Sciences, University of Washington, Box 359911, Harborview Medical Center, 325 9th Avenue, Seattle, WA 98104, USA

In long-term care settings, up to one half of the residents carry a diagnosis of dementia [1]. Behavioral symptoms are common in dementia, associated with caregiver stress, and are often the precipitating factor for nursing home placement [2]. In the coming years, the number of dementia patients in nursing homes will continue to increase. Improving the quality of mental health care in nursing homes will in large part involve effective management of behavioral symptoms in these patients.

Behavioral symptoms, also referred to as "agitation," manifest themselves in a variety of forms, including verbal aggression (yelling and cursing), physical aggression (hitting and biting), purposeless behaviors (packing, hoarding, and wandering), and resistance to care [3,4]. These behaviors in dementia may be the result of an inability to communicate needs in the face of unpleasant environmental conditions (temperature and noise) or physical discomfort (fecal impaction and pain). Behavioral disturbances may also be an inherent part of the disease process. Agitation occurs throughout the course of dementia syndromes and becomes increasingly frequent in later stages [5] when many patients are already residing in long-term care settings. Generally, treatment recommendations emphasize the importance of assessing underlying causes before initiating treatment interventions [6]. However, there are limited data supporting the usefulness of elaborate workups [7]. In the absence of an obvious environmental or physical link, there are a growing number of treatment choices in nursing home settings as interventions continue to be developed and studied.

---

* Corresponding author.
E-mail address: nipali@u.washington.edu (N. Bharani).

0193-953X/05/$ - see front matter © 2005 Elsevier Inc. All rights reserved.
doi:10.1016/j.psc.2005.09.004
psych.theclinics.com

Multiple drug classes are used to treat dementia-related agitation in nursing homes, including anticonvulsants, antidepressants, and, most commonly, antipsychotics. Nursing home clinicians are faced with interesting challenges under the 1987 Omnibus Budget Reconciliation Act nursing home reform policy, which restricts antipsychotic use in patients without specific psychiatric symptoms [8], amid growing concerns about safety profiles of this drug class, particularly the increased risk of mortality and cerebrovascular accidents. Although there is no US Food and Drug Administration (FDA)-approved indication, there are a growing number of randomized controlled trials of drug therapy to treat dementia-related agitation.

In addition, numerous nonpharmacologic interventions for treating agitation in nursing home residents continue to be developed. The interventions most commonly studied in randomized controlled trials include activity and sensory therapies and staff training interventions. This article systematically reviews the literature on pharmacologic and nonpharmacologic treatments for dementia-related agitation in nursing home residents. The intent is to provide clinicians with an evidence-based guide for choosing among pharmacological and nonpharmacologic interventions for behavioral symptoms in nursing home residents with dementia. The limitations of the available evidence and future research needs are also discussed.

Database search

To evaluate the efficacy of pharmacological and nonpharmacologic interventions for dementia-related behavioral symptoms in nursing home residents, systematic searches were conducted of MEDLINE, PsychINFO, EMBASE (for drugs and pharmacology), and CINAHL for reports published from January 2000 to March 2005. The MeSH search terms used were dementia, cognitive impairment, Alzheimer's, agitation, behavior, nursing home, skilled nursing facility, and long-term care. For preceding years, articles were used that were identified in a previous systematic search using the same search terms and database set going back to 1970 [7].

To be included in this review, studies had to be conducted in nursing home settings, and in combination studies at least half of the subjects had to be nursing home residents. Studies presented as letters to the editor and case reports were excluded. A qualitative analysis was conducted of the literature with a focus on the primary outcome measures of behavioral symptoms or agitation. Priority was given to randomized controlled trials, but information from observational trials was summarized as well. Pharmacologic interventions were classified into four categories: antipsychotics, antidepressants, anticonvulsants, and other. Nonpharmacologic interventions were classified into three categories: sensory, training, and activities interventions. A total of 89 articles were reviewed, of which 33 were randomized controlled trials (RCT) (19 in pharmacologic and 14 in nonpharmacologic).

Research on pharmacologic interventions

Antipsychotics

Seven randomized, double-blind, placebo-controlled trials of antipsychotics were reviewed. The trials ranged in length from 4 to 12 weeks. In two studies of conventional agents, both thioridazine and thiothixene demonstrated a significantly superior response in subjects, compared with placebo [9,10]. Four trials that studied atypical agents and had at least 200 subjects demonstrated modest statistically significant effects in favor of antipsychotic therapy [11–14]. The one negative RCT, involving two conventional agents and placebo, was limited by a suboptimal dosing strategy and a smaller sample size (Table 1) [15].

Among atypical antipsychotics, a randomized controlled trial of risperidone (mean dose 1.1 mg) demonstrated a trend-level improvement over placebo in primary outcome measures (30% reduction as measured by the Behavior Pathology in Alzheimer's Disease Rating Scale [BEHAVE-AD]), and significant declines in multiple secondary measures, including the Cohen-Mansfield Agitation Inventory (CMAI) aggression cluster scores and Clinical Global Impression Scale (CGIS) scores. No difference in efficacy was found between haloperidol (mean dose 1.2 mg) and risperidone in this trial [12]. Two randomized, controlled trials found risperidone to be significantly superior to placebo [11,13]. In one study [11], risperidone (mean dose 0.95 mg) was significantly more effective than placebo in reducing CMAI total aggression scores (22% of patients for risperidone versus 9% for placebo). In a subgroup analysis involving patients without psychosis, risperidone remained significantly superior to placebo, suggesting that the effects of risperidone in treating agitation go beyond the reduction of psychotic symptoms. In the other trial, statistically significant improvements over placebo were found with 1- and 2-mg doses of risperidone, but the larger dose resulted in significantly higher adverse events without additional benefit. The improvement with risperidone remained significant after adjusting for the presence of psychotic symptoms [13]. There is additional support for risperidone in observational studies [27,28]. One study suggested risperidone is useful for reducing nighttime wandering hours and increasing nighttime sleeping hours [28].

In a randomized, controlled trial, olanzapine (5-mg and 10-mg doses) significantly reduced Neuropsychiatric Inventory-Nursing Home (NPI-NH) version core symptoms (43%–53% of patients for olanzapine versus 25% for placebo). There was no difference between groups for higher, 15-mg doses of olanzapine [14]. Olanzapine demonstrated sustained significant reductions in NPI-NH core total scores (including agitation and aggressiveness) in an

Table 1
Pharmacologic interventions for treatment of dementia-related agitation in nursing home residents: randomized controlled trials

Study	Agent	Sample (N)	Duration (wk)	Outcome measures (behavioral symptoms)	Results and comments
Antipsychotics					
Stotsky 1984 [9]	Thioridazine	358	4	Hamilton anxiety scale	Statistically significant improvement in anxiety scale scores (including agitation) with active drug (74% vs 42% with placebo)
Finkel et al 1995 [10]	Thiothixene	33	11	CMAI (responder, improvement of ≥5 points on CMAI)	Statistically significant decrease in agitation scores; 69% responders with active drug vs 19% with placebo
Katz et al 1999 [13]	Risperidone	625	12	BEHAVE-AD (response, ≥50% reduction)	Statistically significant greater response with 1 mg (45%) and 2 mg (50%) vs placebo (33%)
De Deyn et al 1999 [12]	Risperidone, Haloperidol	344	12	BEHAVE-AD, CMAI	Trend-level improvement in primary outcome (>30% reduction in BEHAVE-AD) for risperidone compared with placebo 2% lower BEHAVE-AD and 5% lower CMAI scores with risperidone compared with placebo No difference in efficacy between risperidone and haloperidol but extrapyramidal symptoms more common with haloperidol
Brodaty et al 2003 [11]	Risperidone	345	12	CMAI, BEHAVE-AD, CGIC	Statistically significant decline 22% in CMAI total aggression scores with risperidone vs 9% with placebo Secondary outcomes: significant improvement in BEHAVE-AD and CGIC with risperidone Significant decline in agitation in subgroup of patients without psychosis when compared with placebo

Study	Drug(s)	N	Weeks	Outcome measure	Results
Street et al 2000 [14]	Olanzapine	206	6	NPI-NH subsets (agitation, aggression, hallucinations, delusions)	Statistically significant 43% to 53% improvement with active drug vs 25% with placebo
Barnes et al 1982 [15]	Thioridazine, loxapine	60	6	BPRS	No significant differences among groups on behavior scale scores; Small sample size; antipsychotic doses lower than those generally found to be effective.
Lovett et al 1987 [16]	Haloperidol, trifluoperazine	54	6	BPRS	No significant differences between the two drugs; No placebo
Smith et al 1974 [17]	Haloperidol, thioridazine	46	6	BPRS	No significant difference between the two drugs; No placebo
Coccaro et al 1990 [18]	Haloperidol, oxazepam, dipenhydramine	59	8	BPRS	No significant differences among drugs; No placebo
Covington 1975 [19]	Thioridazine, diazepam	40	4	Hamilton anxiety scale	Statistically significant 45% response rate with thioridazine vs 30% with diazepam; No placebo
Stotsky 1984 [9]	Thioridazine, diazepam	252	4	Hamilton anxiety scale	Statistically significant improvement in anxiety scale scores with thioridazine 77% vs 65% with diazepam; No placebo
SSRIs					
Nyth et al 1990 [26]	Citalopram	89	4	Gottfries-Brane-Steen geriatric rating scale	Statistically significant decrease in irritability and depressed mood; Outcomes did not include more typical agitated behaviors
Lanctot et al 2002 [22]	Sertraline	22	4	NPI, CMAI, BEHAVE-AD	No significant difference between groups on NPI and CMAI total; Trend for decreased aggression with sertraline vs placebo on BEHAVE-AD aggression scale, $P = .08$; Small sample size

(continued on next page)

Table 1 (continued)

Study	Agent	Sample (N)	Duration (wk)	Outcome measures (behavioral symptoms)	Results and comments
Anticonvulsants					
Tariot et al 1998 [20]	Carbemazepine	51	6	CGIC, BPRS	Statistically significant global improvement in agitation (21% placebo vs 77% rated improved with carbemazepine) Statistically significant improvement on BPRS for carbamazepine
Porsteinsson et al 2001 [21]	Divalproex	56	6	BPRS	Trend improvement in agitation scores (15.4% for placebo vs 30.8% for divalproex, $P = .08$)
Other agents					
Peskind et al 2005 [23]	Propranolol (augmentation design, ie, active drug added to psychotropics)	31	6	NPI total, CGIC	Statistically significant decline in NPI total scores with propranolol (33% vs 1% with placebo) 6-mo open-label extension with n = 8 patients (markedly or moderately improved on CGIC) showed a decline in ratings to either minimally improved or unchanged compared with pretreatment
Tariot et al 2001 [24]	Donepezil	208	24	NPI-NH	No significant difference of total behavior scores between groups Group selection based on dementia, not agitation
Cantillon et al 1996 [25]	Buspirone, haloperidol	26	10	BPRS, Anxiety status inventory	Decrease in the BPRS tension subscale and anxiety scores No statistical analysis; no placebo.

Abbreviations: BPRS, Brief Psychiatric Rating Scale; CMAI, Cohen-Mansfield Agitation Inventory; NPI-NH, Neuropsychiatric Inventory-Nursing Home version; BEHAVE-AD, Behavioral Pathology in Alzheimer Disease Rating Scale; NPI, Neuropsychiatric Inventory; CGIC, Clinical Global Impression of Change.

uncontrolled 18-week open-label extension of this trial [29]. An analysis conducted on a subgroup of patients from this study focused on the emergence of psychotic symptoms in agitated dementia patients as the primary outcome and demonstrated trend-level decreases in favor of olanzapine [30].

Two randomized trials without placebo compared lower potency, sedating agents to higher potency agents and found no significant difference between groups, which suggests similar efficacy among antipsychotics [16,17]. Three randomized trials without placebo compared antipsychotics with benzodiazepines and found antipsychotics to be equal [18] or significantly superior to benzodiazepines for agitation treatment [19] and anxiety reduction [9].

Anticonvulsants

In a randomized, double-blind, placebo-controlled trial, carbamazepine, 300 mg modal dose, showed significant improvement over placebo in Clinical Global Impression of Change (CGIC) ratings (77% of the patients were rated as "improved" for carbamazepine versus 21% for placebo) and Brief Psychiatric Rating Scale (BPRS) scores. Side effects were significantly more common with the active drug but were generally clinically insignificant [20]. Carbamazepine also significantly reduced agitation scores in an earlier pilot, placebo crossover study [31].

In a randomized, double-blind, placebo-controlled trial, divalproex displayed only statistical trends toward improvement [21]. This result may have been due to a higher placebo response rate than in the carbamazepine study [20] since the response in the divalproex patients was comparable to changes seen in the carbamazepine patients. In a 6-week uncontrolled, open-label extension of this study, there were significant reductions in BPRS scores with divalproex, and 86% of the 43 subjects who completed the study were rated as "improved" on the CGIC [32]. Another 12-week uncontrolled, open-label study of valproate demonstrated a significant 60% reduction in agitation scores but no improvement in a modified CGIS for aggressive behavior [33]. Three additional observational studies of valproate, which include two chart reviews, found mixed results [34–36]. A comparative study of valproate and lorazepam found that significantly more subjects demonstrated improvement with valproate (57% of subjects improved with valproate versus 31% with lorazepam) [37]. In a chart review study of gabapentin, 77% of patients were rated as "much improved" [38], but an open-label trial demonstrated no change in agitation scores with gabapentin [39].

Antidepressants

Two randomized double-blind, placebo-controlled 4-week trials for antidepressants were reviewed. One study focused on outcome measures of irritability, restlessness, anxiety, and depression and found significant reductions in irritability and depressed mood with citalopram [26]. In a placebo-controlled, crossover study of sertraline in 21 subjects, there were no significant differences between groups and only trend-level differences only in favor of sertraline on the BEHAVE-AD aggression subscale [22]. In an observational study of paroxetine, there was a 62% reduction in agitation scale scores, calculated without statistical significance analysis [40].

Other agents

Other studied agents included propranolol, a β blocker. A randomized controlled trial reported significant improvements in total Neuropsychiatric Inventory (NPI) and CGIC scores with propranolol (mean dose 106 mg). However, in a 6-month open-label extension, a majority of subjects receiving the active drug and rated as "moderately to markedly improved" on the CGIC declined to "minimally improved" or "unchanged" in comparison with pretreatment status, suggesting poor long-term effects of propranolol [23]. In a randomized controlled trial, the acetylcholinesterase inhibitor donepezil demonstrated no significant effect on NPI-NH total ratings or any individual item scores when it was compared with placebo [24].

In an observational study, 25 subjects who were unable to communicate complaints of pain were given fixed-dose opiates or placebo. There were no significant differences in CMAI scores between the placebo and treatment phases [41]. In an observational study, melatonin significantly reduced agitation in patients with sundowning-related agitation [42]. An observational study [43] demonstrated no significant improvement of agitation using buspirone; however, in a randomized controlled trial, buspirone was more effective than haloperidol for the reduction of tension and anxiety [25].

Research on nonpharmacologic interventions

Training interventions

Six randomized controlled trials of training interventions were reviewed. Four studies reported no difference between intervention and nonintervention groups (Table 2) [44–47]. These studies involved staff training in combination with treatment plan development, training for care in activities of daily living or psychosocial activities, and training in emotion-oriented care (a multifaceted training program involving validation therapy). One study of training interventions to provide multisensory stimulation to residents demonstrated significant reductions in CMAI aggressiveness behavior scores in the experimental group compared with usual-care controls (34% reduction in experimental group versus 32% increase in control group). In this study, the staff training was supplemented with multiple supervision meetings and feedback sessions to support the implementation of the treatment approach. This study was limited by nonblinded observations and incomplete randomization (two wards were assigned to the experimental group)

[48]. Another study of nurse aide training reported significant declines in verbal agitation but no change in physically aggressive or nonaggressive behaviors [49].

Six observational studies had mixed results. In one study, verbal prompts by certified nursing assistants were no longer associated with increased resident agitation after a communication skills training program, but the study was limited by a lack of validated agitation outcome measures [58]. In another study, the initiation of a behavior management program, which included staff training in addition to environmental interventions (temperature and sound control), significantly reduced the number of agitated behaviors as measured by the Nursing Home-Behavior Problem Scale (NH-BPS) [59]. Two studies of nurse aide training reported decreased incident reports, but one study lacked the statistical analysis of results [60] and the other involved only two subjects [61]. A study of targeted restraint reduction training found decreased restraint use and decreased agitation scores [62]. Finally, a study of staff inservice training found no change in agitated behaviors and an increase in restraint use [63].

Activities interventions

Five randomized controlled trials of activities interventions were reviewed. One study involved planning sensory stimulating and sensory calming activities based on agitation patterns of residents and reported a significant decline in agitation measures for the intervention group compared with the usual-care control group [50]. Another study reporting significant declines in agitation measures for the experimental group over control (a 71% drop in a categorical agitation variable for the experimental group versus a 49% drop in the control group) involved a combination intervention consisting of a group activities therapist, the use of thioridazine, and staff education [51]. One study that compared a physical activity-based intervention with a sleep hygiene improvement control found significant effects in favor of physical activity [52]. In two randomized trials involving a simulated audiotape presence of family members and a walking-talking program, there were no significant differences between control and experimental groups [53,57].

There are numerous observational studies of activities interventions, 14 in all. Two studies [64,65] of animal-assisted therapy reported decreased agitation, but only one study included a statistical analysis and had significant declines (23%) in CMAI scores [65]. One study involving a resident dog on the unit showed a significant decrease in daytime problem behaviors among residents as measured by the NH-BPS [74]. Two simulated audio presence studies reported mixed results [67,68]. Two recreational activities studies demonstrated trend decreases in agitation [69,70]. A pilot study of a moderate intensity exercise program demonstrated significant decreases in some problem behaviors, and a study of a walking program reported a significant decrease in staff incident reports of aggression [71,72]. Overall, six

Table 2
Nonpharmacologic interventions for treatment of dementia-related agitation in nursing home residents: randomized controlled trials

Study	Model and conditions	Sample size (N)	Duration	Outcome measures (behavioral symptoms)	Results and comments
Training					
Finnema et al 2005 [47]	Emotion-oriented care	146	7 mo	CMAI + multiple mood and quality of life outcome measures	No significant difference between groups on agitation measures Non blind observations
Van Weert et al 2005 [48]	"Snoezelen" approach: multisensory stimulation 16-h training (review behaviors, observe preferences, adapt care plan, apply)	129	21 mo	Dutch Behavior Observation scale for psychgeriatric inpatients; subscales CMAI (Dutch version)	Statistically significant reduction in agitation on CMAI aggressive behavior (34% reduction in experimental group vs 32% increase in control); significant treatment effects on subscales of apathetic behavior, loss of decorum, rebellious behavior Nonblind observations; incomplete randomization
Schrijnemaekers et al 2002 [44]	Emotion-oriented care (multifaceted training program); clinical lessons, 6-d training, supervision × 8 mo	151	12 mo	Dutch Behavior Observation scale for psychogeriatric inpatients, subscales	No significant difference between groups on agitation measures Nonblind observations; research subjects 90% female

Study	Intervention	n	Duration	Measure	Results/Comments
Beck et al 2002 [45]	ADL therapy vs psychosocial vs combination; placebo control, no intervention control, 12 wk training	179	20 wk	Disruptive behavior scale, videotape analysis (n = 84)	No significant difference between groups on agitation measures. Video analysis: significantly more positive affect in treatment groups. Nonblind observations, small sample size
Proctor et al 1999 [46]	Training and education	120	6 mo	Crichton Royal Behavioural rating scale	No difference in behavior change scores between groups. Nonblind observations
McCallion et al 1999 [49]	Nurse aide training	105	6 mo	CMAI	Statistically significant 20% decline in verbal agitation; no change in physical agitation. Nonblind observations
Activities					
Kovach et al 2004 [50]	BACE	78	1 wk blocks	Visual analog scale for agitation assessment	Significant decline of agitation scores in BACE group vs control (22% vs 1%; effect size = .7). No measure of psychotropic medication use among residents
Cott et al 2002 [53]	Walking-talking program: 30 min walk + talk vs 30 min talk only vs control	86	16 wks	London psychogeriatric scale	No significant differences between groups. Small sample; Subjects with low MMSE included and unable to participate in program

(continued on next page)

Table 2 (*continued*)

Study	Model and conditions	Sample size (N)	Duration	Outcome measures (behavioral symptoms)	Results and comments
Alessi et al 1999 [52]	Exercise versus sleep hygiene	29	15 wk	Direct observation of behaviors as defined by the CMAI	Statistically significant 22% decrease in agitation with exercise versus 150% increase with control (sleep hygiene alone) Small sample size; nonblind observations
Camberg et al 1999 [57]	Simulated presence audio	54	71 d	SOAPD, SCMAI	No significant differences on agitation scale Significant reduction in SCMAI scores for the treatment group (based on non blind observations)
Rovner et al 1996 [51]	Activities (day program)	89	6 mo	Composite behavior disorder measure based on direct observation or PGDRS behavior subscale and CMAI measurements	Statistically significant 71% reduction in agitation with intervention versus 49% with control Inclusion of both blind and nonblind observations

Sensory

Study	Intervention		Dose	Measure	Results
Woods et al 2005 [54]	Therapeutic touch (using hands to facilitate healing) vs placebo touch vs usual care	57	3 d (intervention given for 5–7 min 2 times per d)	ABRS, modified	No significant differences between therapeutic touch and placebo touch groups Statistically significant decline in total behavioral symptoms scores with therapeutic touch when compared to usual care (no touch)
Ancoli-Israel et al 2003 [55]	Bright-light (2500 lux) qam or qpm or dim (control)	92	18 d	CMAI, total ABRS	No significant treatment effects with light treatment
Remington 2002 [56]	10 min calming music or hand massage or both	68	10 min intervention + immediate observation and 1-h post-observation	CMAI	Significant reduction in agitation for all interventions vs control (53–58% versus 4%); no additive benefit of both interventions; sustained effects 1 h post-intervention ($P \leq .01$) Small sample size; unclear if control included 1:1 contact with caregiver (without intervention)

Abbreviations: ABRS, Agitation Behavior Rating Scale; ADL, activities of daily living; BACE, balancing arousal and controls excesses; CMAI, Cohen-Mansfield Agitation Inventory; MMSE, Mini-Mental State Examination; PGDRS, Psychogeriatric Dependency Rating Scale; SCMAI, short form Cohen-Mansfield Agitation Inventory; SOAPD, Scale for the Observation of Agitation in Persons with Dementia.

[65,68,71–74] studies reported statistically significant results favoring the activities intervention, and two studies reported trend decreases in agitation [68,70]. Four studies of activities, including theory-based activity selection (activity matched to resident skill and premorbid personality style), video activity, therapeutic robocat, and glider swing therapy reported no benefit [75–78].

Sensory therapy

Three randomized controlled trials of sensory therapy interventions were reviewed. Two of the studies involving a specialized therapeutic touch method and bright-light therapy reported no differences on agitation measures between the control and the intervention groups [54,55]. The therapeutic touch study had both usual-care (no touch intervention) and placebo therapeutic touch controls. Although there was no significant difference between specialized versus placebo therapeutic touch, there were significant declines in agitation scores for therapeutic touch over no-touch intervention controls, suggesting some benefit from touch therapies [54]. In another study of calming music or hand massage or both, there were significant reductions in mean CMAI scores favoring the intervention groups over controls, and these effects were sustained 1 hour after treatment [56]. Both studies involving massage or therapeutic touch might have been limited by routine care controls in which the continuous presence of caregivers was not a given, thus making it difficult to identify if it was the touch intervention or the continuous caregiver presence that contributed to decreased agitation.

Observational studies of sensory therapy greatly outnumber randomized trials. Twenty-one observational studies were reviewed. Almost half of the observational studies involved music interventions. Of 10 music intervention studies [79–88], seven [80–84,87,88] reported statistically significant declines in agitation measures. Two studies involving bright-light therapy reported statistically significant declines in agitation scale scores [66,89]. Two observational studies involving massage had results that were mixed [90,91]. Two studies with aromatherapy demonstrated no change in agitated behaviors [92,93]. One pre- and post-test study of sensory air mat therapy and white noise showed significant reductions in CMAI scores, whereas in another study with white noise alone, nine of 13 subjects were noted to be responders by definition, but there was no statistical analysis [94,95].

Discussion

Most pharmacologic studies of treating dementia-related agitation in nursing home patients used validated agitation measures, including NPI subscales, BEHAVE-AD, and CMAI. These scales rate a wide variety of behaviors, including physical and verbal aggression and general activity disturbances (pacing, hoarding, disinhibition, and other behaviors). Most pharmacologic interventions targeted behavioral symptoms as a whole. Several studies used multiple outcome measures to report results. Most studies also included patients with multiple types of dementia. In most medication studies, subjects were required to have some threshold score on an agitation scale for entry into the study. These threshold scores may serve to select a research population that is more likely to demonstrate significant results in response to study interventions. Few studies controlled for the presence of psychotic symptoms. Typically, medication studies did not report whether nonpharmacologic interventions were used during the trial.

Antipsychotic medications have been the intervention most studied in randomized controlled trials. These studies demonstrate modest responses in favor of antipsychotics. The dose response patterns suggest that an increase above fairly moderate doses has no clear additional benefits. Antipsychotics are equal or superior to benzodiazepines, but studies are limited. Studies with anticonvulsants are mixed. Currently, data support the use of carbamazepine over other anticonvulsants. Adverse events with carbamazepine were not considered clinically significant in a typical, frail nursing home patient population. In longer duration observational studies, divalproex has been an effective treatment for agitation, suggesting that the length of current randomized trials may be too short to demonstrate efficacy. In regard to selective serotonin reuptake inhibitors (SSRIs), data support their usefulness in treatment of affective symptoms and irritability rather than typical physical or verbal aggression. Randomized controlled studies of acetylcholinesterase inhibitors in nursing home patients have not shown significant benefits on primary behavioral outcomes measures. Other agents, such as propranolol, which are being investigated, have shown only short-term benefits.

A fair number of nonpharmacologic intervention studies did not use the validated scales found in pharmacologic studies. In some cases, real-time recordings of behavior and video analyses were used to quantify resident behaviors in a specific environmental context. These measures were used to study staff training interventions in which resident–staff interactions could be observed and modified or linked to various outcomes. The benefits of real-time observations are evident. In particular, they allow for the observation of tangible results, which can more easily be understood from a clinical perspective. However, real-time observations are difficult to generalize and compare with scaled measures. In addition, analytic techniques for real-time measures are still under development. Similar to medication studies, few nonpharmacologic studies targeted specific behaviors, and most used multiple outcome measures to report results. During most studies, medications for behavioral symptoms were continued; few studies quantified any changes in medication during the trial.

Studies of training interventions used a variety of approaches. No single approach showed significant supporting data. Generally, studies with positive outcomes included additional supervision for staff or other supportive measures to ensure the implementation of the treatment approach. The several negative studies of training interventions suggest that training alone without such additional measures may be insufficient to produce positive results. Studies of group activities, exercise, and modifying activity schedules based on individual assessments of residents show efficacy in three randomized controlled trials and appear to be more efficacious than simulated presence. Based on observational data only, there is a suggestion of efficacy for animal therapy. In the sensory category, music interventions have the most supporting data, including one positive randomized controlled trial. Hand massage and nonspecific touch therapies have demonstrated efficacy in two randomized controlled trials. Aromatherapy and bright-light therapy have not proved useful.

Summary

Based on this review, both pharmacologic and nonpharmacologic approaches are effective in reducing the severity of dementia-related agitation in nursing home residents. There are insufficient data to prioritize between these approaches because there are no comparison studies. Among pharmacologic approaches, the data support the use of conventional antipsychotics and the atypical agents studied so far. There are too few data in support of other drug classes to consider them as first-line agents. Although acetylcholinesterase inhibitors have demonstrated statistically significant improvements on cognitive measures in several studies [96], the data do not support their use for behavioral symptoms in nursing home residents with dementia. In light of the recent FDA warnings of increased risk of death in subjects treated with atypical antipsychotics for dementia-related agitation and safety alerts indicating the increased incidence of cerebrovascular events in dementia patients treated with these agents, a cautious and conservative approach is recommended when considering antipsychotics for treating agitation in these patients. Coupling nonpharmacologic approaches with pharmacologic approaches may be beneficial, although studies are needed to support this. Among nonpharmacologic approaches, the data support activities and sensory-based interventions. Activities interventions supported by the evidence base include group activities, physical activities, and activity planning based on an evaluation of individual behavior patterns. Sensory interventions supported by the data include music interventions and hand massage. These types of interventions are relatively low cost and fairly straightforward to implement. The cost-benefit ratio of these interventions is low, and a more aggressive use of these treatments is warranted. The data do not support the use of training interventions for the reduction of agitation symptoms in nursing home residents with dementia. Although training interventions may be useful for other purposes, such as reducing staff turnover, these interventions alone are not sufficient to reduce agitation symptoms in this patient population.

Areas that merit further research include comparisons between and within nonpharmacologic and pharmacologic classes of interventions. More high quality studies using standardized outcome measures and reporting adequate data for meta-analyses are necessary to allow for prioritizing treatment approaches. Currently, behavioral symptoms are studied as a whole. However, certain drug types or nonpharmacologic approaches may be more effective for certain behaviors. Behavioral symptoms have been classified into types including verbal and physical aggression and nonaggressive behaviors, suggesting the need for modified treatment approaches based on the type of behavior. In studies, the use of vague target behaviors as outcome measures complicates the practical application of research findings. More specific targets need to be identified in research studies to guide long-term care clinicians. Given the growing dilemma between concern about the side-effect profiles of antipsychotic therapy and the current widespread use of antipsychotics for treating agitation in dementia, clinicians need to be able to adequately weigh the risks and benefits of this intervention. In addition to rigorous studies measuring efficacy of treatments in reducing symptoms and comparison studies, it may be beneficial to include quality of life measures in future studies. Such measures would be a valuable addition in the cost-benefit analyses of medication therapy for agitation.

References

[1] Magaziner J, German P, Zimmerman SI, et al, for the Epidemiology of Dementia in Nursing Homes Research Group. The prevalence of dementia in a statewide sample of new nursing home admissions aged 65 and older: diagnosis by expert panel. Gerontologist 2000;40(6): 663–72.

[2] Yaffe K, Fox P, Newcomer R, et al. Patient and caregiver characteristics and nursing home placement in patients with dementia. JAMA 2002;287(16):2090–7.

[3] Cohen-Mansfield J, Billig N. Agitated behaviors in the elderly: I. a conceptual review. J Am Geriatr Soc 1986;34(10):711–21.

[4] Mega MS, Cummings JL, Fiorello T, et al. The spectrum of behavioral changes in Alzheimer's disease. Neurology 1996;46(1):130–5.

[5] Cummings JL, Back C. The cholinergic hypothesis of neuropsychiatric symptoms in Alzheimer's disease. Am J Geriatr Psychiatry 1998;6(Suppl 1):S64–78.

[6] Howard R, Ballard C, O'Brien J, et al. Guidelines for the management of agitation in dementia. Int J Geriatr Psychiatry 2001;16(7):714–7.

[7] Snowden M, Sato K, Roy-byrne P. Assessment and treatment of nursing home residents with depression or behavioral symptoms associated with dementia: a review of the literature. J Am Geriatr Soc 2003;51(9):1305–17.

[8] Rovner BW, Edelman BA, Cox MP, et al. The impact of antipsychotic drug regulations (OBRA 1987) on psychotropic prescribing practices in nursing homes. Am J Psychiatry 1992;149(1):1390–2.

[9] Stotsky B. Multicenter study comparing thioridazine with diazepam and placebo in elderly, nonpsychotic patients with emotional and behavioral disorders. Clin Ther 1984;6(4): 546–59.

[10] Finkel SI, Lyons JS, Anderson RL, et al. A randomized, placebo-controlled trial of thiothixene in agitated, demented nursing home patients. Int J Geriatr Psychiatry 1995;10:129–36.

[11] Brodaty H, Ames D, Snowdon J, et al. A randomized placebo-controlled trial of risperidone for the treatment of aggression, agitation, and psychosis of dementia. J Clin Psychiatry 2003; 64(2):134–43.

[12] De Deyn PP, Rabheru K, Rasmussen A, et al. A randomized trial of risperidone, placebo, and haloperidol for behavioral symptoms of dementia. Neurology 1999;53(5):946–55.

[13] Katz IR, Jeste DV, Mintzer JE, et al. Comparison of risperidone and placebo for psychosis and behavioral disturbances associated with dementia: a randomized, double-blind trial. J Clin Psychiatry 1999;60(2):107–15.

[14] Street JS, Clark WS, Gannon KS, et al, for the HGEU study group. Olanzapine treatment of psychotic and behavioral symptoms in patients with Alzheimer disease in nursing care facilities: a double-blind, randomized, placebo-controlled trial. Arch Gen Psychiatry 2000; 57(10):968–76.

[15] Barnes R, Veith R, Okimoto J, et al. Efficacy of antipsychotic medications in behaviorally disturbed dementia patients. Am J Psychiatry 1982;139(9):1170–4.

[16] Lovett WC, Stokes DK, Taylor LB, et al. Management of behavioral symptoms in disturbed elderly patients: comparison of trifluoperazine and haloperidol. J Clin Psychiatry 1987;48(6): 234–6.

[17] Smith GR, Taylor CW, Linkous P. Haloperidol versus thioridazine for the treatment of psychogeriatric patients: a double-blind clinical trial. Psychosomatics 1974;15:134–8.

[18] Coccaro EF, Kramer E, Zemishlany Z, et al. Pharmacologic treatment of noncognitive behavioral disturbances in elderly demented patients. Am J Psychiatry 1990;147(12): 1640–5.

[19] Covington JS. Alleviating agitation, apprehension, and related symptoms in geriatric patients: a double-blind comparison of a phenothiazine and a benzodiazepine. South Med J 1975;68(6):719–24.

[20] Tariot PN, Erb R, Podgorski CA, et al. Efficacy and tolerability of carbamazepine for agitation and aggression in dementia. Am J Psychiatry 1998;155(1):54–61.

[21] Porsteinsson AP, Tariot PN, Erb R, et al. Placebo-controlled study of divalproex sodium for agitation in dementia. Am J Geriatr Psychiatry 2001;9(1):58–66.

[22] Lanctot KL, Herrmann N, van Reekum R, et al. Gender, aggression and serotonergic function are associated with response to sertraline for behavioral disturbances in Alzheimer's disease. Int J Geriatr Psychiatry 2002;17(6):531–41.

[23] Peskind ER, Tsuang DW, Bonner LT, et al. Propranolol for disruptive behaviors in nursing home residents with probable or possible Alzheimer disease. Alzheimer Dis Assoc Disord 2005;19(1):23–8.

[24] Tariot PN, Cummings JL, Katz IR, et al. A randomized, double-blind, placebo-controlled study of the efficacy and safety of donepezil in patients with Alzheimer's disease in the nursing home setting. J Am Geriatr Soc 2001;49(12):1590–9.

[25] Cantillon M, Brunswick R, Molina D, et al. Buspirone vs haloperidol: a double-blind trial for agitation in a nursing home population with Alzheimer's disease. Am J Geriatr Psychiatry 1996;4(3):263–7.

[26] Nyth AL, Gottfries CG. The clinical efficacy of citalopram in treatment of emotional disturbances in dementia disorders. Br J Psychiatry 1990;157:894–901.

[27] Goldberg RJ, Goldberg J. Risperidone for dementia-related disturbed behavior in nursing home residents: a clinical experience. Int Psychogeriatr 1997;9(1):65–8.

[28] Meguro K, Meguro M, Tanaka Y, et al. Risperidone is effective for wandering and disturbed sleep/wake patterns in Alzheimer's disease. J Geriatr Psychiatry Neurol 2004;(17)2:61–7.

[29] Street JS, Clark WS, Kadam DL, et al. Long-term efficacy of olanzapine in the control of psychotic and behavioral symptoms in nursing home patients with Alzheimer's dementia. Int J Geriatr Psychiatry 2001;16(Suppl 1):S62–70.

[30] Clark WS, Street JS, Feldman PD, et al. The effects of olanzapine in reducing the emergence of psychosis among nursing home patients with Alzheimer's disease. J Clin Psychiatry 2001; 62(1):34–40.

[31] Tariot PN, Erb R, Leibovici A, et al. Carbamazepine treatment of agitation in nursing home patients with dementia: a preliminary study. J Am Geriatr Soc 1994;42(11):1160–6.

[32] Porsteinsson AP, Tariot PN, Jakimovich LJ, et al. Valproate therapy for agitation in dementia: open-label extension of a double-blind trial. Am J Geriatr Psychiatry 2003;11(4): 434–40.

[33] Sival RC, Duivenvoorden HJ, Jansen PA, et al. Sodium valproate in aggressive behavior in dementia: a twelve-week open label follow-up study. Int J Geriatr Psychiatry 2004;19(4): 305–12.

[34] Gardner ME, Ditmanson LF, Garrett RW, et al. Effectiveness of divalproex sodium in severe dementia-related aggression. Consult Pharm 2001;16:839–43.

[35] Lott AD, McElroy SL, Keys MA. Valproate in the treatment of behavioral agitation in elderly patients with dementia. J Neuropsychiatry Clin Neurosci 1995;7(3):314–9.

[36] Marshall LL, Miller SW. Divalproex sodium for the behavioral manifestations of Alzheimer's disease. Consult Pharm 2001;16:758–66.

[37] Frenchmen IB, Capo C, Kass H. Effect of treatment with divalproex sodium and lorazepam in residents of long-term-care facilities with dementia-related anxiety or agitation: retrospective chart review. Curr Therapeut Res 2000;61:621–9.

[38] Hawkins JW, Tinklenberg JR, Sheikh JI, et al. A retrospective chart review of gabapentin for the treatment of aggressive and agitated behavior in patients with dementias. Am J Geriat Psychiatry 2000;8(3):221–5.

[39] Herrmann N, Lanctot K, Myszak M. Effectiveness of gabapentin for the treatment of behavioral disorders in dementia. J Clin Psychopharmacol 2000;20(1):90–3.

[40] Ramadan FH, Naughton BJ, Bassanelli AG, et al. Treatment of verbal agitation with a selective serotonin reuptake inhibitor. J Geriatr Psychiatry Neurol 2000;13(2):56–9.

[41] Manfredi PL, Breuer B, Wallenstein S, et al. Opioid treatment for agitation in patients with advanced dementia. Int J Geriatr Psychiatry 2003;18(8):700–5.

[42] Cohen-Mansfield J, Garfinkel D, Lipson S. Melatonin for treatment of sundowning in elderly persons with dementia: a preliminary study. Arch Gerontol Geriatr 2000;31(1):65–76.

[43] Cooper JW, Cobb HH, Burfiled AH. Effects of psychotropic load reduction and buspirone conversion on behavioral disturbances and global deterioration in a nursing home population. Consult Pharm 2001;16:358–63.

[44] Schrijnemaekers V, van Rossum E, Candel M, et al. Effects of emotion-oriented care on elderly people with cognitive impairment and behavioral problems. Int J Geriatr Psychiatry 2002;17(10):926–37.

[45] Beck CK, Vogelpohl TS, Rasin JH, et al. Effects of behavioral interventions on disruptive behavior and affect in demented nursing home residents. Nurs Res 2002;51(4):219–28.

[46] Proctor R, Burns A, Powell H, et al. Behavioural management in nursing and residential homes: a randomized controlled trial. Lancet 1999;354(9172):26–9.

[47] Finnema E, Droes R, Ettema T, et al. The effect of integrated emotion-oriented care versus usual care on elderly persons with dementia in the nursing home and on nursing assistants: a randomized clinical trial. Int J Geriatr Psychiatry 2005;20:330–43.

[48] Van Weert JCM, van Dulmen AM, Spreeuwenberg PM, et al. Behavioral and mood effects of snoezelen integrated into 24-hour dementia care. J Am Geriatr Soc 2005;53(1):24–33.

[49] McCallion P, Toseland RW, Lacey D, et al. Educating nursing assistants to communicate more effectively with nursing home residents with dementia. Gerontologist 1999;39(5): 546–58.

[50] Kovach CR, Taneli Y, Dohearty P, et al. Effect of the BACE intervention on agitation of people with dementia. Gerontologist 2004;44(6):797–806.

[51] Rovner B, Steele CD, Shmuely Y, et al. a randomized trial of dementia care in nursing homes. J Am Geriatr Soc 1996;1:7–13.

[52] Alessi CA, Yoon EJ, Schnelle JF, et al. A randomized trial of a combined physical activity and environmental intervention in nursing home residents: do sleep and agitation improve? J Am Geriatr Soc 1999;47(7):784–91.

[53] Cott CA, Dawson P, Sidani S, et al. The effects of a walking/talking program on communication, ambulation, and functional status in residents with Alzheimer disease. Alzheimer Dis Assoc Disord 2002;16(2):81–7.

[54] Woods DL, Craven RF, Whitney J. The effect of therapeutic touch on behavioral symptoms of persons with dementia. Altern Ther Health Med 2005;11(1):66–74.

[55] Ancoli-Israel S, Martin JL, Gehrman P, et al. Effect of light on agitation in institutionalized patients with severe Alzheimer disease. Am J Geriatr Psychiatry 2003;11(2):194–203.

[56] Remington R. Calming music and massage with agitated elderly. Nurs Res 2002;5(51): 317–23.

[57] Camberg L, Woods P, Ooi WL, et al. Evaluation of simulated presence: a personalized approach to enhance well-being in persons with Alzheimer's disease. J Am Geriatr Soc 1999; 47(4):446–52.

[58] Roth DL, Stevens AB, Burgio LD, et al. Timed-event sequential analysis of agitation in nursing home residents during personal care interactions with nursing assistants. J Gerontol B Psychol Sci Soc Sci 2002;57B(5):461–8.

[59] DeYoung S, Just G, Harrison R. Decreasing aggressive, agitated, or disruptive behavior: participation in a behavior management unit. J Gerontol Nurs 2002;28(6):22–31.

[60] Mentes JC, Ferrario J. Calming aggressive reactions: a preventive program. J Gerontol Nurs 1989;15(2):22–7.

[61] Williams DP, Wood EC, Moorleghen F. An in-service workshop for nursing personnel on the management of catastrophic reactions in dementia victims. Clin Gerontologist 1994; 14:47–53.

[62] Werner P, Cohen-Mansfield J, Koroknay V, et al. The impact of a restraint-reduction program on nursing home residents. Geriatr Nurs 1994;15(3):142–6.

[63] Cohen-Mansfield J, Werner P, Culpepper WJ, et al. Evaluation of an inservice training program on dementia and wandering. J Gerontol Nurs 1997;23(10):40–7.

[64] Churchill M, Safaoui J, McCabe BW, et al. Using a therapy dog to alleviate the agitation and desocialization of people with Alzheimer's disease. J Psychosoc Nurs Ment Health Serv 1999;37(4):16–22.

[65] Richeson NE. Effects of animal-assisted therapy on agitated behaviors and social interactions of older adults with dementia. Am J Alzheimers Dis Other Demen 2003;18(6):353–8.

[66] Lovell BB, Ancoli-Israel S, Gevirtz R. Effect of bright light treatment on agitated behavior in institutionalized elderly subjects. Psychiatry Res 1995;57(1):7–12.

[67] Miller S, Vermeersch PE, Bohan K, et al. An audio presence intervention for decreasing agitation in people with dementia. Geriatr Nurs 2001;2(22):66–70.

[68] Woods P, Ashley J. Simulated presence therapy: using selected memories to manage problem behaviors in Alzheimer's disease patients. Geriatr Nurs 1995;16(1):9–14.

[69] Aronstein Z, Olsen R, Schulman E. The nursing assistants use of recreational interventions for behavioral management of residents with Alzheimer's disease. Am J Alzheimer's Dis 1996;May/June:26–31.

[70] Buettner LL, Lundegren H, Lago D. Therapeutic recreation as an intervention for persons with dementia and agitation: an efficacy study. Am J Alzheimer's Dis 1996;September/October:4–12

[71] Landi F, Russo A, Bernabei R. Physical activity and behavior in the elderly: a pilot study. Arch Gerontol Geriatr 2004;(Suppl 9):S235–41.

[72] Holmberg SK. Evaluation of a clinical intervention for wanderers on a geriatric nursing unit. Arch Psychiatr Nurs 1997;11(1):21–8.

[73] Cohen-Mansfield J, Werner P. Management of verbally disruptive behaviors in nursing home residents. J Gerontol A Biol Sci Med Sci 1997;52A:M369–77.

[74] McCabe BW, Baun MM, Spiech D, et al. Resident dog in the Alzheimer's special care unit. West J Nurs Res 2002;24(6):684–96.

[75] Hall L, Hare J. Video respite for cognitively impaired persons in nursing homes. Am J Alzheimer's Dis 1997;May/June:117–121.

[76] Kolanowski AM, Buttner L, Costa PT Jr, et al. Capturing interests: therapeutic recreation activities for persons with dementia. Ther Recreation J 2001;35(3):220–35.

[77] Libin A, Cohen-Mansfield J. Therapeutic robocat for nursing home residents with dementia: a preliminary inquiry. Am J Alzheimers Dis Other Demen 2004;19(2):111–6.

[78] Snyder M, Tseng Y, Brandt C, et al. A glider swing intervention for people with dementia. Geriatr Nurs 2001;22(2):86–90.

[79] Brotons M, Pickett-Cooper PK. The effects of music therapy intervention on agitation behaviors of Alzheimer's disease patients. J Music Ther 1996;33:2–18.

[80] Casby JA, Holm MB. The effect of music on repetitive disruptive vocalizations of persons with dementia. Am J Occup Ther 1994;48(10):883–9.

[81] Clark ME, Lipe AW, Bilbrey M. Use of music to decrease aggressive behaviors in people with dementia. J Gerontol Nurs 1998;24(7):10–7.

[82] Denney A. Quiet music: an intervention for mealtime agitation? J Gerontol Nurs 1997;23(7): 16–23.

[83] Gerdner LA. Effects of individualized versus classical "relaxation" music on the frequency of agitation in elderly persons with Alzheimer's disease and related disorders. Int Psychogeriatr 2000;12(1):49–65.

[84] Goddaer J, Abraham IL. Effects of relaxing music on agitation during meals among nursing home residents with severe cognitive impairment. Arch Psychiatr Nurs 1994;8(3):150–8.

[85] Groene RW. Effectiveness of music therapy 1:1 intervention with individuals having senile dementia of the Alzheimer's type. J Music Ther 1993;30:138–57.

[86] Snyder M, Olson J. Music and hand massage interventions to produce relaxation and reduce aggressive behaviors in cognitively impaired elders: a pilot study. Clin Gerontologist 1996; 17:64–9.

[87] Tabloski PA, McKinnon-Howe L, Remington R. Effects of calming music on the level of agitation in cognitively impaired nursing home residents. American Journal of Alzheimer's Care and Related Disorders and Research 1995;January/February:10–15.

[88] Thomas DW, Heitmna RJ, Alexander T. The effects of music on bathing cooperation for residents with dementia. J Music Ther 1997;34:246–59.

[89] Thorpe L, Middleton J, Russell G, et al. Bright light therapy for demented nursing home patients with behavioral disturbance. Am J Alzheimer's Dis 2000;15:18–26.

[90] Kim EJ, Buschmann MT. The effect of expressive physical touch on patients with dementia. Int J Nurs Stud 1999;36(3):235–43.

[91] Snyder M, Egan EC, Burns KR. Efficacy of hand massage in decreasing agitation behaviors associated with care activities in persons with dementia. Geriatr Nurs 1995;16(2):60–3.

[92] Gray SG, Clair AA. Influence of aromatherapy on medication administration to residential-care residents with dementia and behavioral challenges. Am J Alzheimers Dis Other Demen 2002;17(3):169–74.

[93] Snow LA, Hovanec L, Brandt J. A controlled trial of aromatherapy for agitation in nursing home patients with dementia. J Altern Complement Med 2004;10(3):431–7.

[94] Shalek M, Richeson NE, Buettner LL. Air mat therapy for treatment of agitated wandering: an evidence-based recreational therapy intervention. Am Journal of Recreation Therapy 2004;3(2):18–26.

[95] Burgio L, Scilley K, Hardin JM, et al. Environmental "white noise": an intervention for verbally agitated nursing home residents. J Gerontol B Psychol Sci Soc Sci 1996;51(6):364–73.

[96] Cummings JL. Use of cholinesterase inhibitors in clinical practice: evidence-based recommendations. Am J Geriatr Psychiatry 2003;11(2):131–45.

ELSEVIER
SAUNDERS

Psychiatr Clin N Am
28 (2005) 1007–1038

PSYCHIATRIC
CLINICS
OF NORTH AMERICA

Evidence-Based Caregiver Interventions in Geriatric Psychiatry

Richard Schulz, PhD[a,b,*], Lynn M. Martire, PhD[a,b], Julie N. Klinger, MA[b]

[a]Department of Psychiatry, University of Pittsburgh, 121 University Place, Suite 600, Pittsburgh, PA 15260, USA
[b]University Center for Social and Urban Research, University of Pittsburgh, Pittsburgh, Pennsylvania, USA

Family members are an essential resource to older individuals with chronic illness and disability. Without the care and support provided by relatives, it would be difficult and often impossible for persons with disability to remain in the community. Current estimates indicate that more than 40 million Americans provide assistance annually to an adult relative because of illness and disability. There is strong consensus that caring for an individual with disability is burdensome and stressful to most family members and contributes to psychiatric morbidity in the form of elevated rates of depression and anxiety and, in extreme cases, murder-suicide. Research also suggests that the combination of loss, prolonged distress, physical demands of caregiving, and biological vulnerabilities of older caregivers may compromise their physiologic functioning and increase their risk for physical health problems.

Findings that document the health effects of elder caregiving have been complemented by scores of intervention studies aimed at addressing the burden, distress, and negative health effects associated with caregiving. Although this research has been subjected to periodic review beginning in 1989 [1–11], assessments of the recent literature in this area are lacking. This article examines critically the caregiver intervention studies published between 1999 and 2005. The primary goal was to identify recent randomized controlled trials (RCTs) that evaluated the efficacy toread NIMH P30 of psychosocial and

Preparation of this manuscript was supported in part by grants NIMH P30 MH52247, NHLBI P50 HL65111-65112, NIMH K01 MH065547, NIA K07 AG000923, NIA U01 AG013305, NINR R01 NR008272, NIH P60 MD000207, NHLBI R24 HL076852.
* Corresponding author.
E-mail address: schulz@pitt.edu (R. Schulz).

doi:10.1016/j.psc.2005.09.003
psych.theclinics.com

behavioral interventions for family caregivers of patients often seen by geriatric psychiatrists and to describe and synthesize the findings of these studies. The caregiving studies for Alzheimer's disease, stroke, and mental illness are included that, together, account for a large proportion of the published caregiver intervention studies. Discussion focuses on the intervention studies that involved psychosocial treatment for caregivers and also included environmental and behavioral interventions for the care recipient.

Summary of reviews of the caregiver intervention literature

Early intervention studies were primarily psychosocial and targeted caregivers' appraisals of their resources and situation. These interventions involved mostly support groups, individual counseling, and education approaches. Evidence from this first wave of research was inconsistent and showed modest therapeutic benefits as measured by global ratings of well being, mood, stress, psychologic status, and burden. Recent research based on more rigorous designs has evaluated a broader range of intervention programs involving individual or family counseling, case management, skills training, environmental modification, behavior management strategies, and combinations thereof [9,12–14]. Evidence from these studies suggests that combined interventions that target the multiple sources of caregiving stress and multiple individuals simultaneously (ie, caregiver and patient) produce a significant improvement in caregiver burden, depression, subjective well being, perceived caregiver satisfaction, ability and knowledge, and sometimes care-recipient symptoms [9,14]; that is, interventions that combine different strategies and provide caregivers with diverse services and supports tend to generate larger effects than narrowly focused interventions. Similarly, single-component interventions with a higher intensity (frequency and duration) have a greater positive impact on the caregiver than comparable interventions with lower intensity. Intervention effects tend to be larger for increasing caregiver knowledge and skill than decreasing burden and depression. Also, the intervention effects for caregivers of persons with dementia tend to be smaller than effects for caregivers of other care receivers are.

These conclusions are consistent with a recent meta-analysis of the intervention literature [12] that shows that caregiver interventions produce a statistically significant improvement of .14 to .41 SD units, for outcomes such as depression, caregiver burden, subjective well being, and caregiver satisfaction. Large effect sizes and clinically meaningful outcomes are still relatively rare in the recent literature, but at least some researchers were able to achieve outcomes with strong public health implications. Interventions that result, for example, in delayed institutionalization or in significant improvements for crippling depression represent just two effects with personal and public health significance. Such outcomes have potentially far-reaching consequences for promoting health and wellness for all those affected by chronic disablement.

Compared with earlier reviews of the caregiver intervention literature, these recent analyses have painted a decidedly more positive picture. Beneficial outcomes were more common, and the quality of the science had improved. However, close inspection of these studies also raises methodological concerns, which call into question some of the conclusions reported in this literature. Inasmuch as methodological problems continue to plague even more recent studies, they are discussed later in detail.

Method

The literature search conducted for this article was aimed at identifying recently published evaluations of psychosocial family caregiver interventions, defined as nonmedical interventions that are psychologically, socially, or behaviorally oriented and that involved a member of an older patient's family or both the patient and family member. To identify studies for review, computerized literature searches of numerous electronic databases were performed in May 2005. Studies chosen for initial screening met the following criteria: (1) publication between January 1999 and April 2005; (2) publication in a peer-reviewed, English language journal; (3) evaluation of a psychosocial intervention for family members of older adults (ie, ≥60 years of age) with dementia caused by Alzheimer's disease or a related disorder (eg, Parkinson's disease), stroke, or psychiatric illness; (4) the use of a randomized controlled design; and (5) quantitative outcomes reported for caregiver or caregiver and patient.

Keyword searches of the interlinked search engine OVID included the following databases: MEDLINE (1966–2005), PsychINFO (1967–2005), CINAHL (1982–2005), and evidence-based medicine databases (from 1991–2005 in the ACP Journal Club, the Cochrane Controlled Trials Register, Cochrane Database of Systematic Reviews, and the Database of Abstracts of Reviews of Effectiveness). Combinations of keywords in the following groupings were used for these OVID searches: (1) family, caregiver, caregiving, spouse, or spousal; (2) intervention; (3) dementia, psychiatric, depression, anxiety, bipolar, schizophrenia, stroke, cerebral vascular accident, or substance abuse; and (4) randomized, randomized controlled trial, or controlled. This method yielded 714 citations of studies that met the inclusion criteria. Next, the ancestry method of examining references in review articles or empirical articles was used to identify intervention studies not captured through database searches. An additional 150 citations were obtained through this method, and citations that met the inclusion criteria were extracted for review.

Results

A total of 41 studies focused on dementia caregivers, and 10 studies focused on stroke caregivers met the criteria for this review [15–65]. Studies were excluded primarily because an RCT design was not used or caregivers to older patients were not the focus of the study. The lack of focus on older patients was particularly striking for the studies testing psychosocial interventions for family members of psychiatric patients. Tables 1 and 2 summarize the intervention studies focused on dementia caregivers and stroke caregivers, respectively. These tables describe each study according to baseline sample, number and content of study groups, and statistically significant differences ($P \leq .05$) between groups for caregiver outcomes and patient outcomes (if assessed). In these tables a mathematical notation system is used to indicate that one group showed greater improvement in a study outcome than the comparison group (eg, group 2 $\geq$ group 1). For those studies that had multiple follow-up assessments, findings were summarized for the first follow-up assessment because intervention effects tend to be strongest soon after implementation and dissipate over time.

Recent interventions for dementia caregivers

Table 1 summarizes the findings of 41 dementia caregiver interventions that met the inclusion criteria, including publication in the past 5 years and the use of an RCT design. In this table, the frequency of problem behaviors (usually reported by the caregiver) is classified as a patient outcome, whereas the bother or burden of these behaviors is classified as a caregiver outcome. The placement of the older relative in long-term care also is classified as a patient outcome, although the decision to place a patient is made typically by the caregiver and affects his or her health as well.

Almost all of the interventions tested focused on a mixture of family members (ie, spouses and adult children) and were multicomponent in nature, combining educational materials with some amount of counseling or skills training. Over half of these studies (51%, or 21 of 41) were not statistically powerful enough to detect the small effects that are observed commonly for psychosocial interventions and were not even powered to detect medium-sized effects [66]. The majority (approximately 77%) of these interventions involved only the caregiver and provided no psychosocial treatment to the patient. However, over half of these studies assessed change in outcomes that can be conceptualized as specific to the patient, such as the frequency of memory and behavior problems and placement in long-term care. Overall, this group of recent interventions can be characterized as having their most consistent effects in reducing caregivers' depressive symptoms, burden, and anxiety symptoms.

One of the most ambitious research programs in this group was the Resources for Enhancing Alzheimer's Caregiver Health (REACH) trial, a multisite study designed to test the effectiveness of multiple different interventions and to evaluate the pooled effects of all interventions combined [67–72]. Six sites (Boston, MA, Birmingham, AL, Memphis, TN, Miami, FL, Palo Alto, CA, and Philadelphia, PA) developed and evaluated a variety of multicomponent interventions for family caregivers of persons with Alzheimer's disease at the mild or moderate level of impairment. The multicomponent interventions implemented across the six sites included: (1) individual information and support strategies; (2) group support and family systems therapy; (3) psycho-educational and skill-based training approaches; (4) home-based environmental interventions; and (5) enhanced technology support systems. All of the REACH interventions were guided by detailed treatment manuals and certification procedures that assured that the interventions were delivered consistently over time at each site. Careful attention was also given to the issue of treatment integrity. Each of the sites achieved statistically significant positive outcomes for their intervention on outcomes such as burden and depression (see Table 1). These individual study findings were consistent with a preplanned meta-analysis that showed that being in the treatment group was superior to the control condition, although the magnitude of effects was modest from a clinical perspective [69]. Perhaps most important, this research program was able to link specific elements of a multicomponent intervention to caregiver outcomes, showing that interventions that actively engage the caregiver in skill acquisition aimed at regulating their own behavior result in significant improvements in caregiver depression [72].

Recent interventions for stroke caregivers

A total of 10 published studies meeting the inclusion criteria were focused specifically on the evaluation of an intervention for family caregivers of stroke patients (see Table 2). As found for the dementia caregiver interventions, almost all of the interventions for stroke caregivers were multicomponent in nature. Intervention recruitment and implementation often took place during the patient's inpatient rehabilitation and continued after discharge. Spouses were the most common family members targeted with these interventions.

In contrast to the dementia caregiver interventions, the majority of interventions for stroke caregivers were statistically powered to detect the effects of at least medium size, whereas only a few were not [56–58]. In addition, over half of these studies provided psychosocial treatment to both the caregiver and stroke patient, rather than focusing exclusively on the caregiver. Reflecting this dyadic approach, two thirds of the studies assessed outcomes for the patient as well as the caregiver. Although a few studies were able to demonstrate significant intervention effects on standard mental health indicators such as depressive and anxiety symptoms, most of these studies either did not find effects for these types of outcomes or chose instead to focus on the effects of intervention on skills acquisition, the use of effective coping strategies, and knowledge of stroke and its risk factors. One of the strongest studies in this group, and one of the few caregiving studies that adhered to Consolidated Standards of Reporting Trials CONSORT guidelines for

Table 1
Dementia caregiver intervention studies, randomized clinical trials 1999–2005 (N = 41)

Study	Sample (at baseline)	RCT design[a]	Interventions	Between-group differences for CGs[b]	Between-group differences for PTs[b]
Akkerman 2004 [15]	38 CGs with mild to moderate anxiety	2 groups: UC (intervention waitlist) Group cognitive-behavioral therapy for CG	Nine 2-h weekly meetings of didactic skills training targeted at CG anxiety	2 > 1 for anxiety	No outcomes assessed
Bass et al 2003 [16]	182 CGs	2 groups: UC Integrated AD care for the dyad	Integration of Alzheimer's Association care consultation with managed care services	2 > 1 for depression, utilization of health care services, and satisfaction with services 2 > 1 for relationship strain, for nonspouses only	2 > 1 for case management and direct care svcs, and for non-Association information and support svcs; for PTs w/severe memory problems
Bourgeois et al 2002 [17]	63 spousal CGs	3 groups: General information and support for CG PT-focused skills training for CG CG-focused skills training for CG	12 week interventions: Workshop and weekly in-home visits to provide general information and support Workshop and weekly in-home visits where most frequent and stressful patient behaviors were identified and addressed Workshop and weekly in-home visits focused on increasing pleasant events, problem solving, and relaxation techniques	2, 3 > 1 for mood and depression 2 > 1 for stress	2 > 1 for problem behavior frequency 3 > 1 for total problem behaviors

	Sample	Groups	Description		
Buckwalter et al 1999 [18]	245 CGs (64% spouses)	2 groups: Information and referrals for CG 1 + psychoeducational nursing intervention for CG	2 in-home visits providing general information about AD, community-based referrals, books, and brochures; bi-weekly follow-up phone calls for 6 mo 1+ 3–4 h in-home training in the Progressively Lowered Stress Threshold model, addressing patient symptom clusters, levels of patient behaviors, and disease stages; focus on reducing stress by modifying environmental demands	2 > 1 for depressive symptoms, tension-anxiety, anger-hostility, fatigue-inertia, and confusion-bewilderment	No outcomes assessed
Burgio et al 2003 [19] REACH trial	140 CGs (50% spouses)	2 groups: Minimal support for CG Skills training for CG	15-min telephone contacts composed of empathic statements, active listening and generic written education materials Workshop followed by 16 in-home sessions composed of videotaped demonstrations, behavior management techniques, instruction and support in technical application of specific behavioral and environmental treatments and problem solving techniques	2 > 1 for bother from behavior problems, for African Americans; 1 > 2 for whites 2 > 1 for number of behavior problems, for African American spouses; 1 > 2 for white spouses	No significant differences between groups

(continued on next page)

Table 1 (*continued*)

Study	Sample (at baseline)	RCT design[a]	Interventions	Between-group differences for CGs[b]	Between-group differences for PTs[b]
Burns et al 2003 [20] REACH trial	167 CGs (50% spouses)	2 groups: Behavior care for CG; Enhanced care for CG	Education sessions on behavior management using 25 patient behavior modification pamphlets 1+ stress-behavior management	2 > 1 for general well-being	No outcomes assessed
Castro et al 2002 [21]	100 female CGs (53% spouses)	2 groups: Attention-control (nutrition education for CG); Exercise program for CG	Telephone-based nutrition education for 12 mo; Four 30–40 min exercise sessions per week occurring in a home-based format for 12 mo	2 > 1 for knowledge of exercise benefits and readiness for physical activity	No outcomes assessed
Chang 1999 [22]	65 CG-PT dyads (89% spouses)	2 groups: Attention only for CG; Cognitive-behavioral intervention for CG	Weekly phone calls from nurse to assess general well being; Cognitive-behavioral, video-assisted modeling program (8 wk)	2 > 1 for depressive symptoms	No significant differences between groups
Chu et al 2000 [23]	75 CG-PT dyads	2 groups: Information for CG; Early home care program for the dyad	Information packet on community resources and eligibility for conventional home care; Case management service which featured supportive counseling, referral, skill training, and education over 18 mo	2 > 1 for burden and services used for case management, during the intervention	2 > 1 for rate of long-term care placement over 18 months, for those with mild to moderate cognitive impairment

Corbeil et al 1999 [24]	87 CGs	3 groups: UC Passive cognitive stimulation (dyad) Active cognitive stimulation (dyad)	Passive activities with PT such as TV watching for 12 wk Training in activities to stimulate the mind of the PT for 12 wk	3 > 1, 2 for satisfaction with dyadic interaction	No outcomes assessed
Davis et al 2004 [25]	71 CGs (49% spouses)	3 groups: Friendly calls for CG Telephone training for CG In-home training for CG	Initial home visit and then weekly calls regarding general health and medication regimen 12 weekly skill training sessions focusing on general problem-solving skills, appraisal of behavior problems, writing behavioral programs, and strategies for handling affective responses to difficult situations Same content as above but delivered in the home	3 > 2, 1 for reduced burden and distress	No outcomes assessed
Done and Thomas 2001 [26]	45 CGs	2 groups: Information booklet for CG Communication training for CG	Booklet of advice for communication problems Two therapist-led sessions 1-h to demonstrate successful communication strategies; therapist and group discussion	2 > 1 for awareness of communication strategies	No outcomes assessed

(continued on next page)

Table 1 (*continued*)

Study	Sample (at baseline)	RCT design[a]	Interventions	Between-group differences for CGs[b]	Between-group differences for PTs[b]
Ducharme et al 2005 [27]	137 adult daughter CGs	3 groups: UC Psychoeducation provided by Alzheimer society Group psychoeducation	10 weekly sessions offered by the Quebec Alzheimer Society 10 90-min weekly sessions focused on cognitive appraisal of stressors, empowerment, utilization of coping strategies	3 > 1 for competence dealing with health care staff and perceived challenge of the CG role 3, 2 > 1 for control, perceived threat, social support, role overland, and reframing	No outcomes assessed
Eisdorfer et al 2003 [28] REACH study	225 CGs (65% spouses)	3 groups: Minimal support for CG Structural ecosystems therapy (SET) for CG Structural ecosystems therapy + computer-telephone integrated system (CTIS) for CG	Generic educational materials and telephone calls consisting of active listening and empathic comments for 12 mo Brief strategic family therapy over 12 mo; most were in-home sessions CTIS designed to augment above by providing enhanced access to formal and informal resources	3 > 2, 1 for depressive symptoms; strongest effects for Cuban American husband and daughter CGs	No outcomes assessed
Eloniemi-Sulkava et al 2001 [29]	100 CG-PT dyads	2 groups: UC Nurse care management for the dyad	2-y support program coordinated by a nurse case manager providing advocacy for PTs and CGs, support, counseling, training, follow-up calls, in-home visits, assistance for services, and 24-h hotline	(see next column)	2 > 1 for long-term care placement during first few months

Study	Sample	Groups	Intervention	Results	Outcomes
Fung and Chien 2002 [30]	52 CG-PT dyads (50% couples)	2 groups: Conventional services for CG / Support group for CG	Conventional family services provided by dementia center for 12 wk / 12 1-h weekly sessions of education, psychological support, and problem solving	2 > 1 for distress and quality of life	No outcomes assessed
Gallagher-Thompson et al 2003 [31] REACH study	213 female CGs, Anglo and Latino (38% spouses)	2 groups: Enhanced support for CG / Coping with caregiving class for CG	Weekly peer support group meetings for 10 wk / Psychoeducational group intervention using cognitive-behavioral techniques; emphasized reducing negative affect	2 > 1 for depressive symptoms and use of adaptive coping strategies	No outcomes assessed
Gitlin et al 2001 [32]	171 CGs (25% spouses)	2 groups: UC / Home environmental intervention for CG	Education materials and home environmental safety tips at the conclusion of the study / Multicomponent environmental program over 3 mo led by OT involving education on: impact of environment on dementia-related behaviors and helping CGs to simplify home objects, break down tasks, and involve other supportive persons in daily caregiving activities	2 > 1 for self-efficacy, for female CGs and minority caregivers; 2 > 1 for behavior upset for spousal caregivers	2 > 1 for IADL dependency

(continued on next page)

Table 1 (*continued*)

Study	Sample (at baseline)	RCT design[a]	Interventions	Between-group differences for CGs[b]	Between-group differences for PTs[b]
Gitlin et al 2003 [33] REACH trial	255 CGs (35% spouses)	2 groups: UC Home environmental skill-building program for CG	Systematic needs assessment and targeted plan followed by OT observation, role-playing, walk through home, and education	2 > 1 for upset with memory-related behaviors, need for assistance from others, and affect 2 > 1 for upset with disruptive behaviors, for spouses 2 > 1 for daily oversight, for male CGs 2 > 1 for management ability, well-being, and mastery for female CGs	No significant differences between groups
Grant et al 2003 [34]	55 spousal CGs classified as vulnerable or non-vulnerable	2 groups: UC Respite care for CG	10 days of in-home help (up to 6 h/d) for the CG over a 2-wk period	2 > 1 for plasma epinephrine in the vulnerable CGs	No outcomes assessed
Hebert et al 2003 [35]	158 CGs (84% spouses)	2 groups: Comparison group Psychoeducational group program	Referred to traditional support groups 15 2-h weekly sessions focusing on cognitive appraisal and coping strategies	2 > 1 for negative reactions to behavioral problems	2 > 1 for frequency of behavior problems

Hepburn et al 2001 [36]	117 CGs (66% spouses)	2 groups: No treatment (waitlist) Caregiver training	7 weekly 2-h group sessions focused on education, concept development, role clarification, belief clarification, and mastery-focused coaching	2 > 1 for emotional enmeshment, negative reactions to behavior problems, depressive symptoms, and burden	No significant differences between groups
Logiudice et al 1999 [37]	50 CG-PT dyads (54% couples)	2 groups: UC Memory clinic for the dyad	Complete medical assessment of PTs, advice and counseling for CGs, neuropsychologic assessment of PTs, and a family conference	2 > 1 for overall psychosocial health status and for subscales of alertness behavior and social interaction	No outcomes assessed
Mahoney et al 2003 [38] REACH trial	100 CGs (54% spouses)	2 groups: Information Automated telephone support system for CG	Reference booklet on: strategies for managing disruptive behaviors Year-long access to interactive voice response system, which provided stress monitoring, counseling information, personal voice-mail linkage to AD experts, a voice-mail support group and a distraction call for PTs	2 > 1 for bother, anxiety and depressive symptoms, for those with low mastery	No outcomes assessed
Marriott et al 2000 [39]	42 CG-PT dyads (52% spouses)	3 groups: UC Camberwell Family Interview with CG Cognitive-behavioral intervention for CG	Education, stress management and coping skills training delivered in 14 sessions over 28 wk	3 > 1, 2 for distress, depression and psychiatric caseness	3 > 1 for behavioral disturbance 3 > 1, 2 for ADL disability

(continued on next page)

Table 1 (*continued*)

Study	Sample (at baseline)	RCT design[a]	Interventions	Between-group differences for CGs[b]	Between-group differences for PTs[b]
Martin-Cook et al 2003 [40]	37 CGs	2 groups: UC Psychoeducational group intervention for CG	4 weekly 2-h group psychoeducational sessions	No significant differences between groups	No outcomes assessed
McCurry et al 2003 [41]	22 CG-PT dyads (64% couples)	2 groups: Support for CG Sleep hygiene program for CG	Both groups participated in 6 1-h in-home treatment sessions over a 2-mo period; both groups kept a sleep diary. Nondirective, supportive intervention. CGs developed an individualized sleep hygiene program, given sleep tips and feedback, instructed to exercise and assisted with problem solving	2 > 1 for setting sleep hygiene goals for the PT	2 > 1 for maintaining a consistent bedtime, for patients who were candidates for sleep hygiene changes
Mittelman et al 2004 [42] Mittelman et al 2004 [43]	406 spousal CGs	2 groups: Comparison group Group counseling and support intervention for CG	Availability of normal counseling services offered by Aging and Dementia Research Center. Individual and family counseling, weekly support groups, and ad hoc counseling over 9 mo	2 > 1 for depressive symptoms and negative appraisals of behavior problems	No outcomes assessed
Nobili et al 2004 [44]	69 CG-PT dyads (47% couples)	2 groups: Information control group Counseling and problem solving	Free help line and information about rights of patients and families, legal aspects, state forms, and resources. Separate home visits by a psychologist and an OT; also received information manual and resource contact list	(see next column)	2 > 1 for reduced frequency of problem behaviors

Study	Sample	Groups	Intervention	Result	Other result
Newcomer et al 1999 [45] Miller et al 1999 [46]	5307 CG-PT dyads (50% spouses)	2 groups: UC Case management and community care benefits for CG	Education/training about AD and available community services through 1-on-1 case management and support groups; also received coordination of assistance with CG tasks, family counseling, and transportation to groups and monthly community care benefits up to $699	2 > 1 for burden	No significant differences between groups
Ostwald et al 1999 [47]	117 CG-PT dyads	2 groups: UC Psychoeducational intervention for CG	7 weekly 2-h group sessions which included education and skills building	2 > 1 for caregiver burden and negative reactions to disruptive behaviors	No significant differences between groups
Pillemer et al 2002 [48]	147 CGs (40% spouses)	2 groups: UC Peer Support Project for CG	Emphasized support that persons in the same life situation can provide to one another without professional intervention; community volunteers were trained and met with a caregiver for 8 weekly sessions (approx 2 h each)	No significant differences between groups	No outcomes assessed
Pillemer et al 2003 [49]	932 CGs	2 groups: UC for nursing home PT Workshop for CG and for nursing home staff	Approx 7 h of communication and conflict resolution training delivered separately to CGs and to staff	2 > 1 for perceived empathy of staff	No outcomes assessed

(continued on next page)

Table 1 (*continued*)

Study	Sample (at baseline)	RCT design[a]	Interventions	Between-group differences for CGs[b]	Between-group differences for PTs[b]
Quayhagen et al 2000 [50]	103 CG-PT dyads (all couples)	5 groups: UC (wait-list) Cognitive stimulation for the dyad Dyadic counseling Dual supportive seminar for the dyad Early-stage day care and CG support group	8-wk intervention: Memory, problem solving, conversation Conflict resolution, stress reduction, anger management, communication Group treatment for CG and PT, both together and separately to exchange info, support, problem solving Social, physical, recreational activities and monthly CG support group	4 > 1, 2, 3, 5 for emotion-focused coping	No significant differences between groups
Roberts et al 1999 [51]	77 CG-PT dyads (52% couples)	2 groups: UC Problem-solving counseling for CG	Nurse counseling sessions over 6 mo	No significant differences at first follow-up	No significant differences at first follow-up
Shelton et al 2001 [52]	412 Medicare-eligible CGs (85% spouses)	2 groups: UC Illinois Disease Demonstration and Evaluation project	CGs and PTs received comprehensive in-home, clinical assessments conducted by nurse case managers; care plans were developed and shared with physician and other healthcare providers	2 > 1 lower likelihood of any hospitalization during study period (545 ± 378 d) For those hospitalized no significant difference between treatment and control group in number of hospitalizations, hospital length of stay, or Medicare payments	No outcomes assessed

Study	Sample	Groups	Intervention	Effects[b]	Outcomes
Steffen 2000 [53]	33 CGs (55% spouses)	3 groups: UC (wait list) Home-based anger management intervention Class-based anger management intervention	8 weeks of anger-management videos with weekly telephone check-in sessions 8 weeks of anger-management videos led by trained facilitator	2, 3 > 1 for anger, depression, and self-efficacy	No outcomes assessed
Teri et al 2003 [54]	153 CG-PT dyads (80% couples)	2 groups: UC Exercise program and training for CG	12 1-h in the home Exercise program consisting of aerobic/endurance activities, strength training, balance and flexibility training Caregivers taught to identify and modify patient behavioral problems and precipitants of distress	No significant differences between groups	2 > 1 for exercising at least 60 min/wk, days of restricted activity, physical role functioning and depression
Wishart et al 2000 [55]	24 CGs (32% spouses)	2 groups: UC (wait list) Visiting/walking program for PT	Weekly 2-h visit and walk or outing with PT provided by volunteers for 6 wk	2 > 1 for burden	No outcomes assessed

Abbreviations: AD, Alzheimer's disease; CG, caregiver; OT, occupational therapist; PT, patient; REACH, Resources for Enhancing Alzheimer's Caregiver Health, a multi-site study; UC, usual medical care for the patient; >, greater improvement over time.

[a] Intervention groups also received usual care.

[b] Effects reported are those found at the first follow-up. Differences reported are those that were significant at $P \leq .05$, or at an adjusted probability level set by the study investigators (eg, $P \leq .01$).

Table 2
Stroke caregiver intervention studies, randomized trials 1999–2005 (N = 10)

Study	Sample (at baseline)	RCT design[a]	Interventions	Between-group differences for CGs[b]	Between-group differences for PTs[b]
Clark 2003 [56]	68 CG-PT dyads (all couples)	2 groups: UC Education and counseling intervention for the dyad	Information packet and 3 1-h visits from social worker trained in family counseling, after discharge from inpatient rehabilitation	2 > 1 for perceived family functioning	2 > 1 for perceived family functioning, functional recovery, and social recovery in domestic chores, household maintenance, and social activities
Grant et al 2002 [57]	74 CGs (41% spouses)	3 groups: UC Sham intervention for CG Social problem-solving telephone partnerships for CG	Received weekly and biweekly calls for 12 wk and asked to identify services received since last contact Initial 3-h face-to-face session with a trained nurse who taught positive problem orientation and addressed a safety issue, then weekly and biweekly calls for 12 wk Both delivered after discharge from rehabilitation	3 > 1, 2 for problem-solving skills, preparedness, depression, vitality, social functioning, mental health, and role limitations related to emotional problems	No outcomes assessed
Hartke and King 2003 [58]	88 spousal CGs	2 groups: Comparison group, for CG Group education and support for CG	Written materials on stress management, caregiver stress, and stroke 8 sessions of peer support by teleconference	2 > 1 for competence and burden	No outcomes assessed

Kalra et al 2004 [59] Patel et al 2004 [60]	300 CG-PT dyads (65% couples)	2 groups: Conventional care for CG during PT rehabilitation 1+ CG training during PT rehabilitation	Information on stroke, goal setting for rehabilitation and discharge planning, encouragement to attend nursing and therapy activities, and advice on community svcs Instruction on common stroke-related problems, hands-on training in lifting and handling 3–5 sessions, 30–45 min each; follow-up session at home	2 > 1 for caregiver burden, anxiety, depression, and quality of life, costs of patient care over 1 y	2 > 1 for anxiety, depression, and quality of life
Lincoln et al 2003 [61]	250 CG-PT dyads	2 groups: UC Stroke Association Family Support Organiser service for the dyad	Contact in hospital to provide standard information pack, identify unmet needs; after discharge, home visits to address needs for up to 9 mo; frequency and content left to the discretion of the service	2 > 1 for knowledge about whom to contact for information on stroke, reducing the risk of future PT stroke, and obtaining emotional support; and for satisfaction with information on practical help and emotional support	2 > 1 for knowledge about whom to contact for information on stroke, reducing the risk of future stroke, obtaining community services, and obtaining emotional support; and for satisfaction with information on community services and emotional support

(continued on next page)

Table 2 (*continued*)

Study	Sample (at baseline)	RCT design[a]	Interventions	Between-group differences for CGs[b]	Between-group differences for PTs[b]
Mant et al 2000 [62]	520 CG-PT dyads (87% couples)	2 groups: UC Family support for the dyad	Education, emotional support and liaison with other services through written materials, referrals; provided by family support worker (individual representing national stroke organization); variable number of home and hospital visits (1–5) and telephone contacts (1–7)	2 > 1 for social activities, energy, vitality, mental health, pain, physical function, general health perception, quality of life, and satisfaction with understanding of stroke	2 > 1 for use of physiotherapy after hospital discharge
Rodgers et al 1999 [63]	204 PTs and 176 CGs (44% spouses)	2 groups: UC Stroke education program for the dyad	1-h small-group educational session in hospital followed by 6 1-h educational sessions after discharge from hospital	1 > 2 for social functioning 2 > 1 for stroke knowledge	2 > 1 for stroke knowledge and satisfaction with information received about stroke
Smith et al 2004 [64]	170 PTs and 97 CGs (72% spouses)	2 groups: UC Stroke education program for the dyad	Given stroke information manual and invited to attend educational meetings every two weeks during hospital rehabilitation	No significant differences between groups	2 > 1 for anxiety

van den Heuvel et al 2000 [65]	257 CGs	3 groups: UC Home visits for the CG Group program for the CG	8–10-wk home visit program providing 8 h of education in 4 visits 8-wk group program providing 16 h of education in 8 meetings Interventions focused on information, expressing emotions, and learning how to use active coping strategies	2, 3 > 1 for confidence in knowledge about patient care 2 > 1 for confronting as active coping strategy 3 > 1 for seeking social support as active coping strategy	No outcomes assessed

Abbreviations: CG, caregiver; PT, patient; UC, Usual medical care for the patient; >, greater improvement over time.

a Intervention groups also received usual care.

b Effects reported are those found at the first follow-up. Differences reported are those that were significant at $P \leq .05$, or at an adjusted probability level set by the study investigators (eg, $P \leq .01$).

reporting RCTs, found both statistically significant and clinically meaning-ful outcomes [59,60]. Caregivers assigned to the intervention arm of the study were given instruction on common stroke-related problems and their prevention and hands-on training in lifting, facilitation of mobility and transfers, continence, and communication. In a comparison with caregivers who received conventional care, caregivers who received specialized training reported less burden, anxiety, depression, and a higher quality of life. In ad-dition, the 1-year cost of care for patients in the caregiver training group was $6532 less than for the control group, and patients also reported lower anx-iety, depression, and better quality of life. This study serves as a good exam-ple of how a relatively simple and inexpensive caregiver intervention can achieve meaningful outcomes in both patient and caregiver functioning. In addition, it underscores the importance of hands on training as a key component of successful multicomponent interventions, a finding observed in the dementia caregiver literature as well.

Interventions for caregivers of older adults with late-life mood disorder

Our literature search revealed a significant gap in the empirical knowl-edge base regarding caregiver interventions for older psychiatric patients. Specifically, no recent RCTs have focused on family members of older adults with mood disorders, alcohol problems, or other significant psychiat-ric conditions. The strain that psychiatric illness puts on families is likely to be exacerbated when the patient is older because the patient may have a his-tory of such problems throughout adulthood and may also have physical health problems that complicate the treatment of their psychiatric symp-toms. The lack of focus on older adults with mood disorder and their family caregivers is especially striking given that illnesses such as major and minor depression are among the most common psychologic disorders of late life. Although they are not randomized trials, it is useful to highlight recent interventions that involve particularly promising approaches to family-oriented treatment of late-life depression or bipolar disorder.

Sherrill and colleagues [73] evaluated a psycho-educational workshop for older patients with recurrent major depression who were receiving psychiat-ric treatment through a research study and their close family members. This intervention involved a 2-hour educational session on the nature and treat-ment of depression, followed by separate meetings of clinicians with patients and clinicians with family members to share concerns and experiences and obtain further information. Patients attending this workshop were less likely to discontinue treatment for their depression than patients who could not or preferred not to attend the workshop, and family members reported high levels of satisfaction with the workshop. This type of intervention, perhaps augmented with a series of supportive meetings among caregivers, may re-sult in improved mental and physical health for family caregivers and better treatment response in patients. A randomized controlled study evaluating such an intervention for caregivers and patients is sorely needed. A family focused educational and supportive approach may also benefit older bipolar patients and their family caregivers [74], as suggested by recent work with midlife populations. Miklowitz and colleagues [75] have demonstrated that providing education to family members as an adjunct to patient pharmacotherapy results in fewer patient relapses and longer delays before relapses over a 1-year period, compared with pharmacotherapy alone.

In sum, dementia and stroke caregiver interventions show promise of achieving clinically significant outcomes in improving depressive symptoms and, to a lesser degree, in reducing anxiety, anger, and hostility. Although our ability to improve overall quality of life for caregivers appears to be limited, there is evidence that specific components of quality of life, such as caregiver burden, mood, and perceived stress, are responsive to interventions. Finally, some impressive and clinically meaningful effects have been demonstrated for delayed institutionalization of the care recipient. Such outcomes have potentially far-reaching consequences for promoting health and wellness for all those affected by chronic disablement.

Our review further shows that there is no single, easily implemented, and consistently effective method for achieving clinically significant effects across caregivers. Most intervention studies examined in this review reported some level of success, and as a group, they provided valuable insights about different methods for achieving caregiver impact. There exists strong consensus that all caregivers are likely to benefit from enhanced knowledge about the disease, the caregiving role, and resources available to caregivers. Once the informational needs have been met, caregivers might additionally benefit from training in general problem-solving skills, as well as from interventions that target managing care recipient behaviors or caregivers' emotional response to caregiving. Some studies have taught the caregiver rudimentary behavior management skills, including behavioral assessment techniques and methods for changing antecedents and consequences of disruptive behaviors. Recent intervention studies have also suggested that there may be important synergies achieved by simultaneously treating care recipients (eg, memory retraining) and caregivers, and by altering the social and physical environments through multicomponent interventions.

The recent literature also contains a rich array of methods for delivering interventions to caregivers. Among these are traditional approaches, such as individual and group therapy sessions, as well as newer technologies involving enhanced telecommunication systems, computers, and the World Wide Web. As sophisticated communication technologies become easier to use and more readily available, treatment delivery options will increase.

Limitations of recent studies

Conclusions need to be qualified by a host of methodological problems that still characterize much of this literature. This review is limited to recent studies that used a randomized controlled design because the findings of such studies yield the strongest conclusions regarding efficacy. However, it is important to note that studies can suffer from methodological flaws that are not remedied by an RCT design. Three specific areas of concern are highlighted. First, the random assignment of participants will fail to create equivalent groups if there is a differential attrition across groups during the study. The selection bias that occurs as the result of a higher dropout rate in one group obscures the interpretation of observed differences between groups (eg, did the group with greater attrition receive a less desirable intervention?). High rates of attrition and treatment noncompletion were observed in a number of reviewed studies [65], and researchers often failed to use methods that minimized the bias caused by such events, such as intent-to-treat analyses and techniques for accounting for missing data (eg, last observation carried forward).

Second, the use of a randomized controlled design has no bearing on whether an intervention was fully implemented or fully received by participants. In particular, it was very rare for investigators to report the extent to which patients or family members participated fully in an intervention (eg, number of sessions attended). This lack of information made it difficult to ascertain whether any weak or null effects were caused by participants not receiving the intended intervention or materials (ie, deficits in treatment receipt [76]). Not only were treatment delivery, receipt, and enactment information lacking from many studies, the description of some interventions was so vague they would be extremely difficult to replicate [42,43,61]. These problems are analogous to conducting a randomized trial for a new drug without reporting dose or ascertaining whether the drug was taken.

Third, the assessment procedures used in these studies were often inconsistent with those expected in randomized studies. An important aspect of an RCT design is to keep assessors blind to participant group assignment. It may not always be possible to keep assessors blind to group assignment, but it should be possible to separate the interventionists from the assessors. The extent to which this practice was followed was often not reported in these studies or was violated. For example, in at least one study the interventionist also collected the outcomes data [43]. This would be analogous to doing a therapeutic intervention study in which the therapist assesses the effects of treatment at the conclusion of the study. Not only is the assessor likely to be biased in collecting and reporting such data, the patient is obliged to reinforce the therapist's hard work by reporting positive outcomes. In many of the randomized controlled studies that were reviewed, the extent to which studies suffered from methodological limitations, such as the three highlighted here, were unable to be evaluated because investigators did not report important details regarding participant flow and treatment implementation. The present authors strongly recommend that future studies follow the CONSORT guidelines in conducting and reporting RCTs as one step toward addressing these issues [77].

Although not a methodological limitation per se, many of the dementia caregiver intervention studies that were reviewed did not assess outcomes for the patient. For those studies that evaluated intervention effects for patients, the most common outcome was the occurrence or frequency of memory and behavior problems. It is optimal to assess both the patient and caregiver outcomes to determine the efficacy from the perspective of the dyad (ie, benefits for both or neither individual or benefits for one individual with no change in the other) [78]. Outcomes such as mood and quality of life can and should be assessed for these patients, even in the presence of substantial cognitive impairment [79]. This argument can also be extended to intervention trials that target primarily the patient (ie, drug treatment studies). Inasmuch as the caregiver serves as a primary source of data about the patient and is likely to be affected by patient behavior, it could be argued that the assessment of treatment efficacy should include caregiver outcomes such as burden and depression [80].

Conclusions

Caregivers play a critical role in the treatment of patients with dementia, stroke, and mental illness. Because caregivers often have around-the-clock access to the patient and the knowledge base to identify significant changes in patient functioning, they serve as a critical source of information for the clinical assessment of the patient [81]. In addition, treatments and behavioral interventions for the patient are often implemented or managed by the caregiver who has day-to-day contact with the patient. The centrality of the caregiving role in patient diagnosis and management has resulted in guidelines and recommendations on working with caregivers developed by the major medical societies, including the American Medical Association, the American Psychiatric Association, and the American Association for Geriatric Psychiatry (AAGP). Treating patients with Alzheimer's disease, stroke, or mental illness must be based on a solid alliance with the patient and family. Understanding family caregiver needs and challenges is an essential aspect of effective treatment. The AAGP takes the strong position that family and caregiver counseling is medically necessary for the appropriate treatment of dementia, that counseling may require family or caregiver visits without the patient present, and that caregiver counseling should be considered a reimbursable, covered service. The rationale for this position is based on the observation that caregivers must receive guidance from physicians to observe, monitor, and manage the patient with dementia and that providing this guidance is time consuming and costly. The extant caregiving literature provides useful guidance for operationalizing these guidelines. They help identify caregivers who are at risk for adverse outcomes, methods for addressing identified risk areas, and methods for assessing clinically meaningful outcomes.

Persons who provide high levels of care, live with the care recipient, are older, female, have low levels of social support, low incomes, lower levels of education (ie, less than high school), and feel they had no choice in taking on the caregiving role are at higher risk for adverse outcomes. Developing an intervention strategy for these individuals should include an assessment of safety, depression and anxiety, and self-care health behaviors. The choices of how much and in what way to intervene should be guided by the level of risk identified for each individual. Although this may be the ideal, implementing these recommendations will be challenging. Meeting this challenge will require the development of better ways of quickly and accurately assessing caregiver risk, guidelines on which intervention options are most appropriate for a given individual, and cost-effective methods for monitoring caregiver status over time. Finally, we must identify how best to practically implement this approach and ways in which it can be paid for.

Future directions

The practical value of caregiver intervention research will depend not only on methodological refinements, as discussed earlier, but also on our ability to address some key conceptual issues needed to help move this field ahead. We need to develop a standardized taxonomy for characterizing and measuring multicomponent psychosocial interventions [71]. The application of a clearly articulated and useful taxonomy would enable us to better describe and compare interventions across studies as well as link intervention components to specific outcomes. Closer attention given to the assumed links between an intervention and the proposed outcomes would also be useful. For example, it should not be expected that interventions aimed at reducing caregiver anger or hostility will also delay institutionalization for the care recipient. Furthermore, and this speaks directly to the issue of clinical significance, the choice of study participants must be made more carefully. If caregivers are targeted who are at or near the normal range of depressive symptoms, meaningful improvements with an intervention designed to decrease depression are unlikely to be achieved. In other words, we should be sure that the study participants display the problems targeted by the intervention.

The broad range of outcomes reported in this review is indicative of both the strengths and weaknesses in the caregiver intervention literature. On the one hand, these outcomes point to the multifaceted impact of caregiving and the diversity of intervention effects that can be achieved. On the other hand, this diversity of outcomes along with the diversity of interventions makes it difficult to reach strong conclusions about what has been achieved in this literature. The present authors recommend that a core set of outcomes be included in all intervention studies and that the outcomes represent the major areas of clinical significance identified in the literature [9]. In making this recommendation, these authors are not advocating that all studies need to be designed to achieve clinical significance in all domains, but rather that at least some aspects of all domains be measured. Furthermore, it would be useful to develop consensus-based recommendations regarding specific measures to be used within each category of clinical significance. Once specific measures have been identified, the next step would be to reach consensus on what constitutes a clinically meaningful effect size for a given measure, along with recommended statistical procedures for demonstrating those effects [82].

In addition to recommendations relevant to all intervention studies, this review showed that there is virtually no systematic research on caregiving for late-life mental illness. Despite the important role of family in the course and treatment of late-life psychiatric illnesses, such as major depression, there have been few efforts to address the needs of these family caregivers through psychosocial intervention. The provision of information and support to these caregivers may have beneficial outcomes for the caregiver as well as for the patient (eg, enhanced treatment adherence and response).

Close family members of older adults coping with depression or another psychiatric illness are caregivers, both in a broad sense and often in the more traditional sense as well (ie, provision of assistance with activities of daily living). The family members deal with low mood and suicidality and also provide physical assistance and supervision caused by physical comorbidities and cognitive impairment. The present authors believe that caregiving should be conceptualized as both support and assistance, consistent with the broader social support literature emphasizing the tangible and emotional dimensions of supporting loved ones who are experiencing a chronic stressor such as illness. Adopting this broader conceptualization of family caregiving would allow researchers and policymakers to obtain a more comprehensive picture of the problems faced by families dealing with chronic illness.

Finally, these authors believe it is important to shift focus in caregiving from the physical and organizational challenges of providing care to the less tangible sources of distress caused by the knowledge that someone close to us is suffering and may be on a trajectory toward death. To date, the development of intervention strategies has been guided primarily by the idea that we need to ease the burden of care provision. Thus, intervention strategies such as providing respite, teaching caregiving skills, and enhancing the caregiver's ability to access community resources are common strategies that are consistent with this perspective. Although these types of interventions are clearly useful and important, they ignore the fact that the functional and behavioral disability of the patient account for only a small portion of the variance in the psychiatric and physical morbidity associated with family caregiving. Likewise, identified moderators and mediators of the impact of caregiving on health do not bring us closer to answering the more fundamental question of what is harmful to the health of spouses and adult children of chronically ill older adults. One possible and unexamined factor is the caregiver's perceptions of patient *suffering*, meaning the psychologic distress of the patient, their physical discomfort and pain, and the perception that there is little that can be done about these problems. Virtually none of the measures commonly used to assess emotional or cognitive reactions to caregiving taps into this concept of perceived suffering.

If perceived suffering is in fact a significant predictor of the negative health consequences of family caregiving, interventions may have more impact if they include psychotherapeutic approaches aimed at helping caregivers come to terms with uncertainty regarding their relative's health decline and bolstering the perception that they can act in ways that decrease patient suffering. Another approach to addressing this issue might be to adapt strategies developed for hospice care, where the emphasis is on patient comfort. A better understanding of the impact of patient suffering on caregiver well being may provide new intervention options that get at the heart of the caregiving experience.

References

[1] Bourgeois M, Schulz R, Burgio L. Interventions for caregivers of patients with Alzheimer's disease: a review and analysis of content, process and outcomes. Int J Aging Hum Dev 1996; 43(1):35–92.

[2] Charlesworth GM. Reviewing psychosocial interventions for family carers of people with dementia. Aging Ment Health 2001;5:104–6.

[3] Cooke DD, McNally L, Mulligan KT, et al. Psychosocial interventions for caregivers of people with dementia: a systematic review. Aging Ment Health 2001;5(2):120–35.

[4] Dunkin J, Anderson-Hanley C. Dementia caregiver burden: a review of the literature and guidelines for assessment and intervention. Neurology 1998;51(Suppl. 1):S53–60.

[5] Kennet J, Burgio L, Schulz R. Interventions for in-home caregivers: a review of research 1990 to present. In: Schulz R, editor. Handbook on dementia caregiving: evidence-based interventions for family caregivers. New York: Springer; 2000. p. 61–126.

[6] Knight BG, Lutzky SM, Macofsky-Urban F. A meta-analytic review of interventions for caregiver distress: recommendations for future research. Gerontologist 1993;33(2):240–8.

[7] Pusey H, Richards D. A systematic review of the effectiveness of psychosocial interventions for carers of people with dementia. Aging Ment Health 2001;5(2):107–19.

[8] Roberts J, Browne G, Gafni A, et al. Specialized continuing care models for persons with dementia: a systematic review of the research literature. Can J Aging 2000;19(1):106–26.

[9] Schulz R, O'Brien A, Czaja S, et al. Dementia caregiver intervention research: in search of clinical significance. Gerontologist 2002;42(5):589–602.

[10] Toseland RW, Rossiter CM. Group interventions to support family caregivers: a review and analysis. Gerontologist 1989;29(4):438–48.

[11] Zarit SH, Teri L. Interventions and services for family caregivers. In: Schaie KW, Lawton MP, editors. Annual review of gerontology and geriatrics, volume 11. New York: Springer; 1992. p. 287–310.

[12] Sorenson S, Pinquart M, Duberstein P. How effective are interventions with caregivers: an updated meta-analysis. Gerontologist 2002;42(3):356–72.

[13] Schulz R, editor. Handbook on dementia caregiving: evidence-based interventions for family caregivers. New York: Springer; 2000.

[14] Brodaty H, Green AB, Koschera A. Meta-analysis of psychosocial interventions for caregivers of people with dementia. J Am Geriatr Soc 2003;51:657–64.

[15] Akkerman RL. Reducing anxiety in Alzheimer's disease family caregivers: the effectiveness of a nine-week cognitive-behavioral intervention. Am J Alzheimers Dis Other Demen 2004; 19(2):117–23.

[16] Bass DM, Clark PA, Looman WJ, et al. The Cleveland Alzheimer's managed care demonstration: outcomes after 12 months of implementation. Gerontologist 2003;43(1): 73–85.

[17] Bourgeois MS, Schulz R, Burgio LD, et al. Skills training for spouses of patients with Alzheimer's disease: outcomes of an intervention study. Journal of Clinical Geropsychology 2002;8(1):53–73.

[18] Buckwalter KC, Gerdner L, Kohout F, et al. A nursing intervention to decrease depression in family caregivers of persons with dementia. Arch Psychiatr Nurs 1999; 13(2):80–8.

[19] Burgio L, Stevens A, Guy D, et al. Impact of two psychosocial interventions on White and African American family caregivers of individuals with dementia. Gerontologist 2003;43(4): 568–79.

[20] Burns R, Nichols LO, Martindale-Adams J, et al. Primary care intervention for dementia caregivers: 2-year outcomes from the REACH study. Gerontologist 2003;43(4):547–55.

[21] Castro CM, Wilcox S, O'Sullivan O, et al. An exercise program for women who are caring for relatives with dementia. Psychosom Med 2002;64:458–68.

[22] Chang BL. Cognitive-behavioral intervention for homebound caregivers of persons with dementia. Nurs Res 1999;48(3):173–82.

[23] Chu P, Edwards J, Levin R, Thomson J. The use of clinical case management for early state Alzheimer's patients and their families. Am J Alzheimers Dis Other Demen 2000;15(5): 284–90.

[24] Corbeil RR, Quayhagen MM, Quayhagen M. Intervention effects on demential caregiving interaction. J Aging Health 1999;11(1):79–95.

[25] Davis LL, Burgio LD, Buckwalter KC, Weaver M. A comparison of in-home and telephone-based skill training interventions with caregivers of persons with dementia. J Ment Health Aging 2004;10:31–44.

[26] Done DJ, Thomas JA. Training in communication skills for informal carers of people suffering from dementia: a cluster randomized clinical trial comparing a therapist-led workshop and a booklet. Int J Geriatr Psychiatry 2001;16(8):816–21.

[27] Ducharme F, Levesque L, Lachance L, et al. "Taking care of myself": efficacy of an intervention programme for caregivers of a relative with dementia living in a long-term care setting. The International Journal of Social Research and Practice 2005;4(1):23–47.

[28] Eisdorfer C, Czaja SJ, Loewenstein DA, et al. The effect of a family therapy and technology-based intervention on caregiver depression. Gerontologist 2003;43(4):521–31.

[29] Eloniemi-Sulkava U, Notkola I, Hentinen M, et al. Effects of supporting community-living demented patients and their caregivers: a randomized trial. J Am Geriatr Soc 2001;49: 1282–7.

[30] Fung W, Chien W. The effectiveness of a mutual support group for family caregivers of a relative with dementia. Arch Psychiatr Nurs 2002;26(3):134–44.

[31] Gallagher-Thompson D, Coon DW, Solano N, et al. Changes in indices of distress among Latino and Anglo female caregivers of elderly relatives with dementia: site-specific results from the REACH national collaborative study. Gerontologist 2003;43(4):580–91.

[32] Gitlin LN, Corcoran M, Winter L, et al. A randomized, controlled trial of a home environmental intervention: effect on efficacy and upset in caregivers and on daily function of persons with dementia. Gerontologist 2001;41(1):4–14.

[33] Gitlin LN, Winter L, Corcoran M, et al. Effects of the home environmental skill-building program on the caregiver-care recipient dyad: 6-month outcomes from the Philadelphia REACH initiative. Gerontologist 2003;43(4):532–46.

[34] Grant I, McKibbin CL, Taylor MJ, et al. In-home respite intervention reduces plasma epinephrine in stressed Alzheimer caregivers. Am J Geriatr Psychiatry 2003;11:62–72.

[35] Hebert R, Levesque L, Vezina J, et al. Efficacy of a psychoeducative group program for caregivers of demented persons living at home: a randomized controlled trial. J Gerontol B Psychol Sci Soc Sci 2003;58B:S58–67.

[36] Hepburn KW, Tornatore J, Center B, et al. Dementia family caregiver training: affecting beliefs about caregiving and caregiver outcomes. J Am Geriatr Soc 2001;49(4):450–7.

[37] Logiudice D, Waltrowicz W, Brown K, et al. Do memory clinics improve the quality of life of carers? a randomized pilot trial. Int J Geriatr Psychiatry 1999;14:626–32.

[38] Mahoney DF, Tarlow BJ, Jones RN. Effects of an automated telephone support system on caregiver burden and anxiety: findings from the REACH for TLC intervention study. Gerontologist 2003;43(4):556–67.

[39] Marriott A, Donaldson C, Terrier N, et al. Effectiveness of cognitive-behavioural family intervention in reducing the burden of care in carers of patients with Alzheimer's disease. Br J Psychiatry 2000;176:557–62.

[40] Martin-Cook K, Remakel-Davis B, Svetlik D, et al. Caregiver attribution and resentment in dementia care. Am J Alzheimers Dis Other Demen 2003;18:366–74.

[41] McCurry SM, Gibbons LE, Logsdon RG, et al. Training caregivers to change the sleep hygiene practices of patients with dementia: the NITE-AD project. J Am Geriatr Soc 2003;51: 1455–60.

[42] Mittelman MS, Roth DL, Haley WE, et al. Effects of a caregiver intervention on negative caregiver appraisals of behavior problems in patients with Alzheimer's disease: results of a randomized trial. Journal of Gerontology Psychol Sci 2004;59B:27–P34.

[43] Mittelman MS, Roth DL, Coon DW, et al. Sustained benefit of supportive intervention for depressive symptoms in caregivers of patients with Alzheimer's disease. Am J Psychiatry 2004;161:850–6.

[44] Nobili A, Riva E, Tettamanti M, et al. The effect of a structured intervention on caregivers of patients with dementia and problem behaviors. Alzheimer Dis Assoc Disord 2004;18:75–82.

[45] Newcomer R, Yordi C, DuNah R, et al. Effects of the Medicare Alzheimer's Disease Demonstration on caregiver burden and depression. Health Serv Res 1999;34(3):669–89.

[46] Miller R, Newcomer R, Fox P. Effects of the Medicare Alzheimer's disease demonstration on nursing home entry. Health Serv Res 1999;34(3):691–714.

[47] Ostwald SW, Hepburn KW, Caron W, et al. Reducing caregiver burden: a randomized psychoeducational intervention for caregivers of persons with dementia. Gerontologist 1999; 39(3):299–309.

[48] Pillemer K, Suitor JJ. Peer support for Alzheimer's caregivers. Res Aging 2002;24:171–92.

[49] Pillemer K, Suitor JJ, Charles R, et al. A cooperative communication intervention for nursing home staff and family members of residents. The Gerontologist 2003;43:96–106.

[50] Quayhagen MP, Quayhagen M, Corbeil RR, et al. Coping with dementia: evaluation of four nonpharmacologic interventions. Int Psychogeriatr 2000;12(2):249–65.

[51] Roberts J, Browne G, Milne C, et al. Problem-solving counseling for caregivers of the cognitively impaired: effective for whom? Nurs Res 1999;48(3):162–72.

[52] Shelton P, Schraeder C, Dworak D, et al. Caregivers' utilization of health services: results from the medicare Alzheimer's disease demonstration, Illinois site. J Am Geriatr Soc 2001;49:1600–5.

[53] Steffen AM. Anger management for dementia caregivers: a preliminary study using video and telephone interviews. Behav Ther 2000;31:281–99.

[54] Teri L, Gibbons LE, McCurry SM, et al. Exercise plus behavioral management in patients with Alzheimer disease. JAMA 2003;290:2015–22.

[55] Wishart L, Macerollo J, Loney P, et al. "Special steps": an effective visiting/walking program for persons with cognitive impairment. Can J Nurs Res 2000;31:57–71.

[56] Clark MS. A randomized controlled trial of an education and counselling intervention for families after stroke. Clin Rehabil 2003;17:703–12.

[57] Grant JS, Elliott TR, Weaver M, et al. Telephone intervention with family caregivers of stroke survivors after rehabilitation. Stroke 2002;33:2060–5.

[58] Hartke RJ, King RB. Telephone group intervention for older stroke caregivers. Top Stroke Rehabil 2003;9:65–81.

[59] Kalra L, Evans A, Perez I, et al. Training carers of stroke patients: randomized controlled trial. BMJ 2004;328:1099–104.

[60] Patel A, Knapp M, Evans A, et al. Training care givers of stroke patients: economic evaluation. BMJ 2004;328:1102–4.

[61] Lincoln NB, Francis VM, Lilley SA, et al. Evaluation of a stroke family support organiser: a randomized controlled trial. Stroke 2003;34:116–21.

[62] Mant J, Carter J, Wade DT, Winner S. Family support for stroke: a randomised controlled trial. Lancet 2000;356:808–13.

[63] Rodgers H, Atkinson C, Bond S, et al. Randomized controlled trial of a comprehensive stroke education program for patients and caregivers. Stroke 1999;30:2585–91.

[64] Smith J, Forster A, Young J. A randomized trial to evaluate an education programme for patients and carers after stroke. Clin Rehabil 2004;18:726–36.

[65] van den Heuvel ETP, de Witte LP, Nooyen-Haazen I, et al. Short-term effects of a group support program and an individual support program for caregivers of stroke patients. Patient Educ Couns 2000;40:109–20.

[66] Cohen J. A power primer. Psychol Bull 1992;112(1):155–9.

[67] Schulz R, Burgio L, Burns R, et al. Resources for Enhancing Alzheimer's Caregiver Health (REACH): overview, site-specific outcomes, and future directions. Gerontologist 2003; 43(4):514–20.

[68] Schulz R, Belle SH, Czaja SJ, Gitlin LN, et al. Introduction to the special section on Resources for Enhancing Alzheimer's Caregiver Health (REACH). Psychol Aging 2003;18(3): 357–60.

[69] Gitlin LN, Belle SH, Burgio LD, et al. Effect of multicomponent interventions on caregiver burden and depression: the REACH multisite initiative at 6-month follow-up. Psychol Aging 2003;18(3):361–74.

[70] Wisniewski SR, Belle SH, Coon DW, et al. The Resources for Enhancing Alzheimer's Caregiver Health (REACH): project design and baseline characteristics. Psychol Aging 2003; 18(3):375–84.

[71] Czaja SJ, Schulz R, Lee CC, Belle SH. A methodology for describing and decomposing complex psychosocial and behavioral interventions. Psychol Aging 2003;18:385–95.

[72] Belle SH, Czaja SJ, Schulz R, et al. Using a new taxonomy to combine the uncombinable: integrating results across diverse interventions. Psychol Aging 2003;18(3): 396–405.

[73] Sherrill JT, Frank E, Geary M, et al. Psychoeducational workshops for elderly patients with recurrent major depression and their families. Psychiatr Serv 1997;48:76–81.

[74] Martire LM, Schulz R, Mulsant BH, et al. Family caregiver functioning in late-life bipolar disorder. Am J Geriatr Psychiatry 2004;12:335–6.

[75] Miklowitz DJ, George EL, Richards JA, et al. A randomized study of family-focused psychoeducation and pharmacotherapy in the outpatient management of bipolar disorder. Arch Gen Psychiatry 2003;60:904–12.

[76] Lichstein KL, Riedel BW, Grieve R. Fair tests of clinical trials: a treatment implementation model. Advances in Behavioral Research and Therapy 1994;16:1–29.

[77] Moher D, Schulz KF, Altman D. The CONSORT statement: revised recommendations for improving the quality of reports of parallel-group randomized trials. JAMA 2001;285: 1987–91.

[78] Martire LM, Lustig AP, Schulz R, et al. Is it beneficial to involve a family member? a meta-analytic review of psychosocial interventions for chronic illness. Health Psychol 2004;23: 599–611.

[79] Martire LM, Schulz R. Informal caregiving to older adults: health effects of providing and receiving care. In: Baum A, Revenson T, Singer J, editors. Handbook of health psychology. Mahwah (NJ): Lawrence Erlbaum; 2001. p. 477–93.

[80] Lingler JH, Martire LM, Schulz R. Caregiver-specific outcomes in anti-dementia clinical drug trials: a systematic review and meta-analysis. J Am Geriatr Soc 2005;53:983–90.

[81] Tierney MC, Herrmann N, Geslani DM, et al. Contribution of informant and patient ratings to the accuracy of the mini-mental state examination in predicting probable Alzheimer's disease. J Am Geriatr Soc 2003;51:813–8.

[82] Kendall PC, Marrs-Garcia A, Nath SR, et al. Normative comparisons for the evaluation of clinical significance. J Consult Clin Psychol 1999;67:285–99.

ELSEVIER
SAUNDERS

Psychiatr Clin N Am
28 (2005) 1039–1060

PSYCHIATRIC
CLINICS
OF NORTH AMERICA

Evidence-Based Mental Health Services for Home and Community

Martha L. Bruce, PhD, MPH[a],*,
Aricca D. Van Citters, MS[b],
Stephen J. Bartels, MD, MS[b]

[a]Department of Psychiatry, Weill Medical College of Cornell University,
21 Bloomingdale Road, White Plains, NY 10605, USA
[b]New Hampshire-Dartmouth Psychiatric Research Center, 2 Whipple Place,
Suite 202, Lebanon, NH 03755, USA

The articles elsewhere in this issue describe the large evidence base of effective treatments for the mental health problems commonly experienced by older adults. However, despite the availability of pharmacologic and psychotherapeutic interventions with demonstrated efficacy in geriatric patients, mental illness remains undertreated in older adults [1]. As many as one half of older adults with a recognized mental disorder fail to receive any mental health services, and even fewer receive evidence-based treatments [2]. Bridging this gap between the scientific findings and community-based practice is an explicit goal for the National Institute of Mental Health and the Institute of Medicine [3,4]. In some cases, the lack of mental health treatment reflects decisions made by older adults or their clinicians about the need and preferences for mental health treatment. But in many cases, older adults are unable to access mental health treatment because of barriers posed by the health care system, at both the policy and organization levels.

Timely access to evidence-based mental health treatment for older adults is a key goal of recent reports by the Older Adult Subcommittee of the

This article is revised and updated from: Van Citters AD, Bartels SJ. A systematic review of the effectiveness of community-based mental health outreach services for older adults. Psychiatr Serv 2004;55(11):1237–49; with permission.

* Corresponding author.
  E-mail address: mbruce@med.cornell.edu (M.L. Bruce).

President's New Freedom Commission on Mental Health [5], the Administration on Aging [6], and the Surgeon General [7]. The research literature documents widespread costs of not providing timely access. For older adults with a mental illness and for their families, the lack of access prolongs their suffering. Untreated mental illness in older adults also has a significant impact on health, functioning, and health services use and costs. For instance, late-life mental illness contributes to the risk of decline in cognition and medical status [1], increased disability [8], self-neglect [9], and compromised quality of life [7,8]. Mental illness among older adults is also associated with excess use of health care, increased placement in nursing homes, greater burden to medical care providers, and higher annual health care costs [9–13]. Depression specifically worsens the outcomes of many medical disorders and increases the risk for falls [14], suicide [15], and nonsuicide mortality [16–19].

Access to appropriate mental health care can be especially difficult for homebound and other frail, community-dwelling older adults, who are often isolated from mainstream medical settings such as primary care, where most depression screening now takes place. Common barriers to access, such as lack of transportation, difficulties in identifying mental health symptoms in the context of medical burden, and the disconnect between multiple service providers, are magnified for older adults, whose mobility is compromised and whose ability to navigate complex services is impaired. The need is especially great among homebound seniors. Community-based studies, including population-based surveys and studies of home health care patients, home-delivered meal clients, and other homebound populations, confirm the high rates of many types of mental illness in these groups [20–23]. Depression and other mental health problems are especially insidious among frail or homebound [20,21] community-dwelling older adults, who are made vulnerable by encroaching disability, medical illness, and social isolation, factors associated with both the risk for and outcomes of depressive illness in late life [8,24,25]. The risks associated with the lack of care are also magnified because a quintessential feature of frailty is the inability to withstand acute illness, emotional upheaval, or physical dislocation (Activities of Daily Living (ADL) decline, falls, hospitalizations, institutionalization, and death) [25–28].

Evidence that frail and homebound, community-dwelling older adults have special difficulty accessing adequate mental health care has prompted researchers to test novel strategies for providing mental health services to older adults. The common theme to this growing evidence base is the development of interventions that reach out from traditional health care practice to provide care in the settings where older adults reside or spend a significant amount of time. Elements of home-based and community services may include case finding, assessment, referral, treatment, and care management. These services commonly are multidisciplinary and sometimes integrate social and medical services into mental health care. For instance, outreach programs may offer early intervention, facilitate access to preventive health care services, refer individuals to supportive services, and provide services designed to help keep older adults living longer in the community.

In this article, the growing evidence base surrounding the provision of home and community-based mental health services for homebound and frail older adults is evaluated. Specifically, the focus is whether home-based geriatric mental health services are effective in improving mental health symptoms or outcomes.

Method

To identify relevant articles for this review, the MEDLINE, PsychINFO, CINAHL, and Web-of-Science databases were searched within three topic areas for English language articles indexed through July 2005: community outreach services (keywords outreach, gatekeeper, and consultation and referral), mental illness (keywords mental or "depress" or "psych"), and older adults (keywords geriatric or late-life or elderly). Additional articles were identified through bibliographic review, MEDLINE, and Web-of-Science "related records" searches.

Studies were included that evaluated face-to-face psychiatric outreach and treatment services for older adults (target population age ≥ 65) that provided care in community-based noninstitutional settings such as senior centers, senior housing, and home-based settings. Eligible studies consisted of randomized, controlled trials, quasi-experimental studies, longitudinal outcome studies, and a comparison of two or more interventions.

Studies that evaluated services provided in institutional settings (ie, nursing homes or hospitals) were excluded. Because the goal of this review was to determine the effectiveness of outreach services for primary psychiatric disorders, interventions focused explicitly on persons with dementia or on caregivers of persons with dementia were excluded. Finally, duplicate publications with at least one author in common and only minor differences with respect to study samples and efficacy results were excluded.

This article provides an update to a systematic review evaluating the literature published through May 2004 [29]. Although the updated search strategy identified an additional 21 articles, none of these articles met the eligibility criteria for inclusion in this systematic review of home and community-based mental health services for older adults.

Selection of trials

Approximately 164 articles were identified through the literature search. Ninety-six articles were rejected because of sample selection (ie, nongeriatric population), provision of services in an institutional setting, or the lack of face-to-face contact. The remaining 68 articles were reviewed by examining the abstract or content of the article. Bibliographic and related records searches identified 17 additional articles that were subjected to all review criteria. After these articles were reviewed, an additional 29 were excluded because of sample selection, provision of services in an institutional setting, or a lack of face-to-face contact. Forty articles were excluded based on the quality of data presented; of these, 36 articles contained only model descriptions or descriptive data, and four articles described small case studies. Of the 16 remaining reports, 12 fulfilled all inclusion criteria, but four were published in duplicate. Five studies described results of randomized, controlled trials [30–36]; one reported on a quasi-experimental study [37], four reported on a noncontrolled prospective cohort [38–41], and two reported on a noncontrolled retrospective cohort [42,43].

Data extraction and analysis

Descriptive characteristics and outcome data were abstracted from all of the studies included using a standard data collection form. Data included study type, model description, inclusion and exclusion criteria, sample characteristics, duration, and completeness of follow-up, blinding to intervention and outcome assessment, study measures and outcomes, and strengths and weaknesses. Primary outcomes of interest included the use of mental health services and improvement in psychiatric symptoms. A statistical aggregation of data was not feasible because of the lack of similarity among studies with respect to study design, inclusion criteria, sampling, and outcome measures.

Results

All twelve studies that met full criteria for this review examined the impact of home-based mental health services on improving psychiatric symptoms and community tenure (or reducing the risk of nursing home placement or other institutionalizations). Study designs included five randomized, controlled trials, one quasi-experimental study, and six uncontrolled cohort studies (Table 1). Older adults participating in these studies were predominantly female and between 75 and 85 years old. Three studies focused exclusively on older persons with depression, whereas the other nine studies included individuals with a range of diagnoses. The intervention models generally used a multidisciplinary team of providers to develop a care management protocol, which was implemented in the patient's home. Treatment recommendations varied significantly across individuals and were implemented through a variety of sources.

Four of the five randomized, controlled trials examined the effectiveness of the implementation of a care management protocol developed by a multidisciplinary team, although providers differed across studies. Rabins and colleagues [31] and Waterreus and colleagues [34] used nurses, Banerjee and colleagues [33] used a care manager, and Llewellyn-Jones and colleagues [32] used physicians and residential staff to implement the intervention. The fifth randomized, controlled trial evaluated the effectiveness of problem-solving therapy provided by social workers under the supervision of a psychiatrist in public senior housing [30]. Relative to usual care, all interventions were associated with a significant improvement in depressive symptoms (Table 2). Of note, Rabins and colleagues [31] also found that outreach services were associated with a decrease in overall symptom severity, as measured by the total Brief Psychiatric Rating Scale score, for individuals with a variety of psychiatric disorders.

A recent quasi-experimental study evaluated a multifaceted education and support program administered in a residential care setting, and compared it with usual care. The target population included older persons who were incapable of living independently because of physical, psychiatric, or psychosocial constraints but did not require extensive nursing home care. The intervention included training for caregivers and other employees of the residential home, informational meetings for residents and their relatives, support groups, and discussion and feedback sessions for care providers. Results indicate that an intervention providing education, support, and feedback to residential care providers can reduce depressive symptoms and maintain health related quality of life for older persons [37].

Findings from the small group of longitudinal cohort studies suggest positive effects of multidisciplinary outreach teams in reducing psychiatric symptoms, relative to baseline levels (Table 3). These studies provided in-home assessment followed by interventions ranging from referral and linkage to outpatient treatment to in-home psychiatric care. However, the specific interventions and outcomes differed, limiting cross-study comparisons or pooling of results. These multidisciplinary geriatric mental health outreach interventions were associated with improved global functioning [38], reduced psychiatric symptoms [40,43], and fewer behavioral disturbances [39], relative to baseline measurements of symptoms and functioning. In addition, these interventions were associated with maintained independence [41,42] and were perceived as helpful to caregivers and referring agents [39]. No difference was found in the degree of being homebound [38].

Discussion

This systematic review of the relatively small but growing literature of randomized, controlled trials, quasi-experimental outcome studies, and cohort studies provides qualified support for the effectiveness of home-based mental health services in improving psychiatric outcomes and, in some cases, for extending the ability of older adults to remain in the community. Any general conclusions drawn from these data are necessarily tempered by the varying quality of the different studies and the methodological limitations of specific studies.

Table 1
Studies that evaluated home- and community-based treatment for older adults in noninstitutional settings who are aged 65 and older and have mental illness

Study	Model	N	Setting	Diagnoses	Age (mean ± SD y)	Female (%)	Demographic characteristics
Randomized controlled trials[a]							
Ciechanowski et al [30] 2004	Problem-solving therapy delivered by social workers under a psychiatrist's supervision; intervention delivered in coordination with primary care providers (examines the Program to Encourage Active, Rewarding Lives for Seniors [PEARLS])	138	Senior public housing	Dysthymia, 49%; minor depression, 51%	73 ± 8.5	79	11% were married or lived with partner; 72% lived alone; 58% were white; 36% were African American
Rabins et al [31] 2000	Multidisciplinary development of care protocol; nurse-based outreach (examines the Psychogeriatric Assessment and Treatment in City Housing [PATCH])	298	Senior public housing	Variable	75.4 ± 8.5	85 (intervention group; 70 control group)	8% were married; 50% were widowed; 93% lived alone

Study	Intervention	N	Setting	Diagnosis	Age		Demographics
Llewellyn-Jones et al [32] 1999	Shared care treatment was delivered primarily by the general practitioner	220	Residential facility	Depression	84.3 ± 5.8	85	10% were married; 71% were widowed; 66% lived in a hostel
Banerjee et al [33] 1996	Psychogeriatric team treatment for elderly who receive home care	66	Home	Depression	80.7 ± 6.8	83	16% were married; 64% were widowed; 78% lived alone
Waterreus et al [34] 1994; Blanchard et al [35] 1995	Nurse-based case management; implementation of a care plan that was created by a hospital-based psychogeriatric team	96	Home	Minor depression, 58%; major depression, 23%; dementia, 6%	76 ± 6.8	85	22% were married; 63% were widowed
Quasi-experimental study[a] Cuijpers et al [37] 2001	Training for caregivers and other employees of residential home; information meeting for residents and relatives; group interventions offered	424	Residential facility	All residents; targeted on depressive symptoms	23.7% were 71–80 y, 57.8% were 81–90 y, and 16.4% were ≥90 y	79	10.6% were married; 74.3% were widowed; 33.5% lived in a residential home for 1–3 y; 37.7% lived in a residential home for ≥3 y

(continued on next page)

Table 1 (*continued*)

Study	Model	N	Setting	Diagnoses	Age (mean ± SD y)	Female (%)	Demographic characteristics
Uncontrolled cohort, pre-post study							
Prospective							
Kohn et al [38] 2002	Multidisciplinary outreach team; treatment plan implemented by a social worker	93	Home: study focused on homebound older adults	Affective disorder, 33%; dementia plus depression, 18%; other dementia, 33%	79.7 ± 7 y	76	19% were married; 56% were widowed; 58% lived alone; 66% were white; 18% were African American; 14% were Hispanic
Seidel et al [39] 1992	Multidisciplinary outreach team; management plan implemented by a case manager	100	Residence: 27% lived in their own home, 40% lived in a nursing home, and 33% lived in a hostel or rest home	Major depression, 14%; Alzheimer's disease, 29%; other dementia, 14%; schizophrenia or delusional disorder, 19%	79.2 ± 7.6	63	31% were married; 49% were widowed

Study	Intervention	Setting	%	Diagnosis	Age	%	Demographics
Wasson et al [40] 1984	Multidisciplinary geropsychiatric outreach team; home evaluation and linkage to medical, mental health, and social services	Home	83	Variable	Mean age 77 y; range, 60–94 y	71	63% were white; 35% were African American; 80% were single
Reifler et al [41] 1982	Multidisciplinary outreach team; home evaluation and treatment	Home	100	Depression, 13%; dementia, 21%; alcohol abuse, 9%; schizophrenia, 4%	Mean age 75 y; 25% were 60–69 y, 36% were 70–79 y, and 28% were 80–89 y	69	82% were white; 5% were black; 18% were married; 40% were widowed
Retrospective Brown et al [42] 1996	Multidisciplinary outreach team; case finding followed by home assessment and community support	Home	95	Affective disorder, 42%; organic mental disorder, 40%; schizophrenia, 12%; another diagnosis, 7%	36% were 65–74 y, and 48% were 75–84 y	71	34% lived with their spouse; 44% lived alone
Buckwalter et al [43] 1991	Multidisciplinary rural elderly outreach program; case finding followed by assessment, referral, treatment, follow-up, and coordination	Home and community	30	Depression, 15%; depression was the most common diagnosis	35% were 65–74 y, and 36% were 75–84 y	71	35% were married; 49% were widowed; 43% lived alone

a The comparison group consisted of persons who received usual care.

Table 2
Outcomes of randomized, controlled trials examining home- and community-based treatment of late-life mental illness

Study	Intervention sample size (n)	Control sample size (n)	Follow-up Duration (mo)	Completion rate (%)	Outcomes and results	Limitations
Randomized controlled trials[a]						
Ciechanowski et al [30] 2004	72	66	12	93 (intervention group); 91 (control group)	Intervention group had more improvement in depressive symptoms (HSC). Possible scores of the checklist range from 0–4, with lower scores indicating better functioning. The intervention group had a mean $\pm$ SD score of 1.3 ± 0.5 before the intervention and a mean score of 0.8 ± 0.6 after the intervention. The control group had a mean score of 1.2 ± 0.5 before the intervention and a mean score of 1 ± 0.5 after the intervention; 43% of the intervention group showed a reduction in depression symptoms of (at least 50%) compared with 15% of the control group; 36% of the intervention group had remission of depressive symptoms compared with 12% of the control group. The intervention group had more improvement in functional and emotional well-being (FACTS). Possible scores of the scale range from 0–4, with lower scores indicating better functioning. Mean functional change scores were .52 (CI, .29–.74) for the intervention group and .09 (CI, –.14–.33) for the control group. Mean emotional change scores were .33 (CI, .14–.52) for the intervention group and .11 (CI, –.09–.31) for the control group. No difference was found between the groups in service use or social and physical well-being.	Intervention group had a greater proportion of dysthymia than control group

Rabins et al [31] 2000	131; 393 for weighted sample size	26	50 (intervention group); 58 (control group)	The intervention group had more improvement in psychiatric symptoms (BPRS). Possible scores of the scale range from 1–140, with lower scores indicating better functioning. The intervention group had a mean score of 29.7 ± 8.4 before the intervention and a mean score of 27.4 ± 7.2 after the intervention. The control group had a mean score of 30.1 ± 11.2 before the intervention and a mean score of 33.9 ± 13.6 after the intervention. The intervention group also had more improvement in depressive symptoms (MADRS). Possible scores of the scale range from 1–60, with lower scores indicating better functioning. The intervention group had a mean score of 13.7 ± 9.5 before the intervention and a mean score of 9.1 ± 6.2 after the intervention. The control group had a mean score of 11.7 ± 5.8 before the intervention and a mean score of 15.2 ± 9.5 after the intervention. No difference was found between the two groups in undesirable moves, including evictions or moves to a nursing home or to a board and care home. (Analyses were based on weighted numbers of psychiatric cases: 62 cases in the intervention group and 69 cases in the control group.)	No single standardized treatment was given. Individuals were randomized into groups after identification of mental illness; 33% dropped out of the study because of death or a move; an additional 13% refused to complete the study.
	167; 488 for weighted sample size				

(continued on next page)

Table 2 (*continued*)

Study	Intervention sample size (n)	Control sample size (n)	Follow-up Duration (mo)	Completion rate (%)	Outcomes and results	Limitations
Llewellyn-Jones et al [32] 1999	109	111	9.5	79 (intervention group); 75 (control group)	The intervention group showed greater improvement in depression symptoms than the control group at follow-up. Depression was measured by the GDS; possible scores range from 1–30, with lower scores indicating better functioning. Before the intervention, 44.2% of the intervention group had scores of 14 or higher, 55.8% had scores ranging from 10–13, and none had scores of 9 or lower. After the intervention, 33.7% of the intervention group had scores of 14 or higher, 32.6% had scores ranging from 10–13, and 33.7% had scores of 9 or lower. Before the intervention, 32.5% of the control group had scores of 14 or higher, 67.5% had scores ranging from 10 to 13, and none had scores of 9 or lower. After the intervention, 44.6% of the control group had scores of 14 or higher, 31.3% had scores ranging from 10–13, and 24.1% had scores of 9 or lower. Factors associated with lower GDS scores included low baseline GDS scores, high baseline basic functioning, low neuroticism, younger age, and intervention participation.	Control and intervention periods were not concurrent. The study was conducted in only 1 large residential facility. At follow-up, 75% of participants completed the GDS, but only 58% completed all measures.
Banerjee et al [33] 1996	33	36	6	88 (intervention group); 89 (control group)	The intervention group tended to recover from depression (58% compared with 25% in the control group). The intervention group also had a greater change in the level of depression, as measured by the mean change in score from baseline to the follow-up on the MADRS. Possible scores range from 1–60, with lower scores indicating better functioning. The intervention group showed a mean 18.3 ± 6.5 point reduction; the control group showed a mean 11.6 ± 6.4 point reduction.	There was a possible nonresponse bias. Results may not generalize to non-home care populations. It was difficult to tell which component of the intervention caused the effect.

Source					Findings	Limitations
Waterreus et al [34][b] 1994; Blanchard et al [35] 1995	47	49	3	92 (intervention group); 80 (control group)	The intervention group showed greater improvement in depression symptoms than the control group (SCARE). Possible scores range from 1–18, with lower scores indicating better functioning. The intervention group had mean scores of 8.5 ± 2.5 before the intervention and mean scores of 5.9 ± 2.6 after the intervention. The control group had mean scores of 8.4 ± 2.3 before the intervention and mean scores of 7.2 ± 3.3 after the intervention. No difference was found between the intervention and control group in the number of persons meeting criteria for probable pervasive depression.	There was a lag time between initial assessment and start of intervention. Analyses did not control for baseline factors.
Blanchard et al [36] 1999[b]	47	49	6–14.5	75 (intervention group); 59 (control group)	In an extension of the previous study [34,35], the control and intervention groups received care management protocols provided by the general physician. Individuals with long-term depression did better in the intervention group than the control group (SCARE). Possible scores range from 1–18, with lower scores indicating better functioning. The intervention group had mean scores of 9.3 ± 2.7 before the intervention and mean scores of 6.3 ± 3.5 after the intervention. The control group had mean scores of 9.1 ± 2.7 before the intervention and mean scores of 9.2 ± 3.4 after the intervention. This finding was the only difference that was found between the control and intervention groups.	The study had a small sample, low power, variable follow-up length, and limited implementation of social and antidepressant treatment. In addition, most analyses showed no difference between the two groups.

Abbreviations: BPRS, Brief Psychiatric Rating Scale; FACTS, Functional Assessment of Cancer Therapy Scale; GDS, Geriatric Depression Scale; HSC, Hopkins Symptoms Checklist; MADRS, Montgomery-Asberg Depression Rating Scale; SCARE, Short Comprehensive Assessment and Referral Evaluation.

[a] Comparison group consisted of persons who received usual care.

[b] Study provides longer-term follow-up of the participants in the study by Waterreus and colleagues [34]. In the study by Blanchard and colleagues [36] the investigators provided general practice physicians with care management protocols for all participants, and the nurse case management intervention was discontinued.

Table 3
Outcomes of quasi-experimental and uncontrolled cohort studies examining home- and community-based treatment of late-life mental illness

Study	Intervention sample size (n)	Control sample size (n)	Follow-up Duration	Completion rate (%)	Outcomes and results	Limitations
Quasi-experimental study[a]						
Cuijpers et al [37] 2001	213	211	1 y	59	The intervention group had greater improvement in depression (GDS). Possible scores range from 1–30, with lower scores indicating better functioning. The intervention group had mean scores of 8.1 ± 5.1 before the intervention and mean scores of 7.6 ± 5.2 after the intervention. The control group had mean scores of 9 ± 5.4 before the intervention and mean scores of 9.3 ± 4.2 after the intervention. The intervention group also had greater improvement in health-related quality of life (20-SFHS). Possible scores range from 1–100, with higher scores indicating better functioning. The intervention group had mean scores of 30.4 ± 38.8 before the intervention and mean scores of 29.5 ± 34.9 after the intervention. The control group had mean scores of 37.9 ± 36 before the intervention and mean scores of 21.9 ± 31.5 after the intervention.	The study was not randomized, there was a high dropout rate, and it was unknown which participants received the group therapy component. Also, the change in the GDS score was not clinically significant.

Uncontrolled cohort, pre-post study

Prospective

Kohn et al [38] 2002	93	NA	Variable	100	Participants had improvement in global functioning (GAFS). Possible scores range from 1–100, with higher scores indicating better functioning. Participants had mean scores of 40.5 ± 18.6 before the intervention and mean scores of 48.2 ± 22.3 after the intervention. Participants received more hours per week of homecare services after the intervention (34.6 h compared with 51.6 h), but they did not differ in their degree of being homebound.	The study did not have a control group and had a limited analysis of potential outcomes. The analyses were confounded by unmeasured variables, and there were potential systematic differences between participants who remained in the program.
Seidel et al [39] 1992	100	NA	3 mo	86	Participants had improvement in behavioral disturbances (as measured on a 1 to 4 scale, with higher scores indicating better functioning). Participants had mean scores of 2 ± 0.8 before the intervention and mean scores of 3 ± 0.9 after the intervention; 87% of referring agents and 80% of caregivers perceived the service as helpful or very helpful.	The study did not have a control group and did not evaluate behavioral disturbances among individuals residing in their own home because behavioral disturbances were not a significant problem for that group. The analyses did not adjust for severity of psychiatric symptoms. Cell sizes were too small to be able to accurately detect changes within diagnostic groups.
Wasson et al [40] 1984	83	NA	3 mo	80	Direct psychiatric services were recommended for 77% of the participants; 51% improved at follow-up (decreased symptoms, increased well-being, and reduced tension between participant and significant other).	The study had selection biases; for example, it excluded hospitalized participants from follow-up. Also, the study did not have independent raters, did not have standardized measures, examined few outcome measures, and did not have a control group.

(continued on next page)

Table 3 (*continued*)

Study	Intervention sample size (n)	Control sample size (n)	Follow-up Duration	Completion rate (%)	Outcomes and results	Limitations
Reifler et al [41] 1982	100	NA	3–4 y	74	Limited data were reported. Most participants maintained independence: 69% of participants owned their own home before the intervention, and 62% owned their own home after the intervention. Only 21% of participants used community services.	The study did not have a control group and did not have statistical evaluation or standardized measures. The study reported outcome data that were obtained by the clinicians who provided the interventions. Investigators attempted to contact 400 persons to identify the 100 persons who were included in the study.
Retrospective						
Brown et al [42] 1996	95	NA	6, 12, and 18 mo	100	At 12 and 18 mo, respectively, 13% and 19% had died, 75% and 65% remained in the community, and 13% and 14% lived in long-term care facilities.	The study did not have a control group. Participants who were included in the caseload were more likely than those who were referred but not admitted to the caseload to have affective disorders or schizophrenia. The study was unable to link outcomes to intervention. Discharge locations were unknown. No functional or psychiatric outcomes were given.

Buckwalter et al [43] 1991	30	NA	4 mo	100	Improved psychiatric symptoms (GDS, SPMSQ, and SPES).	No data or statistics were provided. The study had a small sample size and no control group. The study was potentially biased because no description was given of the selection process for the 30 clients in the study. Also, sensitivity of the measures was questionable.

Abbreviations: 20-SFHS, 20-item Short-Form Health Survey; GAFS, Global Assessment of Functioning Scale; GDS, Geriatric Depression Scale; NA, not applicable; SPES, Short Psychiatric Evaluation Schedule; SPMSQ, Short Portable Mental Status Questionnaire.

[a] Comparison group consisted of persons who received usual care.

The considerable variation across studies in types of interventions, designs, and outcome measures precludes conducting meta-analyses of pooled data, prohibits the calculation of an overall effect size, and complicates interpretation of data. There were few randomized, controlled trials, and only one of the nine nonrandomized trials adjusted for symptom severity [37]. Follow-up periods ranged from 3 months to 4 years. Participant characteristics also differed across studies. Although most studies had high proportions of female participants aged 70 to 80, ethnicity and diagnoses differed. Several studies targeted individuals with depression, whereas others included a range of diagnoses, depression and dementia being the most common. Moreover, variability in participant characteristics may limit generalizability to younger male populations or to individuals with psychotic, anxious, or other symptom constellations.

The interventions themselves varied across studies, including the case identification method, type, and intensity of treatment provided and the composition of the treatment team. Two of the twelve outcome studies used gatekeepers to make patient referrals [31,43], two used traditional referral mechanisms [38,41], and most studies screened participants from home and residential care settings or senior service agencies [30,32,34,35, 37,40,44]. The studies also lacked a common taxonomy for characterizing types of mental health service models and associated outcomes.

The strengths of this review include the use of a broad search strategy and standardized inclusion and evaluation criteria to identify candidate studies. One limitation is that the search strategy was limited to published English language articles. In addition, studies that resulted in negative findings might not have been published, so that this review may overly reflect studies with positive outcomes. Home-based mental health care conducted by video was also excluded. Although geriatric telepsychiatry shows promise for improving access to mental health care in underserved areas, literature on the application of this technology remains limited to a small number of feasibility studies [45].

As a group and despite their limitations, these studies represent a significant step toward surmounting the barriers to providing evidence-based mental health care to frail or homebound community-dwelling older adults. The difficulties in meeting the mental health needs of this population mirror those faced by most geriatric mental health services and include concurrent mental health, cognitive, and medical problems, social losses, disability, cultural and ethnic diversity, variations in family resources and involvement, and competency in decision making. These problems can be particularly challenging in homebound older adults because this group tends to have a greater constellation of these concerns than average community-dwelling elders do. Homebound older adults also often do not have the kinds of clinical and professional support available to residents of nursing homes or other institutions. Moreover the health and social needs of frail and homebound older adults change rapidly over time, necessitating greater coordination of care over time and across providers.

An important methodological consideration in further developing this evidence base is the choice of outcome measures, especially in the context of multiple patient needs. Studies need to ensure that their outcomes and specific measures are relevant to age and culture. A similar consideration is the method used to assess outcomes. In the studies reviewed here, outcome measures varied substantially, and many studies failed to use standardized assessment measures [39–42]. Some of the studies reported only outcome data obtained by the same clinicians who provided the interventions, which might have led to biased outcome measures. Among the fourteen studies, nine used independent outcome raters [30–34,37–39,43], two documented inter-rater reliability [32,39], and seven used an intent-to-treat analysis [30–34,37,42]. Generally, uncontrolled cohort studies failed to qualify their conclusions by discussing the possibility that symptom improvement could represent regression to the mean.

Conducting intervention research in the home environment holds its own set of challenges. Difficult aspects include gaining access to potential research subjects, obtaining support from family members, involving appropriate personal clinicians, monitoring intervention fidelity, and ensuring subject safety while respecting individual autonomy, especially when research and services are provided in a person's home. The complexity and time demands of conducting randomized trials in this setting may help to explain the large number of studies in this review that reported qualitative and observational outcome data (as evidenced by 36 descriptive and four case study reports). Although experimental designs offer more support for the association of a causal relationship, there is an inherent difficulty in executing and evaluating randomized, controlled trials in the field of mental health services. As such, the contribution from lower tiers of evidence should not be ignored, especially in an area with potential for improving access and quality of mental health care.

Finally, despite promising evidence in support of interventions that integrate or coordinate care, a potential weakness of many of these models is their lack of sustainability. Only two of the studies reviewed in this analysis included information on the cost of the intervention [30,43], limiting the capacity of policy makers or providers to assess practical considerations associated with implementing and sustaining these treatment models in routine clinical settings. Particularly problematic are models that integrate home-based care by providers from multiple organizations. One hurdle to integrated models is that, to be most effective and sustainable, the intervention must be embraced at the levels of the organization and the frontline practitioner [46].

In summary, the current evidence provides promising support for home-based mental health services for older adults whose access to traditional practice-based models of care is limited. Observational, uncontrolled studies report that mental health outreach services may be associated with greater access for mentally ill older people. More rigorous studies report that home- and community-based treatment is associated with a reduction in psychiatric symptoms. However, additional studies are needed using rigorous, standardized approaches to measure mental health outcomes and to characterize the intervention. Well-designed, controlled studies may help to identify effective and sustainable approaches to providing evidence-based mental health treatment to frail or homebound older adults.

References

[1] Charney DS, Reynolds CF III, Lewis L, et al. Depression and Bipolar Support Alliance consensus statement on the unmet needs in diagnosis and treatment of mood disorders in late life. Arch Gen Psychiatry 2003;60(7):664–72.

[2] Klap R, Tschantz K, Unutzer J. Caring for mental disorders in the United States: a focus on older adults. Am J Geriatr Psychiatry 2003;11(5):517–24.

[3] Report of the National Advisory Mental Health Council's Clinical Treatment and Services Research Workgroup. Bridging science and service. Bethesda, MD: National Institute of Mental Health; 1998. Available at: http://www.nimh.nih.gov/publicat/nimhbridge.pdf. Accessed October 12, 2005.

[4] Institute of Medicine. Crossing the quality chasm: a new health system for the 21st century. Washington, DC: Institute of Medicine; March 2001.

[5] Bartels SJ. Improving the United States' system of care for older adults with mental illness: findings and recommendations for the President's New Freedom Commission on Mental Health. Am J Geriatr Psychiatry 2003;11(5):486–97.

[6] Administration on Aging. Older adults and mental health: issues and opportunities (2001). Washington, DC: Department of Health and Human Services. Available at: http://www.aoa.gov/press/publications/Older-Adults-and-Mental-Health-2001.pdf. Accessed October 12, 2005.

[7] US Department of Health and Human Services. Mental Health: A Report of the Surgeon General, Executive Summary. Rockville, MD: US Department of Health and Human Services, Substance Abuse and Mental Health Services Administration, Center for Mental Health Services, National Institutes of Health, National Institute of Mental Health, 1999. Available at: http://www.mentalhealth.samhsa.gov/features/surgeongeneralreport/home. asp. Accessed October 12, 2005.

[8] Bruce ML, Seeman TE, Merrill SS, et al. The impact of depressive symptomatology on physical disability: MacArthur Studies of successful aging. Am J Public Health 1994;84:1796–9.

[9] Abrams RC, Lachs M, McAvay G, et al. Predictors of self-neglect in community-dwelling elders. Am J Psychiatry 2002;159(10):1724–30.

[10] Sheline YI. High prevalence of physical illness in a geriatric psychiatric inpatient population. Gen Hosp Psychiatry 1990;12:396–400.

[11] Unützer J, Patrick DL, Simon G, et al. Depressive symptoms and the cost of health services in HMO patients aged 65 years and older. JAMA 1997;277(20):1618–23.

[12] Druss BG, Rohrbaugh RM, Rosenheck RA. Depressive symptoms and health costs in older medical patients. Am J Psychiatry 1999;156:477–9.

[13] Luber MP, Meyers BS, Williams-Russo PG, et al. Depression and service utilization in elderly primary care patients. Am J Geriatr Psychiatry 2001;9(2):169–76.

[14] Sheeran T, Brown EL, Nassisi P, et al. Does depression predict falls among home health patients? using a clinical-research partnership to improve the quality of geriatric care. Home Healthc Nurse 2004;22(6):384–9.

[15] Blazer DG. Depression in late life: review and commentary. J Gerontol A Biol Sci Med Sci 2003;58(3):M249–65.

[16] Unützer J, Simon G, Belin TR, et al. Care for depression in HMO patients aged 65 and older. J Am Geriatr Soc 2000;48(8):871–8.

[17] Bruce ML, Leaf PJ. Psychiatric disorders and 15-month mortality in a community sample of older adults. Am J Public Health 1989;79(6):727–30.

[18] Gallo JJ, Bogner HR, Morales KH, et al. Depression, cardiovascular disease, diabetes, and 2-year mortality among older primary care patients. Am J Geriatr Psychiatry 2005; 13(9):748–55.

[19] Bruce ML, Leaf PJ, Rozal GPM, et al. Psychiatric status and 9-year mortality in the New Haven Epidemiologic Catchment Area study. Am J Psychiatry 1994;151(5):716–21.

[20] Bruce ML, McNamara R. Psychiatric status among the homebound elderly: an epidemiologic perspective. J Am Geriatr Soc 1992;40(6):561–6.

[21] Ganguli M, Fox A, Gilby J, Belle S. Characteristics of rural homebound older adults: a community-based study. J Am Geriatr Soc 1996;44(4):363–70.

[22] Bruce ML, McAvay GJ, Raue PJ, et al. Major depression in elderly home health care patients. Am J Psychiatry 2002;159(8):1367–74.

[23] Sirey J, Bruce ML. Prevalence of depression in home delivered meals clients. Poster presented at the 18th National Institutes of Mental Health Services Conference on Mental Health Research (MHSR). Bethesda, MD, July 18–19, 2005.

[24] Bruce ML, Takeuchi DT, Leaf PJ. Poverty and psychiatric status: longitudinal evidence from the New Haven Epidemiologic Catchment Area Study. Arch Gen Psychiatry 1991; 48:470–4.

[25] Bruce ML, Hoff RA. Social and physical health risk factors for first-onset major depressive disorder in a community sample. Soc Psychiatry Psychiatr Epidemiol 1994;29(4): 165–71.

[26] Rockwood K, Howlett SE, MacKnight C, et al. Prevalence, attributes, and outcomes of fitness and frailty in community-dwelling older adults: report from the Canadian study of health and aging. J Gerontol A Biol Sci Med Sci 2004;59(12):1310–7.

[27] Gillick M. Pinning down frailty. J Gerontol A Biol Sci Med Sci 2001;56(3):M134–5.

[28] Rigler SK, Perera S, Jachna C, et al. Comparison of the association between disease burden and inappropriate medication use across three cohorts of older adults. Am J Geriatr Pharmacother 2004;2(4):239–47.

[29] Van Citters AD, Bartels SJ. A systematic review of the effectiveness of community-based mental health outreach services for older adults. Psychiatr Serv 2004;55(11):1237–49.

[30] Ciechanowski P, Wagner E, Schmaling K, et al. Community-integrated home-based depression treatment in older adults: a randomized controlled trial. JAMA 2004;291(13): 1569–77.

[31] Rabins PV, Black BS, Roca R, et al. Effectiveness of a nurse-based outreach program for identifying and treating psychiatric illness in the elderly. JAMA 2000;283(21): 2802–9.

[32] Llewellyn-Jones RH, Baikie KA, Smithers H, et al. Multifaceted shared care intervention for late life depression in residential care: randomised controlled trial. BMJ 1999;319(7211): 676–82.

[33] Banerjee S, Shamash K, Macdonald AJ, et al. Randomised controlled trial of effect of intervention by psychogeriatric team on depression in frail elderly people at home. BMJ 1996; 313(7064):1058–61.

[34] Waterreus A, Blanchard M, Mann A. Community psychiatric nurses for the elderly: well tolerated, few side-effects and effective in the treatment of depression. J Clin Nurs 1994;3(5): 299–306.

[35] Blanchard MR, Waterreus A, Mann AH. The effect of primary care nurse intervention upon older people screened as depressed. Int J Geriatr Psychiatry 1995;10:289–98.

[36] Blanchard MR, Waterreus A, Mann AH. Can a brief intervention have a longer-term benefit? the case of the research nurse and depressed older people in the community. Int J Geriatr Psychiatry 1999;14(9):733–8.

[37] Cuijpers P, van Lammeren P. Secondary prevention of depressive symptoms in elderly inhabitants of residential homes. Int J Geriatr Psychiatry 2001;16(7):702–8.

[38] Kohn R, Goldsmith E, Sedgwick TW. Treatment of homebound mentally ill elderly patients: the multidisciplinary psychiatric mobile team [special issue: Suicidal behaviors in older adults]. Am J Geriatr Psychiatry 2002;10(4):469–75.

[39] Seidel G, Smith C, Hafner RJ, et al. A psychogeriatric community outreach service: description and evaluation. Int J Geriatr Psychiatry 1992;7(5):347–50.

[40] Wasson W, Ripeckyj A, Lazarus LW, et al. Home evaluation of psychiatrically impaired elderly: process and outcome. Gerontologist 1984;24(3):238–42.

[41] Reifler BV, Kethley A, O'Neill P, et al. Five-year experience of a community outreach program for the elderly. Am J Psychiatry 1982;139(2):220–3.

[42] Brown P, Challis D, von Abendorff R. The work of a community mental health team for the elderly: referrals, caseloads, contact history and outcomes. Int J Geriatr Psychiatry 1996; 11(1):29–39.

[43] Buckwalter KC, Smith M, Zevenbergen P, Russell D. Mental health services of the rural elderly outreach program. Gerontologist 1991;31(3):408–12.

[44] Banerjee S, Shamash K, Macdonald AJ, et al. Randomised controlled trial of effect of intervention by psychogeriatric team on depression in frail elderly people at home. BMJ 1996; 313(7064):1058–61.

[45] Jones BN, Ruskin PE. Telemedicine and geriatric psychiatry: directions for future research and policy. J Geriatr Psychiatry Neurol 2001;14(2):59–62.

[46] Rees G, Huby G, McDade L, et al. Joint working in community mental health teams: implementation of an integrated care pathway. Health Soc Care Community 2004;12(6):527–36.

ELSEVIER
SAUNDERS

Psychiatr Clin N Am
28 (2005) 1061–1077

PSYCHIATRIC
CLINICS
OF NORTH AMERICA

Evidence-Based Models of Integrated Management of Depression in Primary Care

Thomas E. Oxman, MD[a],*, Allen J. Dietrich, MD[a], Herbert C. Schulberg, PhD[b]

[a]*Department of Psychiatry, Dartmouth Medical School, One Medical Center Drive, Lebanon, NH 03756, USA*
[b]*Intervention Research Center for Late-Life Mood Disorders, Department of Psychiatry, Weill Medical College of Cornell University, White Plains, NY, USA*

A variety of epidemiologic studies has demonstrated the high prevalence of depressive disorders in primary care [1–4]. Indeed, by patient preference, the majority of treated depressive episodes are in primary care practices [5,6]. This is particularly true for older persons [7,8]. Accordingly, it is not surprising that primary care clinicians place a high priority on recognizing and treating their depressed patients [9,10]. However, formidable obstacles impede appropriate treatment and the prevention of relapse or recurrence, including time pressures, the inclination of both clinicians and patients to focus on presenting symptoms and acute problems, the limits of reimbursement, and the lack of well-organized mental health systems capable of consulting about and treating patients in most primary care settings [9–13].

In response to these obstacles, first-generation health services research has produced multifaceted interventions. The interventions with collaborative care, in which an on-site mental health specialist and the primary care clinician shared the care of depressed patients, most successfully overcame many of

---

The authors have not received pharmaceutical industry support. Dr. Oxman received support from the Substance Abuse and Mental Health Services Administration (as co-investigator for PRISM-E), the John D. and Catherine T. MacArthur Foundation (as co-investigator for RESPECT-D), and the John A. Hartford Foundation (as consultant for IMPACT). Dr. Dietrich received support from the John D. and Catherine T. MacArthur Foundation (as principal investigator for RESPECT-D and consultant for IMPACT). Dr. Schulberg received support from the John D. and Catherine T. MacArthur Foundation (as co-investigator for RESPECT-D) and the John A. Hartford Foundation (as consultant for IMPACT).

* Corresponding author.
E-mail address: thomas.e.oxman@dartmouth.edu (T.E. Oxman).

these systemic obstacles, enhanced the quality care which they provided, and improved the outcomes of patients with major depression [14–16]. The high cost and intensity of collaborative care necessitated a second generation of randomized controlled trials, which were grounded further in the principles and practices of chronic disease care [17,18]. This chronic care model involves the redesign of practice systems, including physician education, patient education, patient registries, and on-site nonspecialist physician extenders supervised by a mental health specialist. This model resulted in an increased frequency of patient contact, with closer monitoring of outcomes and adherence. Compared with the outcomes achieved by usual care, this chronic care model of depression demonstrated significant clinical improvements [19,20]. Contemporary studies incorporating telephone management by nonspecialist physician extenders also demonstrated the effectiveness of off-site interventions by physician extenders [21,22]. Collectively, these second-generation randomized controlled trials (RCTs) demonstrated that when treatment guidelines are integrated into a practice with a multifaceted and longitudinal treatment approach, the intervention systems are superior to usual care practices in terms of treatment adherence, outcomes, and patient satisfaction [23].

The present authors' previous review of second generation RCTs [24] concluded that despite much progress, important concerns remain unresolved. Prominent among them are the following: (1) the interventions often do not persist or disseminate into community practice when the research is completed, or if they do, the effect may not be as strong; (2) it is unclear how well these interventions apply to older persons, given their increased medical comorbidity; and (3) a "voltage drop" occurs when results from efficacy trials are translated into effectiveness trials, particularly when trials have been conducted in nonacademic settings [25]. These and other concerns have stimulated a third generation of related health services studies. This article reviews these four recent studies (Tables 1 and 2), which summarize the design characteristics of the four system-oriented studies. Of particular interest in the following analysis is the manner in which psychiatrists and other mental health specialists can adapt consultation-liaison skills traditionally exercised in general hospitals to the exigencies of primary care practices that subscribe to chronic illness disease management principles. Because of the recent "black box" warnings about suicidal ideation with newer antidepressants [26,27], an important concern in primary care depression management is to maintain primary care clinician comfort with prescribing antidepressants and monitoring for suicidal ideation. Thus, at present, the potential influence of newer caregiving mechanisms on the management of suicidal ideation and behaviors presented by depressed primary care patients must also be considered.

Primary care research in substance abuse and mental health for the elderly

Primary Care Research in Substance Abuse and Mental Health for the Elderly (PRISM-E) is a multisite trial comparing service use, outcomes,

Table 1
Study design of four multisite studies of depression management in primary care

Feature	PRISM-E	IMPACT	PROSPECT	RESPECT-D
Sponsors	Substance Abuse and Mental Health Services Administration; US Veterans Affairs; Health Resources and Services Administration	John A. Hartford Foundation; California Healthcare Foundation; Hogg Foundation; Robert Wood Johnson Foundation	National Institute of Mental Health	John D. and Catherine T. MacArthur Foundation
Health care organizations	10	8	3	5
Practices	30	18	20	60
Primary care clinicians	153	324	186	180
Psychiatrists	18	7	5	6
Care managers	Not applicable	17	16	9
Patients	2022[a]	1801	598	433[b]
Minimum age	65	60	60	18
Recruitment method	Screening	Screening and PCP referral	Screening	PCP referral
Disorders	Maj dep, min dep, dys, GAD, alcohol	Maj dep, dys	Maj dep, min dep	Maj dep, dys
Comparison group	Referral to mental health specialty care	Usual care	Usual care	Usual care
Randomization unit	Patient	Patient	Practice	Practice
Outcome time points	3, 6 mo	3, 6, 12 mo	4, 8, 12 mo	3, 6 mo

Abbreviations: Alcohol, at-risk drinking; dys, dysthymic disorder; GAD, generalized anxiety disorder; maj dep, major depression; min dep, minor depression; PCP, primary care provider.
[a] 1,390 (69% had a depression diagnosis, without at-risk alcohol drinking).
[b] 987 patients were referred and offered treatment, but all did not meet eligibility criteria for the independent evaluation in the RCT.

and costs in integrated versus enhanced referral models of mental health care for older persons with depression, anxiety, or at-risk alcohol consumption. Integrated treatment models have the following features: mental health services are colocated in the primary care setting, with no distinction in terms of signage or clinic names; mental health services are provided by licensed mental health providers from several disciplines (with back-up from a geriatric psychiatrist); verbal or written communication about the clinical evaluation and treatment plan transpires between the mental health and primary care clinicians; and the patient meets with the mental health care

Table 2

Depression management intervention in four multisite studies of depression management in primary care

System change	PRISM-E	IMPACT	PROSPECT	RESPECT-D
	Integrated mental health services	Care smanager	Care manager	Care manager
Treatment algorithm	No	Yes	Yes	No
Care management location	N/A	On site	On site	Off site
Patient education and self-management	Variable	Yes	Yes	Yes
Case management	Yes	Yes	Yes	Yes
Care management to patient contact	N/A	Face to face; telephone	Face to face	Telephone
Psychiatric supervision	N/A	Face to face; telephone	Face to face	Telephone
Care management counseling	N/A	PST-PC	IPT	Supportive
Psychologic supervision	N/A	Telephone	Face to face	N/A
Mental health specialty treatment location	On site	On site	On site	Off site
Geriatrician supervision	No	Yes	No	No
Depression measure for care management	N/A	PHQ-9	HAM-D	PHQ-9
Outcome measure	CES-D change; no depression diagnosis on MINI	HSCL response = 50% drop; remission = score ≤0.5	HAM-D response = 50% drop; remission = score ≤10 or ≤7	HSCL response = 50% drop; remission = score ≤0.5

Abbreviations: CES-D, Center for Epidemiologic Studies Depression Scale; HAM-D, Hamilton Rating Scale for Depression; HSCL, Hopkins Symptom Checklist; MINI, Mini-International Neuropsychiatric Interview; N/A, not applicable.

provider within 2 to 4 weeks after the primary care clinician visit. It is believed that colocating behavioral health care within primary care reduces the stigma associated with traditional mental health systems. Additionally, transportation problems are minimized because visits for physical and behavioral health can be combined. Finally, the colocation of the generalist and specialist can facilitate communication among providers and permit more comprehensive treatment planning.

Enhanced referral models include the following elements: patients are referred to specialty mental health care within 2 to 4 weeks of the primary care clinician appointment; mental health evaluation and treatment occur in a physically separate location by licensed mental health professionals from several disciplinary backgrounds; and specialized mental health clinics coordinate follow-up contacts if the patient fails to attend the first scheduled visit, assure transportation, and facilitate direct or third-party coverage for the costs of the specialty mental health visit. A key advantage of the specialty referral system is its ability to provide a fuller range of services as dictated by patient needs, (eg, individual and group psychotherapeutic options, which are typically unavailable in the primary care setting). Mental health clinics may also be better able than primary care sites to offer the confidentiality sought by patients receiving behavioral health services.

Previous studies of integrated or collaborative care have compared outcomes with usual care, which consists of informing the primary care clinician of the patient's condition and having the clinician treat or refer the patient as appropriate. PRISM-E, however, uniquely uses an enhanced referral process as the comparison arm. Although access to treatment was enhanced under the comparison referral model, it nevertheless resembled a geriatric mental health specialist's usual practice.

With respect to initial engagement in treatment as an outcome measure, the integrated model has been found superior to the enhanced referral model [28]. Seventy-five percent of subjects with depression had at least one mental health visit in the integrated model compared with only 52% in the enhanced referral model (OR 2.86; 95% CI, 2.26%, 3.61%). Although patients in enhanced referral were more likely to be treated by a psychiatrist, there were no significant differences in remission rates in the integrated versus referral model for major depression (28.2% versus 32.7%) or other depression (57.9% versus 54.3%) [29]. These findings endorse integrated services as the preferred mode of psychiatric care entry by older primary care patients with relatively equivalent outcomes to specialty care.

Improving mood: promoting access to collaborative treatment

Improving Mood: Promoting Access to Collaborative Treatment (IMPACT) is a multisite primary care trial of collaborative [14] and stepped care [16] for late-life depression that integrates brief psychotherapy and medication management [30]. IMPACT draws on earlier studies that focused on adults of all ages and that suggested that the barriers to effective treatment of depression might be more problematic for older adults because of stigma, ageism, and the clinical complexities associated with more frequent medical comorbidity. Thus, IMPACT focuses only on late-life depression and incorporates some design features specific to the elderly.

At each of 18 participating primary care clinics, older adults who met structured diagnostic criteria for major depression or dysthymic disorder were randomly assigned to a collaborative stepped-care program or to care as usual. In the intervention program, a depression care manager (a psychologist or a registered nurse with training in brief psychotherapy) based in the primary care clinic worked with patients and their primary care physicians for up to 12 months. These patients received a 20-minute educational videotape and a booklet about late-life depression and were encouraged to have an initial visit with the care manager at the primary care clinic. New cases and those needing treatment plan adjustments were discussed with a supervising team psychiatrist (often a geriatric specialist) and a liaison primary care physician (usually a geriatrician) during a weekly team meeting. The care manager then worked with the patient and the patient's regular primary care clinician to establish a treatment plan according to a stepped-care treatment algorithm. However, the patient and the primary care clinician made the actual treatment choices. The IMPACT treatment algorithm suggests an initial choice of an antidepressant medication (usually a selective serotonin reuptake inhibitor) or a course of Problem-Solving Treatment for Primary Care (PST-PC) [31,32], consisting of 6 to 8 brief sessions of structured psychotherapy for depression, delivered by the care manager at the primary care clinic. Care managers received separate ongoing supervision in PST-PC from academic psychologists who were experts in PST-PC. Care managers also referred patients for additional health or social services, as indicated clinically. Depression outcome was monitored with the Patient Health Questionnaire (PHQ-9) depression scale [33] and an Internet web-based clinical information system [34]. During the acute treatment phase, in-person or telephone follow-up contacts were scheduled at least biweekly.

The IMPACT intervention thus includes key components of evidence-based models for chronic illness care [18,35]: collaboration among primary care providers, patients, and specialists; a personalized treatment plan that includes patient preferences; proactive follow-up and outcome monitoring by the care manager; and a protocol for stepped care that includes the targeted use of psychiatric consultation. In contrast to this planned range of services, usual care patients may receive any primary care or specialty mental health care available to the practice.

The 12-month outcomes have shown consistent and significant differences in favor of the intervention [36]. Forty-five percent of intervention patients achieved a reduction of 50% or greater in baseline depressive symptoms, and 25% had complete remission, compared with 19% and 8%, respectively, of usual care participants. Intervention subjects also experienced higher rates of depression treatment and satisfaction with depression care, lower depression severity, less functional impairment, and greater quality of life than did participants who were assigned to usual care. The fact that all practices in the seven participating organizations obtained these results suggests that collaborative stepped-care management is more effective than usual care for resolving depression in a wide range of older people and diverse types of medical care organizations.

Prevention of suicide in primary care elderly: collaborative trial

The Prevention of Suicide in Primary Care Elderly: Collaborative Trial (PROSPECT) is a multisite collaborative study funded by the National Institute of Mental Health in 1998 and conducted by the Late-Life Mood Disorder Intervention Research Centers at the University of Pittsburgh, the University of Pennsylvania, and Cornell University. PROSPECT was designed to assess whether depression treatment in primary care settings can reduce the risk of suicide in elderly patients. The research design of PROSPECT randomized primary care practices either to an intervention arm or to usual care. In practices randomized to the former, a depression care manager (a nurse, psychologist, or social worker supervised by a geriatric psychiatrist and a psychologist) facilitated adherence to a depression treatment algorithm. The algorithm considered antidepressant medication to be the first-line treatment, and it was provided at no cost to intervention participants. In keeping with the algorithm, the care manager obtained information about the patient's clinical status before the office visit and provided it to the physician. This "on-time, on-target" information was designed to influence guideline adherence by physicians and patients. The physician, who was familiarized previously with Agency for Health Care Policy and Research guidelines, made treatment decisions informed by recommendations from the care manager and in keeping with clinical judgment about the patient's clinical needs. The care manager regularly monitored the patient's clinical status and provided relevant education about depression to patients, families, and physicians. The care managers were trained in interpersonal psychotherapy (IPT) and treated patients who preferred counseling to medications or who did not respond to medications alone. Care managers at each site participated in weekly face-to-face supervision with an academic geriatric psychiatrist and received ongoing supervision in IPT from academic psychologist experts in IPT.

In a comparison of clinical outcomes for patients who were provided with care management versus those who received care as usual, results indicate that the care management group achieved a greater and speedier course of depressive symptom reduction [37]. The pattern was not as robust as in IMPACT for depression response (50% reduction in baseline symptoms as measured by the HAM-D) and depression remission (HAM-D ≤ 7). For all depressed patients (major and minor depression), the intervention patients were more likely than usual care patients to have a response at 4, 8, and 12 months. Remission, however, was significantly more likely only at 4 and 8 months for all depressed patients (32.4% versus 24.8% and 41.1% versus 31.8%) or for just major depression (26.6% versus 15.2% and 36.0% versus 22.5%). A separate substudy comparing clinical outcomes with similar treatment in the specialty mental health sector at one site found that patients in the specialty setting had more severe depression but received more intensive treatment [38].

Re-engineering systems for primary care treatment of depression

In 1995, the John D. and Catherine T. MacArthur Foundation charged leading clinicians and researchers in primary care and mental health to make a national difference in the primary care management of depression. Findings from initial projects [10,39–41] and related first- and second-generation clinical trials spawned a three-component clinical model for primary care depression management and a practice change model to support local adoption of the clinical model [42]. Key elements of the clinical model are: (1) centrally based (rather than on-site) care management providing telephone support for patients and feedback to primary care clinicians; (2) more structured primary care management, including the use of a brief depression severity measure (the PHQ-9); (3) weekly telephone-based psychiatric supervision of care managers; and (4) e-mail or telephone contact by the supervising psychiatrist with primary care clinicians as indicated. The practice change model relies on quality improvement programs existing within each health care organization.

The Re-engineering Systems for Primary Care Treatment of Depression (RESPECT-Depression) project worked with diverse health care organizations to apply its elements in three phases. The first phase pilot tested and refined the models in representative community practices selected by each participating health care organization (HCO). The second phase evaluated the model in a randomized controlled trial conducted in additional practices, seeking to improve depression care. The third phase assessed dissemination of the model to usual care and other additional practices. Because the intervention was applied practice-wide, as with PROSPECT, the practice was the unit of randomization. The local organizational team and research team worked together to build the HCO's capacity to support the clinical and practice change models. The HCO quality improvement program was the locus of practice support in implementing and sustaining the depression care clinical model. The research team led capacity-building efforts with phase-one pilot practices and initially did so in phase two, as well. Each HCO quality improvement program became the central and sustaining source of practice support for most of phase two and for phase three. Throughout this process, primary care practices and clinicians were updated with newsletters, reunion meetings, and academic detailing.

Phase one findings of system uptake and programmatic modifications demonstrated strong clinician participation and excellent short-term clinical response rates [43,44]. Similar to IMPACT and PROSPECT, the RCT results of phase two of RESPECT-Depression demonstrated that intervention patients with major depression or dysthymia achieved significantly greater response rates at 3 (53.0%% versus 34.2%) and 6 months (59.9% versus 46.6%) as well as remission rates at 3 (26.2% versus 16.5%) and 6 months (37.3% versus 26.7%) [45]. The primary research objective of RESPECT-D phase 3 is presently being analyzed to determine how many phase-two practices maintain systemic changes and whether the changes spread to additional practices beyond those participating in the RCT.

Care management and the role of the mental health specialist

The preceding overview of state-of-the-art efforts to systematically modify the management of depression in primary care practice highlights the diverse factors affecting the success of these efforts. The three trials comparing system change with usual care included different depression diagnoses and used different outcome time points and different depression measures. Nevertheless, the results were all positive, with effect sizes in the small to medium range. Given the small number of studies and the differing design features, a summary effect size is not useful. However, taken together, all four of these large, multisite RCTs provide an evidence base that strongly supports the clinical value of systematic changes in primary care to manage depression.

From the perspective of a mental health specialist seeking to optimize the management of depression medical settings, two factors warrant particular attention as the shift continues from efficacy and effectiveness research to wide spread clinical implementation. These factors are care management and the mental health specialist's relationship to this process.

Care management is an intrinsic element of the chronic care model and is used commonly by primary care practices, with patients who experience high rates of chronic illnesses such as asthma, diabetes, and congestive heart failure. Only recently has the relapsing and recurring clinical course of depression raised consciousness to the need to manage this disorder in a manner akin to that used with other chronic illnesses. More specifically, it must now be acknowledged that even when they desire to do so, primary care physicians may be constrained from performing all of the clinical tasks pertinent to managing a depressive episode. The constraint of insufficient time for needed appointments is particularly critical during the acute phase of depression. The problem of managing depression in primary care practice is complicated further by the fact that depressed patients are at high risk for not adhering to the treatments that primary care physicians prescribe for them.

Given these difficulties, increased attention is being devoted to findings that demonstrate that care management can ensure a treatment plan is being followed, symptoms and side effects are being monitored to determine the need for a modified treatment plan, and patients are being educated about their disease and its treatment, including self-management techniques [46,47]. For depression, these studies reveal a spectrum of care management, varying in intensity and cost. The spectrum ranges from a fixed and limited number of highly structured contacts [21,22] to Master's degree level specialists who provide case management and even acute phase versions of time-limited psychotherapy [30,48]. Table 2 shows the variability in the management of care of chronic depression in the reviewed third-generation studies.

Care management may be delivered through a central telephone resource serving multiple practices or directly within the practice, using internal or shared personnel. Care management that is limited to a basic level of telephone contact requires less mental health training and can be applied to chronic diseases other than depression. However, it may not achieve the same degree of improvement in clinical outcomes as face-to-face care management with psychotherapy. Conversely, internal and face-to-face care management, even if more effective, is more costly. Relieving internal personnel of their previous responsibilities often proves difficult. Without changes in reimbursement policy, externally funded on-site personnel are more likely to be terminated when a research or demonstration program is completed.

Despite these realities, care management is emerging as a meaningful primary care intervention for depression, given the relative shortage of doctoral level mental health specialists trained to work in medical settings, the higher costs of such personnel, and the absence of a clinical need for every depressed patient to see a mental health specialist. Goldberg and Gournay [49] recommended, therefore, that "link workers" serve as intermediaries between mental health providers and primary care clinicians. The care manager, indeed, performed the linkage function effectively in these third-generation health services primary care depression studies.

The present authors suggest that to provide this link with confidence and safety, care managers require regular and systematic supervision by a mental health specialist. Depending on the complexity of the case mix assigned to the care manager and his or her experience with depression, 10 to 30 cases can be reviewed in an hour of psychiatric supervision. This rate compares quite favorably with the one to four cases possibly seen by a psychiatrist in an hour when providing individual therapy or medication management. The third-generation studies indicate that a significant number of depressed primary care patients experience complex psychosocial problems and can benefit from consultation or co-treatment with a mental health specialist. Although better and speedier outcomes may be achieved with specialty sector treatment, the PRISM-E study demonstrates that particularly older patients are the most reluctant to seek help in the specialty sector. It is significant, therefore, that the IMPACT and PROSPECT studies have found that care managers, under specialist supervision, can provide much of the care recommended by contemporary guidelines for managing depression. When a specialist consultation is needed, it can be completed successfully in the primary care clinic. The combination of the care manager and the supervising mental health specialist, therefore, constitutes a potent enabling force. The resources and back-up they provide permits the primary care clinician to fulfill depression screening recommendations more comfortably [50], formulate depressive diagnoses more aggressively, and manage depressive episodes more effectively.

Assessing and managing suicidality

Considering the care manager's role in assessing and treating depression in the primary care sector, can this person also serve as a resource in managing the suicidal ideation and behaviors presented by a subgroup of depressed ambulatory care patients? The significance of this question is highlighted by a growing awareness that the primary care sector potentially can play a crucial role in resolving the public health crisis of suicide [51,52]. Because approximately 45% of persons who killed themselves had contacted their physicians in the month preceding the life-ending act [53], these health care providers and their staff are possibly well positioned to identify, treat, or refer persons at high risk for self-harm. Given this perspective, do the four RCTs described previously provide data regarding the prevalence of suicidal ideation and its course in primary care facilities to gauge the levels of suicide-related efforts that will be required from primary care physicians and depression care managers?

The proportion of patients who are assigned the diagnosis of major depression or dysthymia and who experience suicidal ideation is not comparable directly across the four RCTs, given their differing criteria for defining thoughts of death and self-harm and procedures for assessing such ideation. The PROSPECT investigators [37] determined that 25% of older patients recruited to their treatment trial scored more than zero on the Scale For Suicidal Ideation. The varying risk levels associated with elevated scores, however, were not specified. The RESPECT [34,45,54] researchers did classify such risk levels in a range from none to mild-moderate to severe and even to critical and those patients who required immediate intervention. With regard to the prevalence of clinically significant suicidal ideation at the higher ends of this severity continuum, the three RCTs derived rates of 10%, 11%, and 14%, respectively.

These closely similar prevalence rates across both mid- and late-life populations indicate that primary care practices should be concerned about the small but highly distressed subgroup of depressed individuals whose suicidal psychopathology requires urgent or emergent psychiatric care. The significance of focusing on this subgroup is highlighted by Bartels and colleagues' [54] finding that older patients who experience suicidal ideation tend to withdraw rather than increase contacts with their physicians and other potential sources of support. At any single point in time, primary care physicians and their collaborating depression care managers typically will be responsible for no more than one or two depressed patients at serious risk for self-harm. Given this distribution, the identification and management of high-risk suicidality is likely feasible in primary care practices that choose to assume this clinical responsibility. The potential value to a practice in doing so is emphasized by the finding of the 2001–2003 National Comorbidity Survey Replication [55] that the most serious cases of suicidality ironically experienced smaller treatment increases during the 1990s than did less serious cases of such psychopathology.

In addition to clarifying the prevalence of suicidal ideation in primary care practices, do the RCTs reviewed previously explicate the clinical course of such ideation in ambulatory medical settings that use depression care managers? The nature of depression care management with suicidal patients remains to be detailed and cause-effect imputations are premature. It is of interest, nevertheless, that the PROSPECT and IMPACT treatment trials with older primary care patients both found suicidal ideation reduced significantly more frequently in practices offering depression care management than in practices offering the physician's usual care. The PROSPECT investigators [37] found this favorable outcome to pertain at 4 and 8 months post-baseline, whereas the IMPACT investigators [34] found it to persist even during the 12-month follow-up period after the 12-month intervention. The RESPECT study design did not permit the comparison of suicidal ideation's course in the face of depression care management versus usual care. However, 76% of the study's mid-life patients who were classified initially at the intermediate level of suicide risk had low or no suicidal ideation 3 months later. Continued improvement on this measure was evident at 6 months as well [56].

The epidemiologic and evidence-based clinical data generated by the four RCTs conducted within primary care practices lead to two important findings. First, the prevalence of suicidal ideation among depressed mid- and late-life patients at the urgent and emergent severity levels is at a sufficiently low rate as to make its management feasible within practices willing to undertake this clinical responsibility. Second, suicidal ideation at these severity levels responds to treatment, and the depression care manager's contribution, supported by a psychiatrist, results in greater reduction of suicidal ideation than in usual care. This additional evidence supports the clinical and policy value of disseminating such models, especially in light of the latest "black box" warnings on suicidal ideation and newer antidepressants.

Discussion

The sizeable number of primary care practices, clinicians, and patients that have participated in three generations of health services research on the management of depression is impressive. The most recent generation of this research focuses extensively on the elderly, and its findings deserve the attention of geriatric mental health specialists. The study results published to date suggest that these system changes produce better outcomes than usual care for depression in a wide range of patients and health care organizations. The findings, thus, have important implications for clinical practice and challenges for health services policy.

Although three of the studies described in this report focused on older people, the totality of findings from this line of health services research suggests that usual care for major depression or dysthymia in primary care is no longer acceptable for any age group. Although more intensive and expensive treatment in the mental health specialty setting would conceivably produce superior clinical outcomes, most older and primary care patients are more likely to accept depression treatment when it is integrated within primary care. The consistency of this finding suggests that primary care providers and practice administrators need to examine how best to improve depression management. Depending on the size and resources of a practice, at least some components of the chronic disease model, such as care management, could be implemented. For mental health specialists, these studies emphasize the importance of seeking out and being integrated into primary care consultative and supervisory roles so that they can indirectly but effectively serve a larger number of patients. The present authors would also emphasize that for any system change to be successful, it is vital to have substantial administrative support, strong physician leadership advocating the change, and credible data available for feedback [57,58]. Mental health specialists, thus, should prominently ally themselves with administrators and physician leaders in health care organizations delivering primary care.

Although the preliminary findings of these third-generation clinical trials are encouraging, they contain potentially disturbing trends as well. The relatively low remission rates, even with relatively intensive and closely supervised interventions, are disconcerting. It may be tempting to recommend a national policy, which shifts more depression care to the specialty sector, but there will continue to be an insufficient number of geriatric mental health specialists to meet all clinical needs. Accordingly, it is incumbent on geriatric specialists to lobby government and organizational policy makers to offer fair and reasonable reimbursement for care management services and for the telephone or in-person consultation that mental health professionals provide to care managers and primary care physicians.

From a health services perspective, it is remarkable how far the field of primary care depression treatment has come. Nevertheless, service delivery and knowledge gaps remain to be filled, and advocacy for fiscal and administrative policy changes should be of the highest priority. With respect to future health services research that addresses knowledge gaps, it is of paramount importance that investigators help health care organizations test and find the costs of the various components of the chronic care model as it pertains to depression. Research that replicates findings about the better patient outcomes achieved by altered structures of care is no longer a significant need. Investigators, instead, should now help health care organizations and health plans to identify the chronic disease system components and intensity levels at which they can proceed practically and fiscally with needed change. In this context, structuring the collaborative relationship of depression care managers and mental health specialists is a continuing challenge, as is the mental health specialist's optimal manner of collaborating with primary care physicians. For example, some practices may use their own employees as care managers and require psychiatric consultation or clinical back up on only certain aspects of their caseload once the care managers are experienced.

With overall remission effect sizes proving to be small to medium in magnitude, cost effectiveness may become a barrier to successful dissemination. Accordingly, at least four approaches, used alone or in combination, are recommended in the next generation of studies. The first approach would be to emphasize stepped care, reserving the more expensive service (care management with weekly mental health supervision) for more complex, severe, or resistant cases of depression [16]. Initially a full model might be applied to all depressed patients while the practice becomes comfortable with a structured, disciplined care process. When the practice is "prepared" after a certain number of treated cases, the primary care clinician could more selectively use the costlier full model when patients are identified as nonadherent or treatment resistant. More adherent patients could be taught to pro-actively and systematically self-report progress and side effects. A second approach is to include care management as part of the quality improvement division of larger group practices, in order not to count against the small margin of the individual primary care practice. By maintaining or improving quality indicators such as those of Health Plan Employer Data and Information Set, this budget justification would be reasonable. The third approach would be to combine different chronic diseases. The same care manger can be involved in the process of care for different chronic diseases but supervised by different specialists. This approach could focus alternatively on persons having two separate but interacting chronic diseases, such as diabetes and depression. A fourth approach is to form a partnership with health plans and employers to broaden the scope and thus improve cost effectiveness by documenting the effects of these interventions on work absenteeism and productivity [59–61].

In conclusion, the majority of primary care clinicians accept the responsibility for treating depression across the life span [9,10]. Mental health specialists must respect and foster this responsibility. Primary care clinicians are ready to entertain more organized monitoring, follow-up, and collaboration with mental health specialists, as long as the issues of care complexity, role clarification, and costs can be resolved. Disseminating the concepts and tools of systems of depression management to primary care practices while simultaneously addressing policy implications at the level of payers and regulators holds considerable promise for translating this evidence-based research into improved care for the large numbers of depressed patients in primary care.

References

[1] Barrett J, Barrett J, Oxman T, et al. The prevalence of psychiatric disorders in a primary care practice. Arch Gen Psychiatry 1988;45:1109–15.

[2] Coyne J, Fechner-Bates S, Schwenk T. Prevalence, nature, and comorbidity of depressive disorders in primary care. Gen Hosp Psychiatry 1994;16:267.

[3] Hoeper E, Nycz G, Cleary P, et al. Estimated prevalence of RDC mental disorder in primary medical care. Int J Ment Health 1979;8:6.

[4] Schulberg H, Saul M, McClelland M, et al. Assessing depression in primary medical and psychiatric practices. Arch Gen Psychiatry 1985;42:1164.

[5] Fortney J, Rost K, Zhang M. A joint choice model of the decision to seek depression treatment and choice of provider sector. Med Care 1998;36:307.

[6] Shepherd M. Primary care psychiatry: the case for action. Br J Gen Pract 1991;41:252.

[7] Mickus M, Colenda CC, Hogan AJ. Knowledge of mental health benefits and preferences for type of mental health providers among the general public. Psychiatr Serv 2000;51:199.

[8] Shapiro S, Skinner E, Kessler L, et al. Utilization of health and mental health services. Arch Gen Psychiatry 1984;41:971.

[9] Solberg L, Korsen N, Oxman T, et al. Depression care: a problem in need of a system. J Fam Pract 1999;48:973.

[10] Williams J, Rost K, Dietrich A, et al. Primary care physicians' approach to depressive disorders: effects of physician specialty and practice structure. Arch Fam Med 1999;8:58.

[11] Institute of Medicine. Crossing the quality chasm: a new health system for the 21st century. Washington (DC): National Academy Press; 2001.

[12] Klinkman MS, Schwenk TL, Coyne JC. Depression in primary care–more like asthma than appendicitis: the Michigan Depression Project. Can J Psychiatry 1997;42:966.

[13] Nutting P, Rost K, Dickinson M, et al. Barriers to initiating treatment for depression in primary care practice. J Gen Intern Med 2002;17:103.

[14] Katon W, Robinson P, Von Korff M, et al. A multifaceted intervention to improve treatment of depression in primary care. Arch Gen Psychiatry 1996;53:924.

[15] Katon W, Von Korff M, Lin E, et al. Collaborative management to achieve treatment guidelines: impact on depression in primary care. JAMA 1995;273:1026.

[16] Katon W, Von Korff M, Lin E, et al. Stepped collaborative care for primary care patients with persistent symptoms of depression. Arch Gen Psychiatry 1999;56:1109.

[17] Von Korff M, Goldberg D. Improving outcomes in depression: the whole process of care needs to be enhanced. BMJ 2001;323:948.

[18] Wagner E, Austin B, Vonkorff M. Organizing care for patients with chronic illness. Millbank Quarterly 1996;74:511–44.

[19] Rost K, Nutting P, Smith J, et al. Improving depression outcomes in community primary care practice: a randomized trial of the QuEST Intervention. J Gen Intern Med 2001;16:143.

[20] Wells KB, Sherbourne C, Schoenbaum M, et al. Impact of disseminating quality improvement programs for depression in managed primary care: a randomized controlled trial. JAMA 2000;283:212.

[21] Hunkeler EM, Meresman JF, Hargreaves WA, et al. Efficacy of nurse telehealth care and peer support in augmenting treatment of depression in primary care. Arch Fam Med 2000;9:700.

[22] Simon GE, Von Korff M, Rutter C, et al. Randomised trial of monitoring, feedback, and management of care by telephone to improve treatment of depression in primary care. BMJ 2000;320:550.

[23] Badamgarav E, Weingarten S, Henning J, et al. Effectiveness of disease management programs in depression: a systematic review. Am J Psychiatry 2003;160:2080.

[24] Oxman T, Dietrich A, Schulberg H. The depression care manager and mental health specialist as collaborators within primary care. Am J Geriatr Psychiatry 2003;11:507–16.

[25] Eisenberg JM, Power EJ. Transforming insurance coverage into quality health care: voltage drops from potential to delivered quality. JAMA 2000;284:2100.

[26] Fergusson D, Doucette S, Glass KC, et al. Association between suicide attempts and selective serotonin reuptake inhibitors: systematic review of randomised controlled trials. BMJ 2005;330:396.

[27] Gunnell D, Saperia J, Asby D. Selective serotonin reuptake inhibitors (SSRIs) and suicide in adults: meta-analysis of drug company data from placebo controlled, randomised controlled trials submitted to the MHRA's safety review. BMJ 2005;330:385.

[28] Bartels SJ, Miles KM, Van Citters AR, et al. Improving mental health assessment and service planning practices for older adults: a controlled comparison study. Ment Health Serv Res, in press.

[29] Krahn D. Depression and at-risk alcohol use outcomes for older primary care patients in integrated care and enhanced specialty referral. Presented at the Academy of Health Annual Research Meeting, Boston, MA, June 26–28, 2005.

[30] Unützer J, Katon W, Williams JW Jr, et al. Improving primary care for depression in late life: the design of a multicenter randomized trial. Med Care 2001;39:785.

[31] Hegel M, Barrett J, Oxman T. Training therapists in problem-solving treatment of depressive disorders in primary care: lessons learned from the Treatment Effectiveness Project. Fam Syst Health 2000;18:423.

[32] Hegel M, Barrett J, Oxman T, et al. Problem-solving treatment for primary care (PST-PC): a treatment manual for depression. Lebanon (NH): Whitman Press; 1999.

[33] Spitzer R, Kroenke K, Williams J. Validation and utility of a self-report version of PRIME-MD: the PHQ Primary Care Study. JAMA 1999;282:1737.

[34] Unützer J. Reducing suicide risk by treating late-life depression in primary care: outcomes from the IMPACT trial. Paper presented at the Annual Meeting of the American Association for Geriatric Psyciatry. San Diego, CA, March 3–5, 2005.

[35] Wagner EH. The role of patient care teams in chronic illness management. BMJ 2000; 320:569.

[36] Unützer J, Katon W, Callahan CM, et al. Collaborative care management of late-life depression in the primary care setting: a randomized controlled trial. JAMA 2002;288:2836.

[37] Bruce ML, Ten Have TR, Reynolds C, et al. Reducing suicidal ideation and depression symptoms in depressed older primary care patients. JAMA 2004;291:1081.

[38] Thomas L, Mulsant BH, Solano FX, et al. Response speed and rate of remission in primary and specialty care of elderly patients with depression. Am J Geriatr Psychiatry 2002;10:583.

[39] Cole S, Raju M, Gerrity M, et al. MacArthur Foundation depression education for primary care physicians: background, participant's workbook, and facilitator's guide. Gen Hosp Psychiatry 2000;22:299.

[40] Brody D, Dietrich A, deGruy F. The Depression in Primary Care Tool Kit. Int J Psychiatry Med 2000;30:99.

[41] Williams J, Barrett J, Oxman T, et al. Treatment of dysthymia and minor depression in primary care: a randomized controlled trial in older adults. JAMA 2000;284:1519.

[42] Oxman TE, Dietrich AJ, Williams JW, et al. A three component model for re-engineering systems for primary care treatment of depression. Psychosomatics 2002;43:441.

[43] Dietrich AJ, Oxman TE, Burns MR, et al. Application of a depression management office system in community practice: a demonstration. J Am Board Fam Pract 2003;16:107.

[44] Korsen N, Scott P, Dietrich AJ, et al. Implementing an office system to improve primary care management of depression. Psychiatr Q 2003;74:45.

[45] Dietrich AJ, Oxman T, Williams JW, et al. Re-engineering systems for the primary care treatment of depression: a cluster randomized controlled trial. BMJ 2004;329:602.

[46] Haynes R, McKibbon K, Kanani R. Systematic review of randomised trials of interventions to assist patients to follow prescriptions for medications. Lancet 1996;348:383.

[47] Riegel B, Carlson B, Kopp Z, et al. Effect of standardized nurse case-management telephone interventions on resource use in patients with chronic heart failure. Arch Intern Med 2002;161:707–12.

[48] Schulberg HC, Bryce C, Chisk K, et al. Managing late-life depression in primary care practice: a case study of the health specialist's role. Int J Geriatr Psychiatry 2001;16:577.

[49] Goldberg D, Gournay K. The general practitioner, the psychiatrist, and the burden of mental health care. In: Maudsley Discussion. London: Institute of Psychiatry, 1988.

[50] US Preventive Services Task Force. Screening for depression: recommendations and rationale. Ann Intern Med 2002;136:760–4.

[51] Goldsmith S, Pellman T, Bunney W, editors. Reducing suicide: a national imperative. Washington (DC): National Academies Press; 2002.

[52] Schulberg H, Bruce M, Lee P, et al. Preventing suicide in primary care patients: the primary care physician's role. Gen Hosp Psychiatry 2004;26:337.

[53] Luoma J, Martin C, Pearson J. Contact with mental health and primary care providers before suicide: a review of the evidence. Am J Psychiatry 2002;159:909.

[54] Bartels SJ, Coakley E, Oxman TE, et al. Suicidal and death ideation in older primary care patients with depression, anxiety, and at-risk alcohol use. Am J Geriatr Psychiatry 2002; 10:417.

[55] Kessler R, Berglund P, Borges G, et al. Trends in suicide ideation, plans, gestures, and attempts in the United States, 1990–1992 to 2001–2003. JAMA 2005;293:2487.

[56] Schulberg H, Lee P, Bruce M, et al. Suicidal ideation and risk levels among primary care patients with uncomplicated depression. Ann Fam Med, in press.

[57] Berwick D. Disseminating innovations in health care. JAMA 2003;289:1969.

[58] Bradley E, Holmboe E, Mattera J, et al. A qualitative study of increasing beta-blocker use after myocardial infarction: why do some hospitals succeed? JAMA 2001;285:2604.

[59] Crosson F, Madvig P. Does population management of chronic disease lead to lower costs of care? Health Aff 2004;23:76.

[60] Rost K, Smith JL, Dickinson M. The effect of improving primary care depression management on employee absenteeism and productivity: a randomized trial. Med Care 2004;42: 1202.

[61] Stewart RA, North FM, West TM, et al. Depression and cardiovascular morbidity and mortality: cause or consequence? Eur Heart J 2003;24:2027.

ELSEVIER
SAUNDERS

Psychiatr Clin N Am
28 (2005) 1079–1092

PSYCHIATRIC
CLINICS
OF NORTH AMERICA

From Establishing an Evidence-Based Practice to Implementation in Real-World Settings: IMPACT as a Case Study

Jürgen Unützer, MD, MPH, MA[a],*,
Diane Powers, MA[a], Wayne Katon, MD[a],
Christopher Langston, PhD[b]

[a]Department of Psychiatry and Behavioral Sciences, University of Washington,
Box 356560, Seattle, WA 98195, USA
[b]John A. Hartford Foundation, Inc., 55 East 59th Street, New York, NY 10022, USA

Little is known about how to disseminate efficacious treatments from the research stage to real-world practice, other than perhaps the area of proprietary knowledge of pharmaceutical companies regarding new medicines. Crowley and colleagues [1] outline how treatment research moves from basic science to treatment efficacy studies and, ultimately, to health services studies that evaluate the effectiveness of evidence-based treatments. Fixsen and colleagues [2] describe the implementation of evidence-based treatment programs in real-world health care systems, a final step in the trajectory from treatment development to improving health outcomes in the real world.

This article presents the IMPACT (Improving Mood: Providing Access to Collaborative Treatment for Late-Life Depression) model as a case study in moving from the development of an evidence-based model of care for late-life depression to the implementation of the model in diverse health care settings. Four steps in this implementation process are discussed: (1) research regarding the clinical epidemiology of late-life depression; (2) the development of a feasible, evidence-based intervention strategy; (3) the

Funding support for dissemination of the IMPACT model of care is provided by the John A. Hartford Foundation. Funding for the original research trial was provided by the John A. Hartford Foundation and the California HealthCare Foundation.

* Corresponding author.
E-mail address: unutzer@u.washington.edu (J. Unützer).

evaluation of the effectiveness and cost-effectiveness of the intervention in diverse settings; and (4) moving from research to practice.

Clinical epidemiology of late-life depression

Between 5% and 10% of older adults who visit a primary care provider suffer from a major depression or dysthymic disorder [3–7]. Late-life depression is associated with an increased symptom burden from medical illnesses, losses in functioning and quality of life, mortality, and increased health care costs [8–10]. Although late-life depression can be treated successfully with psychotherapy, medication, or other somatic therapies (see articles by Mackin, Shanmughan, and Cole elsewhere in this issue) [11], few older adults receive adequate trials of such evidence-based treatments in primary care or are seen by a mental health specialist [12–17]. The past 10 years have seen a substantial increase in the prescription of antidepressant medications to older primary care patients [18–21], but the outcomes of depression treatment in primary care remain poor. In the care as usual arm of the IMPACT trial, only one in five depressed older adults experienced a substantial improvement in depression over a 12-month follow-up period, despite the fact that the majority received treatment with antidepressants [22].

Several barriers contribute to poor treatment outcomes in primary care [23–29]. Patients and providers may assume that depression is a natural consequence of aging and that treatment may not help. Primary care providers caring for comorbid medical problems often lack the time and resources to treat depression or to provide adequate follow-up to patients who have been started on antidepressants [25]. Additional barriers include the stigma associated with depression [29], the physical, organizational, and cultural separation of primary and specialized mental health care, and the comparatively lower reimbursement for the treatment of mental versus physical disorders [12,14,16,30,31].

Developing a feasible and effective intervention strategy based on the existing evidence base

In 1997, the John A. Hartford Foundation commissioned a 1-year effort to review the evidence base for treatments of late-life depression and lay the foundation for the development of a treatment program that could be effective in diverse practice settings [14,32,33]. Experts reviewing the available evidence noted that the results of clinical efficacy studies may not always be generalizable to real-world treatment settings [34,35] where there are multiple barriers to the use of evidence-based treatments [14] and where treatments often do not perform as well as they do in efficacy trials [34]. Reviewers also noted that most successful quality improvement programs for depression had been tested with mixed age populations in managed care settings, whereas the majority of older adults remained in fee-for-service Medicare.

The clinical epidemiology of late-life depression strongly suggested that efforts to improve care for depressed older adults should be based, or at least initiated, in primary care because this is where most older adults receive their health care. The IMPACT investigators based their intervention strategy on 15 years of research showing that collaborative interventions that are founded on evidence-based treatment guidelines and that assist primary care providers in providing evidence-based treatments are more effective than care as usual [7,30,36–42]. Effective models often use a stepped-care treatment approach in which the treatment selection and intensity of services are guided by evidence-based treatment algorithms and clinical outcomes of individual patients [43,44].

IMPACT is a collaborative, stepped-care program for the treatment of late-life depression [22,45]. Key program components include (1) patient education about depression; (2) measurement and proactive tracking of depression; (3) treatment plans based on an evidence-based treatment algorithm [45], patient preference, treatment history, medication formularies in participating organizations, and financial and other considerations; (4) evidence-based treatments such as antidepressant medications and psychotherapies such as behavioral activation or problem solving; (5) adjustment of treatment plans according to clinical outcomes; (6) a depression care manager in primary care; and (7) consultation from a team psychiatrist and primary care expert and referral to specialized mental health services, as indicated clinically.

Investigators consulted closely with clinical and operational leaders at eight participating, diverse health care organizations to make sure that the interventions were feasible and to optimize the chances of successful implementation. Intervention services were delivered by a depression care manager (DCM) who worked closely with the patient's regular primary care provider. Participating organizations hired nurses (at the bachelor and masters degree level) with and without previous mental health experience and psychologists (at the masters and doctoral degree levels) as DCMs [45,56]. Caseloads for full-time DCMs ranged from 75 to 100 patients [46–48]. DCMs were trained according to intervention manuals [49–52] during a 2-day orientation session and two subsequent refresher-training meetings. Each DCM treated five training patients with four to six sessions of problem-solving treatment for primary care (PST-PC) and received supervision based on videotaped sessions from a PST-PC expert. DCMs also participated in monthly telephone conference calls to help standardize the intervention across sites. DCMs used an internet-based clinical information system [53] to record patient contacts, track patient progress, and support the implementation of the stepped care treatment model.

Evaluating the effectiveness and cost-effectiveness of the intervention in diverse health care settings

A randomized control trial compared the IMPACT intervention with care as usual at each of the eight participating health care organizations. An ethnically diverse sample of 1801 depressed older adults (age ≥ 60) who had high rates of comorbid medical disorders, anxiety disorders, or cognitive impairment were assigned randomly to the IMPACT program for 12 months or to care as usual [22,45]. This study design was chosen to balance internal validity with the ability to generalize study findings across diverse practice settings. Attempts to maximize the internal validity of the study included random assignment at the patient level, standardized inclusion criteria, independent assessments by blinded interviewers, and standardized implementation of a well-specified treatment protocol across sites. This emphasis on internal validity was intended to increase the quality of the evidence and its future persuasiveness to a variety of audiences; however, these criteria tended to limit potential participating sites to those that were more willing to accept the burdens of scientific rigor. For example, a highly desirable, real-world applicant site from a rural community withdrew its proposal in the face of these requirements. Another participating nonacademic site insisted on financial indemnification from possible unreimbursed patient visits.

Because primary care clinics vary substantially in their patient populations, staffing, and care for depressed older adults, the funding organizations and investigators believed that it was important to include diverse health care organizations in the trial. Eight health care organizations representing 18 primary care clinics were selected to participate in the trial [22,45]. Over a 2-year recruitment period, IMPACT enrolled between 2% and 3% of all older adults served by the participating study organizations, resulting in a representative sample of depressed older adults [22,45].

Patients assigned to care as usual were informed of their depression diagnosis and encouraged to follow-up with their primary care providers, who were notified that the patient screened positive for depression. Usual care participants were observed under naturalistic conditions, allowing them and their providers to use all available primary care or specialized mental health treatments without any restrictions. The majority of care as usual participants underwent at least one trial of an antidepressant medication, prescribed usually by their primary care provider, and a smaller number (≤ 20%) used specialized mental health care or psychotherapy.

As an effectiveness study, the trial was not intended to compare the efficacy of specific treatments, such as antidepressant medications or psychotherapy with placebo, but rather to see if an organized disease management model that attempts to maximize the use of evidence-based treatments leads to better outcomes than care as usual. Details about the IMPACT intervention program and study evaluation methods can be found elsewhere [22,45].

Compared with the care as usual group, IMPACT participants were more likely to receive evidence-based treatments such as antidepressant medications or psychotherapy and expressed higher satisfaction with depression care, lower depression severity, lower rates of major depression [22], better physical and social functioning [54], less functional impairment from pain [55], and better overall quality of life [22]. Significant effects on depression and functioning persisted even during the second year of the trial, 1 year after intervention resources were no longer available in participating clinics [56]. Cost-effectiveness analyses found that although IMPACT participants had slightly higher health care costs during the initial year of the intervention, these increases were largely offset by lower health care costs in the second year of the study [57]. The overall cost effectiveness of IMPACT care compares favorably with many medical interventions such as the use of statin drugs, hypertension screening, or coronary artery bypass grafting.

IMPACT is one of several recent trials [16,58] (see the article by Oxman elsewhere in this issue) that adds to the evidence base for effective primary care-based interventions for late-life depression. The IMPACT model was found to be feasible and more effective than care as usual at each of eight health care organizations (Fig. 1) [22], providing robust evidence to support the dissemination of the model in diverse practice settings.

Moving from research to practice

Publications in peer reviewed journals and media coverage can help disseminate research findings, but they are not sufficient to facilitate the successful adoption, implementation, or sustainability of evidence-based programs [2]. One condition of the original grant to the trial sites was to

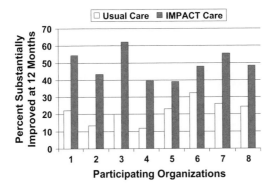

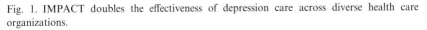

Fig. 1. IMPACT doubles the effectiveness of depression care across diverse health care organizations.

make a good faith effort to maintain the intervention model if it were to prove its cost effectiveness. Despite this commitment, maintaining the model at the trial sites after the initial grant period proved to be challenging and required a modification of the program in several cases [59]. To meet the challenges of moving from a successful effectiveness trial to the implementation in the real world, IMPACT investigators developed a 5-year plan to disseminate the model with ongoing support from the John A. Hartford Foundation. Investigators searched available literature on the successful translation from research to practice and developed a dissemination framework based on the available literature [2,16,60–71] and previous experience working with diverse health care organizations [66,68,72,73].

The IMPACT dissemination framework (Fig. 2) begins by articulating the clinical epidemiology and barriers to evidence-based care for late-life depression to diverse audiences. The strategy then focuses on describing and marketing the IMPACT program to key stakeholders, including patients, family members, consumer advocacy groups, primary care and specialized mental health care providers, health care administrators, and policy makers. This step requires detailed specifications of the intervention model, including information about the start-up costs associated with implementing IMPACT in diverse health care organizations. The information presented in peer-reviewed medical journals is helpful for some decision-makers, but information about IMPACT also is presented in the form of photos, videos and digital media, brochures, and newsletters to reach diverse audiences. The IMPACT website (www.impact.ucla.edu) has proven to be a particularly valuable tool. The website provides (1) an overview of the model, including key components; (2) information about the research evidence for IMPACT; (3) links to print and broadcast media coverage and information for interested journalists; (4) a bulletin board to facilitate interaction among clinicians and organizations in implementing the model; (5) implementation tools; and (6) training opportunities. Goodman (www.agoodmanonline.com) emphasizes the importance of story telling, and we have found stories from patients and participating clinics to be helpful in communicating key aspects of the IMPACT model.

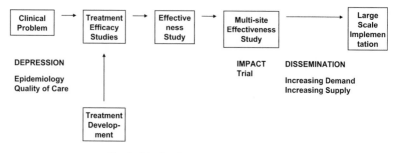

Fig. 2. Moving from research to practice.

The IMPACT dissemination framework attempts, first, to increase the demand for evidence-based effective care models such as IMPACT and, second, to increase the supply of practitioners and organizations that are capable of delivering such care. These efforts are pursued in partnership with key stakeholders and organizations that share the goal of improving health care for older adults (eg, the John A. Hartford Foundation and the AARP) and organizations that have distribution channels to make the program available to large numbers of depressed older adults (eg, insurance companies, disease management firms, and large health care organizations).

Efforts to increase demand include working with federal, state, and local governments, private purchasers, and employers to reduce policy and financial barriers to evidence-based programs such as IMPACT. Examples of such efforts include "piggy backing" on recent federal and state policies to fund evidence-based treatments for mental health and federal and private pay-for-performance initiatives. Another example is a recent initiative by the Substance Abuse and Mental Health Services Administration (SAMHSA), which provides funding for implementing evidence-based mental health services for older adults. Over 10 service delivery agencies from around the country contacted the IMPACT coordinating center for support with implementing the IMPACT model as part of this initiative.

Efforts to increase supply include consulting with interested health care organizations and developing tools to facilitate program implementation. These tools include an implementation toolkit with intervention manuals, educational materials, the 9 item Patient Health Questionnaire (PHQ-9), and tracking systems such as the Internet web-based Clinical Information System developed for IMPACT [53]. Other tools include detailed specifications of the intervention model and its core components, information on start-up and operating costs, a needs assessment and implementation guide, and business models for the IMPACT model under different financing arrangements.

Successful program implementation also requires training of clinical staff in the use of these tools. The IMPACT coordinating center offers a comprehensive training program for DCMs and consulting mental health professionals. This program includes presentations of the model at national and regional conferences, 1- and 2-day training conferences organized by the IMPACT coordinating center or partnering health care organizations, and an Internet web-based training program that can be accessed from the IMPACT website. In addition to initial training, ongoing consultation and support are provided to DCMs and consulting mental health professionals as well as suggestions to program administrators for adjustments of the model as needed.

National experts in IMPACT care also provide consultation to organizations that wish to adapt the model for new types of health care systems (eg, home health care) or new clinical populations. Several health care organizations, for example, have adapted core elements of the IMPACT model as part of disease management programs for diabetes and heart disease. In addition to direct consultation, the IMPACT coordinating center also facilitates peer consultation with other organizations that have successfully implemented the program or that face similar challenges (eg, creating a viable business plan in a fee-for-service billing environment).

The IMPACT model or key components of the model have been successfully sustained in several of the organizations that participated in the original study [59]. In one large health maintenance organization, the program was not only sustained but also adapted and expanded to two additional primary care clinics. A program evaluation of the sustained program showed that the same positive clinical and cost results were achieved as during the original study, and these strong results helped to convince senior health care executives at this organization to expand the program to 12 large regional medical centers serving a population of approximately 3 million insured members. Presently, clinicians from over 50 organizations in the United States and Canada have been trained in the IMPACT model, and several new organizations are implementing core components of the entire model. These organizations include a large health care system in northern California, a multiclinic health system in New York City, several primary care clinics affiliated with the US Veterans Affairs Administration, and a large home health care agency in southern California. Other organizations have adapted the IMPACT program and are conducting newly funded research on the effectiveness of the program in new populations of depressed patients (eg, patients who have had myocardial infarctions, multiple sclerosis, or Parkinson's disease, patients in disease management programs for diabetes and congestive heart failure, and depressed older African Americans in rural settings).

Discussion

This case study provides one example of moving from the development of an evidence-based care model to the implementation of the model in diverse health care settings. Although the trial is now complete, efforts to move IMPACT from research to practice are relatively recent and thus constitute a work in progress. The focus over the next several years is to draw on systematic observations from this second phase of IMPACT to add to the limited but growing evidence base on implementing successful research interventions in the real world.

The experience to date suggests that the relationship between treatment research and practice change to implement evidence-based treatments in real-world health care settings is, at best, tenuous. Real-world cynics may argue that researchers have little interest in implementing research findings but rather move on to the next research question, "chasing the next grant" (including grants testing the IMPACT model in new populations).

Academics, on the other hand, may argue that real-world practice seems to be largely reactive to reimbursement policies (or "chasing the money") rather then research evidence and that most of the care provided in the real world is not based on evidence. It is not clear whose job it is in the medico-academic industrial complex to disseminate evidence-based practices and whose job it is in the real world of health care delivery to adopt proven innovations, particularly when market forces do not drive such behavior.

The literature on innovation in service systems [70,71] suggests certain characteristics of innovations that favor diffusion, such as relative advantages, compatibility, low complexity, trialability, and observability. This approach favors relatively simple interventions, such as new medications, and presents substantial challenges for complex organizational innovations in mental health services that require changes in the organization of health care and substantial start-up costs, even if costs clearly add value in terms of health outcomes and have the potential for long-term cost savings.

Experience confirms the importance of engaging key stakeholders, decision makers, change agents, and communicators (eg, experts, opinion leaders, and local champions) in the efforts to disseminate and implement evidence-based programs [71]. Stakeholders also include clinical leaders, operations staff (eg, clinic managers), and budget managers who must support and facilitate program start-up and ongoing operations. In addition to engaging such key individuals, substantial ongoing consultation, support, and feedback on progress are needed to help organizations adapt the program to their unique settings, to train staff, and to successfully implement and sustain the program.

Although the IMPACT model was developed to fit diverse health care environments, additional adaptation has been required for the successful implementation of the model in diverse health care settings. Such adaptations can make it challenging for researchers to track the fidelity of new programs to the interventions tested in the original research. Attempts to deal with this challenge have used a two-pronged strategy. First, a set of core components has been developed to help evaluate the fidelity of adapted programs to the original model. Second, organizations are advised to closely track several key process and clinical outcomes (eg, the number of clients treated in the program and PHQ-9 scores of enrolled patients over time). As long as the observed clinical improvements are comparable to the original trial, it is reasonably certain that modifications made to the protocol for implementation purposes do not excessively dilute or weaken the effectiveness of the model.

In addition, although the dissemination framework (see Fig. 2) suggests a linear process, this process can be far from linear. The capacity of organizations for adopting new knowledge and the receptivity for such change can change rapidly based on changes in leadership or organizational relations or changes in the environment (eg, changes in financial incentives, norms, or external mandates) [71]. For example, an organization that has invested recently in an electronic medical records system suddenly has the capacity to track PHQ-9 depression scores, one of the key requirements of successful disease management for depression. Attempts are made to work with leaders in participating organizations to build on such local opportunities. At times, unexpected external opportunities develop that facilitate the dissemination and implementation process; examples of such opportunities for IMPACT have included

1. Funding and financial incentives: Examples include the SAMHSA funding opportunity and new funding generated in California by Proposition 63 [74]. Another example is the introduction of Hierarchical Condition Categories as the basis of calculating Centers for Medicare and Medicaid Services payments to Medicare Advantage plans. This type of risk-adjusted payment methodology provides powerful incentives for organizations to improve documentation and treatment of depression in their Medicare populations.
2. "Captive audiences": The Chronic Care Initiative Program (also known as the Medicare Health Support Program) was created by the Medicare Modernization Act; the program seeks to evaluate the effects of care management for congestive heart failure and complex diabetes on patient outcomes and costs. This program will enroll over 250,000 Medicare recipients in eight United States markets and provides an excellent opportunity for demonstrating the effects of improving depression care in the context of chronic disease management on health outcomes and health care costs.
3. Outcome accountability and pay for performance initiatives: Government and private purchasers are demanding increasingly that services be evidence based, and several large payors have initiated pay-for-performance programs to improve health outcomes. Purchaser coalitions such as the National Business Coalition on Health are negotiating with health insurers for evidence-based cost-effective depression care programs. This represents an exceptional opportunity for programs such as IMPACT because relatively few mental health programs for older adults are evidence-based.
4. Calls to action: Recommendations promoting evidence-based mental health treatments that are issued by respected bodies such as the President's New Freedom Commission [44] and the Institute of Medicine can increase visibility and lend credibility to evidence-based care programs such as IMPACT.

It may be more difficult to widely disseminate and implement an evidence-based model of care than to develop the model and establish its effectiveness in a large research trial. The task of helping an organization implement an evidence-based program such as IMPACT can feel as overwhelming as working with a depressed older person who faces multiple medical, social, and psychologic barriers to recovery. To confront these challenges, it useful to draw on many of the problem-solving and stepped-care skills that have been developed and tested in the IMPACT trial. Organizations are helped to establish clear goals for implementation and then helped to break down what can appear to be overwhelming challenges into specific problems to help identify solutions. Ongoing support is provided to help implement such solutions or to make changes in implementation plans if initial efforts do not succeed, and partnering organizations are strongly encouraged to keep track of key process and clinical outcomes (eg, PHQ-9 scores) to help guide these efforts.

Finally, the present authors want to join others [2,71] in making a strong argument for more research on the translation from successful intervention research to large-scale program implementation. Such work is crucially important if the kinds of evidence-based treatments and programs described in this issue of the *Psychiatric Clinics of North America* are to reach the older adults who most need them. Going beyond the research, the development and funding of effective mechanisms are needed to help promote the effective translation of research findings into the real world.

References

[1] Crowley WF Jr, Sherwood L, Salber P, et al. Clinical research in the United States at a crossroads: proposal for a novel public-private partnership to establish a national clinical research enterprise. JAMA 2004;291(9):1120–6.

[2] Fixsen DL, Naoom SF, Blase KA, et al. Implementation research: a synthesis of the literature. Tampa (FL): University of South Florida; 2005 [FMHI Publication no 231].

[3] Lebowitz BD. Depression and treatment of depression in late life: an overview of the NIH consensus statement. Am J Psychiatry 1996;4:S3–6.

[4] Barry KL, Fleming MF, Manwell LB, et al. Prevalence of and factors associated with current and lifetime depression in older adult primary care patients. Fam Med 1998;30(5):366–71.

[5] Gurland B, Cross P, Katz S. Epidemiological perspectives on opportunities for treatment of depression. Am J Geriatr Psychiatry 1996;4:7–14.

[6] Lyness JM, Caine ED, King DA, et al. Psychiatric disorders in older primary care patients. J Gen Intern Med 1999;14(4):249–54.

[7] Schulberg HC, Block MR, Madonia MJ, et al. Treating major depression in primary care practice: eight-month clinical outcomes. Arch Gen Psychiatry 1996;53(10):913–9.

[8] Alexopoulos GS, Vrontou C, Kakuma T, et al. Disability in geriatric depression. Am J Psychiatry 1996;153(7):877–85.

[9] Unützer J, Patrick DL, Simon G, et al. Depressive symptoms and the cost of health services in HMO patients aged 65 years and older: a 4-year prospective study. JAMA 1997;277(20):1618–23.

[10] Penninx BW, Geerlings SW, Deeg DJ, et al. Minor and major depression and the risk of death in older persons. Arch Gen Psychiatry 1999;56(10):889–95.

[11] Lebowitz BD, Pearson JL, Schneider LS, et al. Diagnosis and treatment of depression in late life: consensus statement update. JAMA 1997;278(14):1186–90.

[12] Callahan CM, Hendrie HC, Dittus RS, et al. Improving treatment of late life depression in primary care: a randomized clinical trial. J Am Geriatr Soc 1994;42(8):839–46.

[13] Unützer J, Katon W, Russo J, et al. Patterns of care for depressed older adults in a large-staff model HMO. Am J Geriatr Psychiatry 1999;7(3):235–43.

[14] Unützer J, Katon W, Sullivan M, et al. Treating depressed older adults in primary care: narrowing the gap between efficacy and effectiveness. Milbank Q 1999;77(2):174, 225–56.

[15] Unützer J, Simon G, Belin TR, et al. Care for depression in HMO patients aged 65 and older. J Am Geriatr Soc 2000;48(8):871–8.

[16] Bartels SJ, Coakley EH, Zubritsky C, et al. Improving access to geriatric mental health services: a randomized trial comparing treatment engagement with integrated versus enhanced referral care for depression, anxiety, and at-risk alcohol use. Am J Psychiatry 2004;161(8): 1455–62.

[17] Klap R, Unroe KT, Unützer J. Caring for mental illness in the United States: a focus on older adults. Am J Geriatr Psychiatry 2003;11(5):517–24.

[18] Crystal S, Sambamoorthi U, Walkup JT, et al. Diagnosis and treatment of depression in the elderly Medicare population: predictors, disparities, and trends. J Am Geriatr Soc 2003; 51(12):1718–28.

[19] Harman JS, Crystal S, Walkup J, et al. Trends in elderly patients' office visits for the treatment of depression according to physician specialty: 1985–1999. J Behav Health Serv Res 2003;30(3):332–41.

[20] Sambamoorthi U, Olfson M, Walkup JT, et al. Diffusion of new generation antidepressant treatment among elderly diagnosed with depression. Med Care 2003;41(1):180–94.

[21] Coyne J, Katz IR. Improving the primary care treatment of late life depression: progress and opportunities. Med Care 2001;39(8):756–9.

[22] Unützer J, Katon W, Callahan CM, et al. Collaborative care management of late-life depression in the primary care setting: a randomized controlled trial. JAMA 2002;288(22): 2836–45.

[23] Brown SL, Salive ME, Guralnik JM, et al. Antidepressant use in the elderly: association with demographic characteristics, health-related factors, and health care utilization. J Clin Epidemiol 1995;48(3):445–53.

[24] Gallo JJ, Anthony JC, Muthen BO. Age differences in the symptoms of depression: a latent trait analysis. J Gerontol 1994;49(6):251–64.

[25] Glasser M, Gravdal JA. Assessment and treatment of geriatric depression in primary care settings. Arch Fam Med 1997;6(5):433–8.

[26] Rabins P. Barriers to the diagnosis and treatment of depression in elderly patients. Am J Geriatr Psychiatry 1996;4:79–84.

[27] Thompson TL 2nd, House RM. Geriatric psychiatry patients' care by primary care physicians. Psychosomatics 1989;30(1):65–72.

[28] Cole SC, Raju JF, Feldman M. Depression. In: Behavioral medicine in primary care: a practical guide. Stamford (CT): Appleton and Lange; 1997.

[29] US Department of Health and Human Services. Mental health: a report of the surgeon general. Rockville (MD): USDHHS, Substance Abuse and Mental Health Services Administration, Center for Mental Health Services, NIMH; 1999.

[30] Paveza GC. D. Treatment of mental health problems in the elderly. In: Levin LP, editor. Mental health services: a public health perspective. New York: Oxford University Press; 1996.

[31] Rubenstein LV, Jackson-Triche M, Unützer J, et al. Evidence-based care for depression in managed primary care practices. Health Aff (Millwood) 1999;18(5):89–105.

[32] Callahan CM. Quality improvement research on late life depression in primary care. Med Care 2001;39(8):772–84.

[33] Unützer J. Diagnosis and treatment of older adults with depression in primary care. Biol Psychiatry 2002;52(3):285–92.

[34] Wells KB. Treatment research at the crossroads: the scientific interface of clinical trials and effectiveness research. Am J Psychiatry 1999;156(1):5–10.

[35] Wells KB. The design of Partners in Care: evaluating the cost-effectiveness of improving care for depression in primary care. Soc Psychiatry Psychiatr Epidemiol 1999;34(1):20–9.

[36] Katon W, Von Korff M, Lin E, et al. Collaborative management to achieve treatment guidelines: impact on depression in primary care. JAMA 1995;273(13):1026–31.

[37] Katon W, Robinson P, Von Korff M, et al. A multifaceted intervention to improve treatment of depression in primary care. Arch Gen Psychiatry 1996;53(10):924–32.

[38] Katon W, Von Korff M, Lin E, et al. Stepped collaborative care for primary care patients with persistent symptoms of depression: a randomized trial. Arch Gen Psychiatry 1999; 56(12):1109–15.

[39] Wells KB, Sherbourne C, Schoenbaum M, et al. Impact of disseminating quality improvement programs for depression in managed primary care: a randomized controlled trial. JAMA 2000;283(2):212–20.

[40] Hunkeler EM, Meresman JF, Hargreaves WA, et al. Efficacy of nurse telehealth care and peer support in augmenting treatment of depression in primary care. Arch Fam Med 2000;9(8):700–8.

[41] Gilbody DS. Review: disease management programmes improve detection and care of people with depression. Evid Based Ment Health 2004;7(3):80.

[42] Gilbody S, Whitty P, Grimshaw J, et al. Educational and organizational interventions to improve the management of depression in primary care: a systematic review. JAMA 2003; 289(23):3145–51.

[43] Von Korff M, Tiemens B. Individualized stepped care of chronic illness. West J Med 2000; 172(2):133–7.

[44] Unützer J, Schoenbaum M, Druss B, et al. Transforming mental health care at the interface with general medicine: report for the President's New Freedom Commission for Mental Health. Psychiatr Serv, in press.

[45] Unützer J, Katon W, Williams JW Jr, et al. Improving primary care for depression in late life: the design of a multicenter randomized trial. Med Care 2001;39(8):785–99.

[46] Oishi SM, Shoai R, Katon W, et al. Impacting late life depression: integrating a depression intervention into primary care. Psychiatr Q 2003;74(1):75–89.

[47] Saur CD, Harpole LH, Steffens DC, et al. Treating depression in primary care: an innovative role for mental health nurses. J Am Psychiatr Nurses Assoc 2002;8:159–67.

[48] Harpole LH, Stechuchak KM, Saur CD, et al. Implementing a disease management intervention for depression in primary care: a random work sampling study. Gen Hosp Psychiatry 2003;25(4):238–45.

[49] Unützer J for the IMPACT Study Investigators. IMPACT intervention manual. Los Angeles (CA): Center for Health Services Research, UCLA Neuropsychiatric Institute; 1999.

[50] Hegel MB, Oxman JE, Mynors-Wallis TE, et al. Problem-solving treatment for primary care (PST-PC): a treatment manual for depression. 1999.

[51] Arean PH, Unützer J. Problem-solving therapy for older primary care patients: maintenance group manual for Project IMPACT. Los Angeles: UCLA Neuropsychiatric Institute, Center for Health Services Research. 1999.

[52] Arean PH, Unützer MJ. Problem-solving treatment in primary care: addendum to PST-PC treatment manual for Project IMPACT. 1999.

[53] Unützer J, Choi Y, Cook IA, et al. A web-based data management system to improve care for depression in a multicenter clinical trial. Psychiatr Serv 2002;53(6):671–3, 8.

[54] Callahan CM, Kroenke K, Counsell SR, et al. Treatment of depression improves physical functioning in older adults. J Am Geriatr Soc 2005;53(3):367–73.

[55] Lin EH, Katon W, Von Korff M, et al. Effect of improving depression care on pain and functional outcomes among older adults with arthritis: a randomized controlled trial. JAMA 2003;290(18):2428–34.

[56] Hunkeler E, Katon W, et al. Two years of IMPACT: long term effects of collaborative care for depression among older adults in primary care. Presented at the 57th Annual Meeting of the Gerontological Society of America. Washington, DC, November 2004.

[57] Katon W, Schoenbaum M, Fan My, et al. Cost-effectiveness of improving primary care treatment of late-life depression. Arch Gen Psychiatry, in press.

[58] Bruce ML, Ten Have TR, Reynolds CF III, et al. Reducing suicidal ideation and depressive symptoms in depressed older primary care patients: a randomized controlled trial. JAMA 2004;291(9):1081–91.

[59] Blasinsky M, Goldman HH, Unützer J, et al. Project IMPACT: a report on barriers and facilitators of sustainability. Adm Policy Ment Health. in press.

[60] Goldman HH, Ganju V, Drake RE, et al. Policy implications for implementing evidence-based practices. Psychiatr Serv 2001;52(12):1591–7.

[61] Glasgow RE, Magid DJ, Beck A, et al. Practical clinical trials for translating research to practice: design and measurement recommendations. Med Care 2005;43(6):551–7.

[62] Casalino L, Gillies RR, Shortell SM, et al. External incentives, information technology, and organized processes to improve health care quality for patients with chronic diseases. JAMA 2003;289(4):434–41.

[63] Rosenheck R. Stages in the implementation of innovative clinical programs in complex organizations. J Nerv Ment Dis 2001;189(12):812–21.

[64] Bradley EH, Webster TR, Baker D, et al. Translating research into practice: speeding the adoption of innovative health care programs. Issue Brief (Commonw Fund) 2004;(724): 1–12.

[65] Berwick DM. Disseminating innovations in health care. JAMA 2003;289(15):1969–75.

[66] Kilbourne AM, Schulberg HC, Post EP, et al. Translating evidence-based depression management services to community-based primary care practices. Milbank Q 2004;82(4):631–59.

[67] Schoenwald SK, Hoagwood K. Effectiveness, transportability, and dissemination of interventions: what matters when? Psychiatr Serv 2001;52(9):1190–7.

[68] Dietrich AJ, Oxman TE, Williams JW Jr, et al. Going to scale: re-engineering systems for primary care treatment of depression. Ann Fam Med 2004;2(4):301–4.

[69] Gotham H. Diffusion of mental health and substance abuse treatments: development, dissemination, and implementation. Clin Psychol Sci Prac 2004;11:160–76.

[70] Rogers E. Diffusion of innovations. New York: Free Press; 1995.

[71] Greenhalgh T, Robert G, Macfarlane F, et al. Diffusion of innovations in service organizations: systemic review and recommendations. Milbank Q 2004;82(4):581–629.

[72] Dietrich AJ, Oxman TE, Williams JW Jr, et al. Re-engineering systems for the treatment of depression in primary care: cluster randomised controlled trial. BMJ 2004;329(7466):602.

[73] Meredith L, Unützer J, Mendel P, et al. Success of implementation and maintenance of quality improvement for depression. Psychiatr Serv, in press.

[74] Scheffler RM, Adams N. Millionaires and mental health: proposition 63 in California. Health Aff (Millwood) 2005. Vol. W5. p. 212–24.

ELSEVIER
SAUNDERS

Psychiatr Clin N Am
28 (2005) 1093–1121

PSYCHIATRIC
CLINICS
OF NORTH AMERICA

Cumulative Index 2005

Note: Page numbers of article titles are in **boldface** type.

0193-953X/05/$ - see front matter © 2005 Elsevier Inc. All rights reserved.
doi:10.1016/S0193-953X(05)00107-3

psych.theclinics.com

United States Postal Service

Statement of Ownership, Management, and Circulation

1. Publication Title	2. Publication Number	3. Filing Date
Psychiatric Clinics of North America	0 1 9 3 - 9 5 3 X	9/15/05

4. Issue Frequency	5. Number of Issues Published Annually	6. Annual Subscription Price
Mar, Jun, Sep, Dec	4	$170.00

7. Complete Mailing Address of Known Office of Publication (Not printer) (Street, city, county, state, and ZIP+4)

Elsevier Inc.
6277 Sea Harbor Drive
Orlando, FL 32887-4800

Contact Person
Gwen C. Campbell

Telephone
215-239-3685

8. Complete Mailing Address of Headquarters or General Business Office of Publisher (Not printer)

Elsevier Inc., 360 Park Avenue South, New York, New York, NY 10010-1710

9. Full Names and Complete Mailing Addresses of Publisher, Editor, and Managing Editor (Do not leave blank)

Publisher (Name and complete mailing address)

Tim Griswold, Elsevier Inc., 1600 John F. Kennedy Blvd., Suite 1800, Philadelphia, PA 19103-2899

Editor (Name and complete mailing address)

Sarah Barth, Elsevier Inc., 1600 John F. Kennedy Blvd., Suite 1800, Philadelphia, PA 19103-2899

Managing Editor (Name and complete mailing address)

Heather Cullen, Elsevier Inc., 1600 John F. Kennedy Blvd., Suite 1800, Philadelphia, PA 19103-2899

10. Owner (Do not leave blank. If the publication is owned by a corporation, give the name and address of the corporation immediately followed by the names and addresses of all stockholders owning or holding 1 percent or more of the total amount of stock. If not owned by a corporation, give the names and addresses of the individual owners. If owned by a partnership or other unincorporated firm, give its name and address as well as those of each individual owner. If the publication is published by a nonprofit organization, give its name and address.)

Full Name	Complete Mailing Address
Wholly owned subsidiary of	4520 East-West Highway
Reed/Elsevier Inc., US holdings	Bethesda, MD 20814

11. Known Bondholders, Mortgagees, and Other Security Holders Owning or Holding 1 Percent or More of Total Amount of Bonds, Mortgages, or Other Securities. If none, check box. ☒ None

Full Name	Complete Mailing Address
N/A	

12. Tax Status (For completion by nonprofit organizations authorized to mail at nonprofit rates) (Check one)
The purpose, function, and nonprofit status of this organization and the exempt status for federal income tax purposes:
☐ Has Not Changed During Preceding 12 Months
☐ Has Changed During Preceding 12 Months (Publisher must submit explanation of change with this statement)

(See Instructions on Reverse)

13. Publication Title	14. Issue Date for Circulation Data Below
Psychiatric Clinics of North America	June 2005

15.	Extent and Nature of Circulation	Average No. Copies Each Issue During Preceding 12 Months	No. Copies of Single Issue Published Nearest to Filing Date
a.	Total Number of Copies (Net press run)	3050	2700
b. Paid and/or Requested Circulation	(1) Paid/Requested Outside-County Mail Subscriptions Stated on Form 3541. (Include advertiser's proof and exchange copies)	1696	1510
	(2) Paid In-County Subscriptions Stated on Form 3541 (Include advertiser's proof and exchange copies)		
	(3) Sales Through Dealers and Carriers, Street Vendors, Counter Sales, and Other Non-USPS Paid Distribution	359	317
	(4) Other Classes Mailed Through the USPS		
c.	Total Paid and/or Requested Circulation [Sum of 15b. (1), (2), (3), and (4)]	2055	1827
d. Free Distribution by Mail (Samples, complimentary, and other free)	(1) Outside-County as Stated on Form 3541	89	123
	(2) In-County as Stated on Form 3541		
	(3) Other Classes Mailed Through the USPS		
e.	Free Distribution Outside the Mail (Carriers or other means)		
f.	Total Free Distribution (Sum of 15d. and 15e.)	89	123
g.	Total Distribution (Sum of 15c. and 15f.)	2144	1950
h.	Copies not Distributed	906	750
i.	Total (Sum of 15g. and h.)	3050	2700
j.	Percent Paid and/or Requested Circulation (15c. divided by 15g. times 100)	96%	94%

16. Publication of Statement of Ownership
☐ Publication required. Will be printed in the **December 2005** issue of this publication. ☐ Publication not required.

17. Signature and Title of Editor, Publisher, Business Manager, or Owner

[signature]

Kari Fenucci - Executive Director of Subscription Services

Date
9/15/05

I certify that all information furnished on this form is true and complete. I understand that anyone who furnishes false or misleading information on this form or who omits material or information requested on the form may be subject to criminal sanctions (including fines and imprisonment) and/or civil sanctions (including civil penalties).

Instructions to Publishers

1. Complete and file one copy of this form with your postmaster annually on or before October 1. Keep a copy of the completed form for your records.
2. In cases where the stockholder or security holder is a trustee, include in items 10 and 11 the name of the person or corporation for whom the trustee is acting. Also include the names and addresses of individuals who are stockholders who own or hold 1 percent or more of the total amount of bonds, mortgages, or other securities of the publishing corporation. In item 11, if none, check the box. Use blank sheets if more space is required.
3. Be sure to furnish all circulation information called for in item 15. Free circulation must be shown in items 15d, e, and f.
4. Item 15h., Copies not Distributed, must include (1) newsstand copies originally stated on Form 3541, and returned to the publisher, (2) estimated returns from news agents, and (3), copies for office use, leftovers, spoiled, and all other copies not distributed.
5. If the publication had Periodicals authorization as a general or requester publication, this Statement of Ownership, Management, and Circulation must be published; it must be printed in any issue in October or, if the publication is not published during October, the first issue printed after October.
6. In item 16, indicate the date of the issue in which this Statement of Ownership will be published.
7. Item 17 must be signed.

Failure to file or publish a statement of ownership may lead to suspension of Periodicals authorization.